ARTHRITIS

WHAT WORKS

By the same authors:

Backache Relief

An Arthritis Survey™ Publication

ARTHRITIS

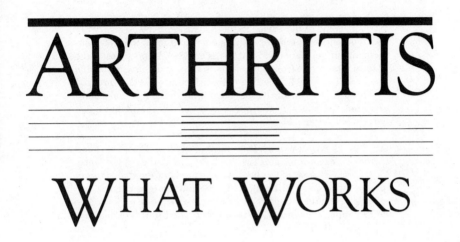

WHAT WORKS

Dava Sobel and Arthur C. Klein

St. Martin's Press   New York

NOTICE: Some of the advice in this book can be traced directly to the thousands of medical practitioners who treated the 1,051 participants in our nationwide Arthritis Survey™, and some of the information comes from our own constantly updated search of the medical literature. But neither of these facts implies that this book is a substitute for medical care. Read it for the things your doctor may not tell you—for the discoveries and the possibilities that could change your life.

ARTHRITIS: WHAT WORKS. Copyright © 1989 by Dava Sobel and Arthur C. Klein. All rights reserved. Printed in the United States of America. No part of this book may be used or reproduced in any manner whatsoever without written permission except in the case of brief quotations embodied in critical articles or reviews. For information, address St. Martin's Press, 175 Fifth Avenue, New York, N.Y. 10010.

Editor: Jared Kieling
Production Editor: Mark H. Berkowitz
Book design: Judith Stagnitto

Library of Congress Cataloging-in-Publication Data

Sobel, Dava.
    Arthritis: what works / Dava Sobel and Arthur C. Klein; foreword by Willibald Nagler.
      p. cm.
    Bibliography: p.
    Includes index.
    ISBN 0-312-03289-7
  1. Arthritis—Popular works. I. Klein, Arthur C. II. Title.
RC933.S615 1989 616.7'2206—dc20 89-30422

First Edition
10 9 8

Copies of this book are available in quantity for promotional or premium use. Please see page 477 for details.

Printed in the United States of America on acid-free ∞, recycled paper

For Zoë and Isaac

CONTENTS

SECTION IV: WHAT YOU NEED TO KNOW ABOUT UNCONVENTIONAL TREATMENTS FOR ARTHRITIS

21. How to Go About Your Everyday Activities with Minimum Pain and Maximum Ease   403

■ *Smart tips for joint protection* ■ *Gadgets that get things done* ■ *Scheduling activities and rest to help you accomplish more* ■ *New ways to keep doing what you need to do, what you love to do*

ACKNOWLEDGMENTS

Our thanks to Regina Gload, most of all, and also to Bridget MacSweeney and Eva Collins, for handling all the clerical work involved in conducting the Arthritis Survey™;

To Kathleen Pratt, M.S., R.D., for turning the dietary suggestions of survey participants and researchers into the Arthritis Survey™ Diet and Thirty-Day Meal Plan;

To Anthony F. Hitchcock and Jean Lindgren, for their help with the on-line searches of the medical literature;

To rheumatologists Barry L. Gruber, M.D., and Michael V. Sobel, M.D., for their expert opinions and advice;

To Willibald Nagler, M.D., and Irene von Estorff, M.D., of the Department of Rehabilitation Medicine at The New York Hospital–Cornell Medical Center, for their careful review of the exercise recommendations;

To Jared Kieling of St. Martin's Press, for pursuing and endorsing this project; and

To the 1,051 Arthritis Survey™ participants, for sharing their knowledge and experiences with us.

FOREWORD

Experienced physicians know that medical knowledge derives as much from observing patients closely and listening to them carefully, as from studying and analyzing a multitude of scientific facts. There is much to be learned from people who live every day with a chronic condition, such as osteoarthritis or rheumatoid arthritis, and the authors of this book do an excellent job of capturing these people's insights and their resourcefulness. *Arthritis: What Works* looks at arthritis treatment from all angles, presenting clear and practical discussions of pharmacological agents, exercise, and diet.

Over one thousand people from around the country with osteoarthritis or rheumatoid arthritis filled out carefully designed questionnaires and were also given free rein to comment on their experiences. The criteria for inclusion in this analysis appear to be as strict as for any clinical study which encompasses a large number of participants.

Much progress has been made in the treatment of arthritis, in its various forms, with improved anti-inflammatory agents and joint-replacement techniques. But this book also points out the crucial importance of a close partnership between patient and physician, who together must face the challenge of dealing with the persistent presence of an uninvited guest. The rheumatologist and orthopedic surgeon are found to play an especially important role in the overall care of the arthritis patient. The physiatrist's expertise in prescribing exercise is also recognized, as is the role of the physical or occupational therapist who helps the patient remain as active as possible within a given environment.

Much work still needs to be done to improve and refine what we know about exercise programs for each individual, but one thing is clear: very well stretched and strong muscles, as well as sound "body machines," are the joint's best friends!

Some of the less conventional approaches to arthritis that are found helpful by the subjects of this study are not accepted in academic circles. I do think, however, they are deserving of closer analysis. After all, for a long time no one thought diet could have any effect on arthritis, and now we know that it does.

I recommend this book to anyone who must live with, or who is involved in the treatment of, osteoarthritis or rheumatoid arthritis. Dava Sobel and Arthur C. Klein are to be praised for their efforts.

Willibald Nagler, M.D.
Jerome and Anne Fisher Physiatrist-in-Chief
The New York Hospital
Professor of Rehabilitation Medicine
Cornell Medical College
March 1989

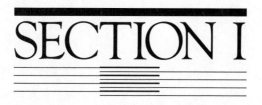

SECTION I

NEW FINDINGS AND A NEW SOURCE OF HELP

To move freely without restriction due to pain, disability, or weakness is among the most basic of human rights. Any disorder that impairs mobility; limits the capacity to touch, embrace, or protect; and interferes with personal hygiene, physical labor, or recreation threatens a person's sense of dignity and self worth.

—Stephen R. Kaplan, M.D., and Edward V. Lally, M.D., from an article on arthritis treatments in *The Journal of Musculoskeletal Medicine* (September 1986)

May the work you do to help the suffering and educate the public be blessed by God.

—Survey Participant #440, a Canadian psychologist, minister, and mother of four

1

YOU HAVE GOOD REASONS
TO BE HOPEFUL

■ A new kind of knowledge about helpful treatments for arthritis ■ Startling findings from an unprecedented nationwide survey ■ Questions you dare not ask your doctor—answered here

If you've read only this far, you already know something about arthritis. Maybe you know how it feels to lie imprisoned in bed each morning by knees and hips that have hardened to cement during the night. Or maybe you know the ringing noise that aspirin blares in your ears after you've swallowed your tenth or twelfth tablet of the day, or the fatigue that knocks you down in mid-morning, before you've had a chance to do half the things you used to accomplish with ease, or the anger that flares up when television commercials describe your ailment as "minor aches and pains."

No doubt you would like a *different* sort of knowledge about arthritis. What would help most to kill the pain? Would a change in diet help? Which experimental treatments hold real promise? Is surgery worth the risk? Can exercise slow the deterioration of the joints? Who gives the best care for arthritis? Which drugs fight inflammation best? Is there any harm in wearing a copper bracelet or drinking cod liver oil? How does one carry on—homemaking, making a living, making love—in spite of arthritis?

Your doctor may lack the time or the information to address these questions as fully as you might wish. Indeed, you dare not even ask some of the questions, for fear your doctor will laugh at you. And so you are left to ferret out the answers on your own.

This is a book of answers—a guide to the practitioners, treatments, and self-help strategies that can change your life for the better. It is based on the collective experience of more than one thousand people with osteoarthritis or rheumatoid arthritis* who took part in our nationwide Arthritis Survey, and who have, among them, tried literally everything.

This is *not* a book of anecdotes, although as you read it, you will hear people telling their stories in their own words. Instead, it is a detailed report of *what's out there,* with a painstaking analysis of *what works.*

Because this book draws heavily on people's actual experiences, it covers everything from the orthodox to the outlandish. Rather than dismiss alternative approaches and so-called "quack" remedies with a sneer, we explore them in detail, since some of our participants tried them—and since you may be tempted to try them, too.

Because this book *also* draws on the rich store of information in the current medical literature, it introduces you to a few of the experimental therapies that are too new to be widely available yet, and some of the revolutionary developments in nutrition research that suggest how changes in diet may benefit people with arthritis.

In fact, so many treatments work to relieve arthritis pain that the real challenge is to discover *which* ones will work best for you. You can use the information in this book to help you:

*Osteo- and rheumatoid are the two most common forms of arthritis. Osteoarthritis is the "wear and tear" disease—the breakdown of cartilage inside one or more joints. Rheumatoid arthritis is a whole-body disease that inflames many different tissues, but especially the membranes that line the joints.

- Find the kind of doctor best qualified to treat your arthritis

- Get extra help from nonmedical practitioners who can significantly improve the quality of your care

- Discover which practitioners are best avoided

- Put together a new diet plan that may relieve pain and control inflammation

- Minimize the risks of the prescription medications and over-the-counter drugs you take

- Replace the vitamins and minerals that medications may rob from your body

- Enjoy pain relief from simple techniques you can use at home or at work

- Learn how to exercise safely and effectively to preserve the natural motion of your joints

- Prepare for joint surgery so as to improve the likelihood of a successful outcome

- Manage your emotional reactions to arthritis and control pain-aggravating stress

- Explore the value of some unorthodox approaches, such as acupuncture and Yoga

- Continue to carry on your everyday activities with the help of a wealth of practical tips

You may want to go through the material from start to finish, or turn immediately to the topics that intrigue you the most. The text is full of cross-references, so you can be sure to find all the information on any given subject, even if you don't read the chapters in order.

The voice that speaks to you from this book is a far cry from the entreaties of those around you who *insist* that you try what they tried or go to the foreign clinic where Aunt So-and-So was cured.

It isn't the voice, or rather the countless disparate voices, of alternative health-care providers who have a cause to promote, or product manufacturers with a gimmick to sell. Nor is it the voice of the Arthritis Foundation. For all its good work in funding research and providing many kinds of services to people with arthritis (including about one-third of our survey participants), the Foundation wears the blinders of establishment medicine. It lauds drug therapy and surgical techniques but rejects out of hand many other approaches that often prove helpful to our participants, especially nutritional and nonallopathic therapies.

The voice that speaks to you from these pages is broadly informed and charged with the encouragement, support, and advice of a thousand other people who have at least one thing in common with you—arthritis. But what makes this book a voice of authority?

Arthritis: What Works is based on a nationwide survey we conducted of 1,051 people with arthritis, *and* on a rigorous search of the medical literature that pertains to arthritis. It is at once people-centered and scientifically supported. The individuals who took part in the survey shape the book by virtue of their interests and experiences. *The medical literature validates their views in most cases,* helps explain why they reacted as they did to various kinds of treatment, and shows you the surprising new directions that arthritis research is taking today.

Our participants are a microcosm of the 37 million Americans with arthritis. As a group, they match the national arthritis picture in terms of their age, sex, and the kinds of treatment they've received. What's more, the pooled experiences of the participants repeatedly mirror the results of medical studies on some of the topics covered here. For example, forty-eight of our survey-group members have tried methotrexate, a treatment borrowed from cancer therapy for use against particularly destructive cases of rheumatoid arthritis, and only recently approved for this use by the Food and Drug Administration. Fifty percent of these participants (twenty-four individuals) told us they enjoyed dramatic improvement on the methotrexate therapy—virtually the same rate of significant relief reported in a 1984 study of 189 patients at the University of Utah.

In telling us their honest opinions of prescription anti-inflammatories for arthritis, to cite another example, our participants suffered headaches from **Indocin** (indomethacin) and diarrhea from **Meclomen** (meclofenamate) with precisely the same frequency as subjects in clinical trials of these drugs. The difference here, of course, is that our participants also tell what *else* happened—how they resolved the difficulties, what other things they tried, and with what success. The survey participants can function as your national self-help group in print. You can compare your experiences with theirs and use their collective advice to guide your next choices.

Nor is their advice limited to the kinds of things your doctor might tell you. It has a broader range, addressing the whole gamut of arthritis care, from over-the-counter to under-the-counter and everything in between. Anything hyped on television or claimed in catalogs to be an arthritis "cure" is subject to scrutiny here—because all treatments offered and all promises made about arthritis are of potential interest to people who have arthritis. As a result of our survey, we can use our participants' assessments of chiropractic care, for example, to rate and compare what these doctors achieve to what medical doctors and other health-care practitioners have to offer you. We can take a serious look at the likes of copper bracelets, DMSO, bee venom, honey, cod liver oil, and apple-cider vinegar, and appraise their relative risks and benefits. In some of these areas, where respectable research has not been done, our participants' advice may be the *only* source of unbiased information available to you.

On the question of nutrition—and there isn't a person with arthritis who doesn't have some question about nutrition—most practicing physicians either laugh or flatly declare that there is no connection between nutrition and arthritis. Many of our participants say there *is* a connection, having found that a change in diet amounts to a measure of pain relief or a reduction of inflammation. Many *researchers* agree and are busying themselves with landmark studies that show how certain foods can aggravate arthritis, while others apparently ameliorate the symptoms. Fascinating findings about fasting, about vitamins, and about specific food intolerances are spelled out here, both from the perspective of the individual survey participant, who has perhaps replaced red meat with fish, and the researcher in the hospital setting, who has watched patients with severe chronic rheumatoid arthritis *respond* to dietary therapy.

Many of our participants volunteered extra information we hadn't asked for—the probable *cause* of their arthritis, for example, the history of arthritis in their families, or the effects of the weather (dampness, cold, changes in humidity) on their pain. A few even took us to task for not probing these topics. But we intentionally avoided such questions in order to focus on purely practical matters. We were after the tools and strategies that worked to make our participants feel better—not the root cause of their problems. It was beyond the scope of our project to consider the influence of genetic or environmental factors in causing arthritis, and surely the weather is beyond anyone's control.

Our aim—and we achieved it—was to learn what works best for the most people: what stops pain, what reduces inflammation, what gets stiff joints moving in the morning, what practitioners offer the most help, what diet makes the most sense, what exercises can improve joint function, what techniques allow people to do what they must in spite of disability. If this is the kind of information you've been looking for, please read on.

2

THESE PEOPLE CAN HELP YOU

▪ How early proper treatment changed a family history of arthritis ▪ How gold reclaimed one woman's life ▪ Surgery banished this man's pain ▪ Experimental drug to the rescue ▪ Diet makes a difference after all ▪ Stories of people who helped themselves with exercise, grit, and guts

You are about to read a few case histories selected from the 1,051 stories in our Arthritis Survey. We chose these particular vignettes because each one of them recounts an experience shared by tens, scores, or hundreds of other individuals in the group. The accounts present some of the most important elements of arthritis care—and they introduce the people who help make this book a message of hope and encouragement.

When M.W. was a little girl, she saw her father stricken and then crippled by arthritis before his thirty-fifth birthday. He walked on crutches for the rest of his life, she recalls. "I knew I didn't want to go through what I saw him go through." And so, three years ago, when M.W. began to feel pain herself in her knees, elbows, and fingers, she suspected arthritis and sought treatment immediately, even though she was just twenty-eight at the time.

"When I began seeing the rheumatologist, I was naturally concerned and more worried than some people might have been. The rheumatologist was a real help to me. He was a good listener and took the time to talk to me, so I could get through that rough period and become determined to do what I needed to. He stressed the importance of a doctor and a patient working together for the patient's benefit. He helped me to believe that medications would help me resume a normal life, and I have found that to be so."

M.W.'s father never saw a rheumatologist, nor did he know that there was such a thing as an arthritis specialist. These doctors were extremely helpful to our participants, as you can see in Chapter 3 by the way they compare to other kinds of M.D.s. Chapter 4 describes the non-M.D. practitioners, such as physical therapists, who offer the best help for arthritis.

"I took aspirin in the beginning," M.W. continues, "and it helped a little, but I am doing much better with my arthritis since I have been using a prescription anti-inflammatory drug called **Feldene**. The arthritis no longer interferes with my shopping and cooking and taking care of my three children."

Feldene and most other drugs like it did not exist when M.W.'s father was a young man. Today they are a mainstay of treatment, and drug companies keep coming out with new ones. You can read a full account of their pain-killing and anti-inflammatory effects in Chapter 5. Nonprescription drugs, including aspirin, are covered in Chapter 6.

H.L. was also young—thirty-five—when rheumatoid arthritis came on suddenly, invading all her joints with pain so intense she could barely function. And although her doctor tried to help her with several of the new anti-inflammatory drugs, including **Feldene**, she got no relief from any of them.

"When he saw that the arthritis was not getting better, he sent me to a rheumatologist who started me on gold injections and physical therapy," she writes. "Then I began to get better in a hurry." She felt her first moment of pain relief while soaking in the warm water of a hospital's whirlpool bath. She used the whirlpool every day for the next two weeks, and got hot-wax wraps for her hands from the physical therapist, as well as hand splints to wear while resting or sleeping. These things all helped her feel better while she waited for the gold salts, called **Solganal**, to build up in her body with each weekly injection.

"The rheumatologist told me the gold shots would take at least three months to work, maybe six months, but I felt about 100 percent better in six *weeks.* After only two months on gold, I found I could do almost anything I had been able to do before I got sick. I have little discomfort at all, now. When I do, I take two aspirin a day. A warm bath helps a lot, too. Other times I might get that drained feeling and need to lie down for a few minutes. But the gold injections work so well I can do whatever I want."

H.L. no longer sees the rheumatologist who helped her so much. Her family doctor has taken over her care again and gives her the necessary injection of **Solganal** twice each month.

Gold injections, which have been used as rheumatoid arthritis treatment on and off for the last sixty years, have recently been joined by gold in pill form, to be swallowed instead of injected. You can see how the two compare in the second half of Chapter 5, and size them up against other specialized treatments that come into play when anti-inflammatory drugs fail to help.

L.F., an English professor, talks about his arthritis in the past tense, thanks to two total hip replacements he had six years ago, at the age of sixty-five. "I do have a little arthritis in my thumbs," he concedes, "and I can't turn my neck very far, but I have *no* constant aches anymore, and I take *no* pain medications."

After discovering he had osteoarthritis, L.F. relied on aspirin, then switched to the newer anti-inflammatory drugs. He also joined a health club, where he found *"great* relief and help" from swimming and using the Jacuzzi about three times a week. But his rheumatologist and orthopedist agreed at the end of seven years that he could be dramatically improved with surgery.

L.F.'s two operations were scheduled six months apart, and he had the benefit of physical therapy twice a day, including exercise instruction, during each hospital stay. The result? "I have no pain! I suppose it took months to *fully* recover from the surgery, but I remember that I drove to the health club after two weeks. Now that I've retired, I work in the yard and do all my own housework. I can only have praise for my doctors and my therapist because I am pain-free. If my hips come 'unglued' in the future, I'll go back to my surgeon."

Because his artificial hips were cemented in place, which is still standard procedure, there is a chance that they may loosen sometime in the next ten years, or "come unglued," as L.F. aptly describes the possibility. However, new surgical techniques, described in Chapter 7, make use of "cementless" joints that encourage your own bone to grow into the replacement parts and form a living, lasting fusion. In Chapter 8, you can find out about a dozen "extra" measures, including many forms of physical therapy, that can ensure the best possible outcome from surgery—or from any other treatment, for that matter.

"Two years ago I could hardly move my wrists, elbows, shoulders, ankles, or knees," writes C.E., a forty-five-year-old high school guidance counselor. "Just walking from the chair to the kitchen was a *major,* painful chore. I cried every day because it all seemed so futile. I was getting no sleep, I couldn't make love, and I was about to give up and just 'sit.'" The drug treatment that brought C.E. out of this terrible state was considered experimental at the time, and has only recently been approved for use in some cases of severe rheumatoid arthritis. It is called methotrexate, and until now its major use has been in the treatment of cancer.

Every Monday, at 8 A.M., 3 P.M., and 10 P.M., C.E. swallows one small yellow tablet of methotrexate, in addition to the anti-inflammatory drug she takes every day. "Now, three and a half years after my rheumatoid arthritis began, I am in semiremission with the methotrexate therapy."

C.E. is one of the more than seventy members of our survey group who have used experimental arthritis treatments under medical supervision, and whose experiences are the substance of Chapter 11. Another three hundred or so "experimented" on themselves by trying various unproven approaches—the ones typically denounced as "quackery," which are rated and described in Chapter 9, from bee venom to DMSO. Chapter 10 documents the extremely high rate of effectiveness of several traditional yet unconventional treatments, including acupuncture and Yoga.

As though he hasn't had enough to do, helping to care for his thirty-one-year-old brain-damaged son and managing his own rheumatoid arthritis for the past twenty-six years, P.D. has had three episodes of cardiac arrest and lives with a constant reminder of his years as a coal miner—the respiratory disease called black lung. For his arthritis, P.D. has taken aspirin, anti-inflammatory drugs, and prednisone. He's had steroid injections, physical therapy, and surgery to replace his left hip and knee. And while he speaks well of the help he's received in all these avenues, the thing that makes the biggest difference to him now is the dietary change he prescribed for himself. "I eat a lot less meat, bread, and sweets, and drink less coffee and cola. I eat more raw fruits and vegetables. I don't know how this diet would affect others, but I've found, beyond a doubt, that the closer I stick to it, the better I feel."

The internist who first diagnosed P.D.'s arthritis didn't say anything about nutrition, beyond the standard advice to eat a balanced diet. Since that time, P.D. has been around enough doctors to know what most of them think of nutritional approaches to arthritis care. "I know this is against everything that has been told to people, but I believe that a diet without animal products, wheat products, sugar, salt, and cola can be of great benefit to the arthritic. To eat fresh raw fruit and vegetables will cause even further improvement."

P.D. will be very surprised to learn that several mainstream specialists are at last seriously exploring the role of nutrition in arthritis prevention and treatment—*and* calling for an intensified research effort in this area, as you will see in

Chapter 12. P.D.'s diet specifics are spelled out in Chapter 13, with other advice from the more than one hundred participants who say they have reduced their pain by changing the way they eat. Their suggestions, together with findings from new medical research on nutrition's role in arthritis, form the basis for the thirty-day meal plan that comprises Chapter 14. The vitamins and minerals that you may be missing, either because of your arthritis or the drugs you take to treat it, are discussed in Chapter 15, with specific recommendations.

R.D. had shrugged off minor arthritis pain in his knees for nearly thirty years, but when the arthritis settled in his spine, the pain became agonizing and relentless. Although he had only recently retired at age sixty-six, the pain was beginning to make R.D. think that he had perhaps lived long enough. He certainly didn't feel he had anything good to look forward to, and he still vividly remembers the night the pain sent him to the local hospital emergency room, begging for a strong pain-killer or anything else that might help him find relief. Then his doctor encouraged him to lose weight and got him started on an exercise program with a physical therapist. Today, forty pounds lighter and the veteran of eight years of regular exercise, R.D. controls his arthritis pain with nothing more than an occasional tablet of **Advil**.

"I do two sets of exercises for my back—one for the upper spine and shoulders, and another for the lower back and legs. These are standard exercises recommended by doctors and registered physical therapists. They take, on average, not over fifteen minutes each day. And yet I am confident that the exercises did *more than anything else* to relieve the terrible pain I was having."

Exercise has proven to be so beneficial for treating arthritis that no one questions its value any longer—although there are still many practitioners who do not prescribe exercise because they don't know what to suggest. Less than half of our survey participants who exercise regularly say they were taught or urged to do so by their doctors. The others learned about exercise from a physical therapist, an arthritis self-help class, or their own determined searching. If you don't already have an exercise regimen, you can turn to Chapters 18 and 19 for a rundown of the best overall fitness activities, as described and rated by our participants, as well as specific exercises for specific joints.

For all the help she has received from doctors—and there's been a lot for which she's thankful—G.N. has boosted herself over some of the worst times by her own grit. Other survey participants also find that a positive outlook and some well-chosen strategies for reducing stress, controlling pain, and working around their limitations, as described in Chapters 16, 17, 20, and 21, make them feel in control of their lives again.

"My vanity has been very helpful to me," G.N. writes. "At the onset of the disease, when I couldn't comb my hair until two o'clock in the afternoon, I steadfastly refused to cut it off, and decided that I must learn to look good. I've continued to do this, and although people's comments imply that I can't have a chronic disease when I look so well, it's a source of pride to know that the 'outside' looks good even when the 'inside' is a mess.

"One of the most annoying aspects of living with arthritis is people's attitudes toward it. I, for one, look perfectly normal (except for the splint I wear), and I find that most people either do not understand the physical limitations that I have, or don't really believe they exist. I feel it is of the greatest importance to admit what one cannot do and learn to adapt or ask for help. My attitude is that there are many people who enjoy helping others, so why deprive them? I've also found that asking for help (when it's needed) helps others understand the limitations that the disease imposes.

"Another thing I've had to learn to do is express *feelings* to those who are close, so they can understand my mood shifts. This was so difficult for me at one time that I started out by putting notes on the refrigerator. Gradually, I was able to *say,* 'I'm having a _____ day.' (Put in any four-letter word you like.)

"I've also learned that love doesn't stop because I have a chronic disease, and that I can be a valuable person despite my physical limitations. Ironically, it was my rheumatoid arthritis that taught my older son the sensitivity to cope successfully with his wife's disease when she learned she had multiple sclerosis. And it has taught me that people can continue to have intimate relationships and be needed by the able-bodied."

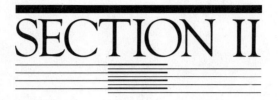

SECTION II

HOW TO GET
SIGNIFICANTLY BETTER
RESULTS FROM
PROFESSIONAL CARE

May I never forget that the patient is a fellow creature in pain. May I never consider the patient merely a vessel of disease.

—from the Code of Maimonides, an oath taken by graduates of Mount Sinai Medical School

I will remember that there is art to medicine as well as science, and that warmth, sympathy and understanding may outweigh the surgeon's knife or the chemist's drug.

—from "A Modern Hippocratic Oath," by Dr. Louis Lasagna, taken by graduates of Tufts University School of Medicine

Anyone with arthritis needs many warm fuzzies and insights that are not available in doctors' offices.

—Survey Participant #238, a freelance writer from New Mexico

3

MEDICAL DOCTORS:
Which Ones to See,
Which Ones to Avoid

■ Why rheumatologists and orthopedists are so effective ■ How to find an arthritis specialist ■ The advantages of a family doctor ■ Where to get medical advice on exercise ■ How to talk to your doctor

Most of the 1,051 participants in our Arthritis Survey consulted at least two or three medical doctors for help with their arthritis, and some of them saw as many as nine or ten. The searching paid off, because about two-thirds of our participants say they are satisfied with the care they're receiving now. The experiences of the group as a whole point up the best and worst of medical care and can steer you to the most likely sources of help—right from the beginning.

Getting the correct professional help right away is extremely important. Unfortunately for them, a number of our participants accepted what they called the "inevitability" of arthritis and ignored the pain and stiffness as long as possible before seeking medical attention. Now they look back at the time they spent being stoical or philosophical and curse themselves for the delay. "I self-doctored myself until about two years ago," writes a disabled printer from California. "I feel now that this has been much to my downfall, and I would *not* recommend it to anyone. What helped me the most was finally admitting that I could not handle the arthritis by myself. Now I am seeing a specialist in this field, and I have full confidence in him, so I follow his instructions to the letter. And I am no longer bedridden, thanks to his treatments and advice."

Other participants *tried* to get help right away, but got nowhere because the doctors they saw had some serious misconceptions about arthritis. For example, the myth that arthritis is a disease of old age persists in the minds of some medical professionals. As a result, a few of our participants in their twenties or thirties weren't taken seriously, because they were "too young" to have arthritis. Now they have one or more artificial joints, even though they're "too young" for those, too.

This chapter names and rates the various types of doctors who treat arthritis. As you will see, there are a few kinds of specialists who far outstrip the others in achieving dramatic success. If you haven't been examined by one of these practitioners and you are not satisfied with your present care, you owe yourself a trial visit. Also, check the tips at the end of the chapter for suggestions on how to make *any* visit to the doctor more productive.

Our participants saw more than 2,100 M.D.s. (They also saw more than 1,100 non-M.D.s; we'll tell you about them in Chapter 4.) They rated their doctors by judging the kind of help they'd received from each one, whether it was dramatic long-term relief, for example, moderate long-term relief, temporary relief, or no relief, which meant that the practitioner was ineffective. As you'll see, some practitioners only succeeded in making our participants feel *worse*, either because of the treatment they provided or the negative attitude with which they offered their advice. Some survey participants did not rate this or that practitioner because they had started treatment too recently to make a judgment, or because they'd seen the doctor only for diagnostic tests or a second opinion about surgery.

The following evaluations are arranged in order of popularity, beginning with the physicians most frequently consulted by our survey participants. First on our list are the rheumatologists, who turn out to be the most sought-after practitioners in our survey—and the most effective ones as well.

Rheumatologists

- These arthritis specialists get praise for providing long-term relief, especially for rheumatoid arthritis.

- Aside from being the most knowledgeable about arthritis treatments, including experimental approaches, they may teach you a lot about self-care.

Rheumatologists, together with orthopedists (see pages 32–35), are the popular heroes in the battle against arthritis. Rheumatologists are doctors of internal medicine who have gone on for at least two years of special training in the many different types of arthritis and related conditions. This extra measure of education and experience makes them the reigning experts on the disease and most aspects of its treatment. "My rheumatologist is top-drawer," writes a housewife from Maryland. "He's up on the latest data, sees more actual cases of arthritis, and thus he inspires more confidence. He listens more, cares more, due to his very choice of rheumatology as a specialty. He advises correctly and adds caution where necessary."

In cold, hard statistics, rheumatologists top the charts. Nearly *half* of those rated in our survey are credited with helping participants attain *dramatic* long-term relief. Here are the figures.

Total number of **rheumatologists** seen	482	
Number rated by participants	456*	(95%)
Outcome of treatment:		
Dramatic long-term relief	217	(48%)
Moderate long-term relief	77	(17%)
Temporary relief	97	(21%)
No relief (ineffective)	49	(11%)
Made participant feel worse	16	(3%)

*Although we list the total number of practitioners seen in each specialty, we use the number *rated* to calculate the outcome of care. In other words, the 217 rheumatologists who provided dramatic long-term relief account for 48% of the 456 who were rated. (And these 456 rheumatologists account for 95% of the total 482 who were seen by our participants.)

What do these numbers mean? They mean that your chances of finding help with a rheumatologist are better than four out of five, since 86 percent of those rated were able to provide *at least* temporary relief. Much of this relief comes in the form of drugs, including aspirin and other anti-inflammatory pills and shots that *could* be dispensed by any M.D. or osteopath (see pages 35–37). But rheumatologists are probably better acquainted with these drugs than other practitioners because they use them all the time, observing their good effects and their not-so-good side effects in hundreds or thousands of patients every year. It follows that rheumatologists are also more conversant with the less familiar treatments for arthritis, such as gold injections and penicillamine (see Chapter 5). And, if you have a particularly painful, disabling case of rheumatoid arthritis, for example, that defies all of these approaches, then the rheumatologist is the one who will try to attack the disease with more potent, possibly experimental, therapies (see Chapter 11).

More than medicine

The best rheumatologists, however, don't limit their advice to what they can write on a prescription pad. They are firm believers in patient education. They explain what they're going to do and why, enlisting you as a partner in your own care. They teach exercise, or refer you to someone who can, such as a physical therapist. They offer advice about ways to protect your joints and perform your day-to-day activities, or recommend an occupational therapist or self-help course teaching these strategies. If you need joint replacement or other surgery for arthritis, the rheumatologist will help you find an orthopedist to perform those operations. And if you are overweight, the rheumatologist will no doubt tell you that losing a few pounds will minimize the stress on your joints. "The rheumatologist was the most helpful," says a New York actress who appears in TV commercials, "since he advised exercise and weight loss as being the best treatment. He instructed me on daily exercises that would strengthen my muscles and reduce the stress on my joints, and these have given me excellent help."

The good rheumatologist is also a crackerjack diagnostician. Over and over, we heard our participants tell of months or years spent wondering what their problem was—until they either were referred to a rheumatologist or wound up in one's office through sheer persistence. "The acceleration of my osteoarthritis is the result of an inherited blood disease," reports a fifty-year-old chemist from California. "Before this was diagnosed, my advanced arthritis condition puzzled the following practitioners: internist, acupuncturist, body worker, podiatrist, and orthopedic surgeon. Finally, a rheumatologist identified the primary cause and much of the picture fell into place."

"It took going to four different doctors before finally getting to this rheumatologist and getting proper treatment," recalls a thirty-seven-year-old radio disc jockey from Louisiana. "In that six-month searching period, I became totally disabled. Despite continued misdiagnosis, I kept trying different doctors until I got to this specialist."

Ideally, the rheumatologist not only recognizes the problem but understands the other problems arthritis can cause, from the stress of living with pain to the fear of not being able to continue working or caring for a family. "My present rheumatologist," writes a clinical laboratory supervisor from Ohio, "knows the pain is real, not imaginary. He is compassionate, encouraging, and sympathetic, while also reassuring me that I will be able to cope and adapt." A retired teacher from South Carolina thanks her rheumatologist for being "not only extremely helpful, but a great morale booster, too."

A slight advantage in treating rheumatoid arthritis

Although rheumatologists are highly regarded by our whole survey group, the fact is they do better treating people with rheumatoid arthritis than those with osteoarthritis. This is because of the so-called "second-line" or "remittive therapies"—**Plaquenil** is one example—that they can offer to their patients with rheumatoid arthritis, but which are generally considered useless in treating osteoarthritis. Looking just at the reports from survey participants with rheumatoid arthritis, we find that 57 percent of rheumatologists treating them are able to give dramatic long-term help. The comments from these participants are likewise more glowing: "I can honestly say my rheumatologist was a godsend," writes a nursing-home administrator from Pennsylvania, whose rheumatologist is treating her with an experimental drug. "I was in so much pain, and he knew exactly what to try and what to do to help. If I'd found him sooner, I would never have lost any joints."

For those participants with osteoarthritis, on the other hand, "only" 34 percent of rheumatologists achieved dramatic long-term results. This is still an extremely good track record. What's more, when we add on the figures for moderate long-term improvement and temporary help, it turns out that fully 79 percent of our participants with osteoarthritis who saw a rheumatologist also saw some improvement.

As specialists, rheumatologists are in relatively short supply. There are only about 2,000 rheumatologists in the United States who are certified by the American Board of Internal Medicine, and about another 1,400 doctors who, though they don't have all the credentials, spend as much as half their time treating people with arthritis and other rheumatic diseases. That makes some 3,400 practitioners who are uniquely qualified to treat arthritis—and there are nearly 40 million Americans with one form of arthritis or another who might request their services. In other words, it may be hard for you to find a rheumatologist or hard to get an appointment to see one, or both. "There are only three rheumatologists practicing in our whole state," observes an elementary school principal from Delaware. In some places, especially rural areas, the shortage is keenly felt. "To go to a rheumatologist here," writes a high school aide from Ontario, "you have to be referred by your doctor. The wait to get an appointment is three to four months, and then he is so busy, you are in and out before you know it."

In other places, rheumatologists practically have to go begging for patients with arthritis, and they fill many office hours seeing people who have other medical problems. A retail buyer from Connecticut tells us that she had a rheumatologist for her family doctor but wasn't even aware of his specialty until she developed arthritis symptoms herself.

Specialists may charge more for office visits, which puts them beyond the reach of some participants. "I cannot afford a rheumatologist," writes a retired advertising director from

Illinois. "The only one in the city charges seventy dollars for the first office visit—and that's just to get your history."

The trouble with some rheumatologists

As you can see from the ratings, 11 percent of the rheumatologists in our survey were ineffective, and 3 percent of them made their patients—our participants—feel worse. The problems all had to do with bad reactions to certain drugs, insensitivity, and personality mismatches between doctors and participants.

"My rheumatologist has always been very supportive," explains a computer operator from Missouri. "But I had to fault him when I was having problems with allergic reactions and unusual side effects to medications, because I couldn't convince him these were serious problems. I remember that **Methotrexate** caused nausea, hair loss, severe swelling of my lower legs and feet, and red quarter-sized lesions with white centers of pus on my legs. Yet it took six weeks of suffering on my part to convince him that this wasn't working. On one other occasion, I finally refused to continue my medication, despite his objections, because of its side effects."

There's no question that most rheumatologists rely on drug treatments. "The rheumatologist prescribed many drugs," a New Jersey homemaker recalls, "which gave me severe rashes, nausea, and diarrhea, and I also found myself becoming depressed. But the doctor was not very concerned about depression, and told me there was another new drug I could try. After that visit, I decided not to expose my system to further side effects. I asked the doctor whether a change in diet would help, but he said there was no connection between nutrition and arthritis."

Asking some rheumatologists about nutrition can be as inflammatory as anything going on in your joints. Many of them are rigidly opposed to the concept of dietary help for arthritis because it smacks of quackery. Some have watched patients follow fad diets that turned out to be useless, or harmful, and that left them feeling duped. What's more, rheumatologists, like most doctors, receive little or no formal training in nutrition and may not know what counsel to offer—other than the casual advice to eat a balanced diet and keep the weight down. A few rheumatologists, however, are involved in exciting new research showing that certain foods and supplements can indeed have a positive effect, while other foods can aggravate arthritis in allergic or sensitive individuals. (See Section V for a full discussion of nutrition and arthritis, including the Arthritis Survey Diet and Thirty-Day Meal Plan in Chapter 14.)

Every rheumatologist is a human being first, and some doctors' personal skills just don't measure up to their technical expertise. This is a no-win situation for someone treating people with a chronic disease, patients who may require regular, even frequent, doctor visits over a period of years. A writer from North Carolina expresses the sentiments of many participants when she says, "It has been important to me to be treated as an intelligent human being of worth, and to be included as a thinking participant in my treatment. I have left doctors who did not inform me or consult me."

"As with any profession," concludes a twenty-nine-year-old Texas teacher, "I have seen some great rheumatologists and some quacks. The doctors who truly helped me spent time with me, made me feel good about myself. The doctors who did the most damage belittled my self-confidence, spent zero time with me, and were impatient in answering my questions. One doctor told me I'd probably become a quadraplegic and that I might as well accept the fact that I could never have what normal people have due to my arthritis." This woman, we are pleased to report, has since improved tremendously through a combination of physical therapy and drug treatment from her present rheumatologist.

How to find a rheumatologist

If you want to see a rheumatologist but don't know how to find one, here are some suggestions:

1. If it seems appropriate, ask your present doctor for a referral.

2. If you have no doctor or don't want to mention the subject, call your county medical society for a list of rheumatologists practicing in your area.

3. Call your local chapter of the Arthritis Foundation for names of rheumatologists near you. The number should be available from your phone book, your county medical society, or from the national headquarters of the Arthritis Foundation, 1314 Spring St., N.W., Atlanta, GA 30309, telephone (404) 872–7100.

4. Consult the "Physicians" listing in the Yellow Pages of your telephone directory, where these doctors may be listed under "Arthritis" or "Rheumatology."

5. As a last resort, write to the American College of Rheumatology, 17 Executive Park Drive, Suite 480, Atlanta, GA 30329.

Internists (Doctors of Internal Medicine)

- Internists do quite well with nondisabling cases of arthritis.

- As "total care" practitioners, internists can treat your arthritis with an eye to your other health problems.

Internists are the least specialized specialists, and arthritis is one of the many diseases they "specialize" in treating. More than three-quarters of our participants who saw an internist for arthritis treatment got at least temporary relief. But it's also true that more of them came away with temporary help than dramatic long-term improvement. Here are the actual figures.

Total number of internists seen	473	
Number rated by participants	446	(94%)
Outcome of treatment:		
Dramatic long-term relief	107	(24%)
Moderate long-term relief	113	(25%)
Temporary relief	134	(30%)
No relief (ineffective)	77	(17%)
Made participant feel worse	15	(4%)

Medically speaking, internists can do almost everything rheumatologists do. They can prescribe drugs, give injections, make referrals, and tell their patients to exercise and lose weight. "My internist gave me a drug that helped and sent me to a water aerobics class at the YMCA," writes a fifty-two-year-old aircraft mechanic from Alabama. "The drug has been good—no side effects, and the water exercise has helped more than anything." Participants with osteoarthritis and those with rheumatoid received the same quality of care from internists.

Doctors like to distinguish between mild and severe cases of arthritis. "But anybody with arthritis," points out a telephone company supervisor from Arizona, "knows that a mild case is what someone *else* has." Nevertheless, an internist may use these criteria to decide whether to treat you or to send you on to a rheumatologist or an orthopedic surgeon. "I am indebted to my internist," swears a New York credit analyst, "for suspecting rheumatoid arthritis in the first place and referring me to a rheumatologist before the disease was out of control."

If you are seeing an internist, and you are pleased with your care, there is no reason to think you'd be better served by a rheumatologist. Some participants, who have gone to both types of practitioners, actually favor the internist over the rheumatologist. "Once when I was laid up for six weeks," says a chauffeur from South Carolina, "it was the internist who helped me get back to where I could walk again."

Although we didn't ask for this information, 256 participants mentioned that they had another medical problem in addition to arthritis, such as heart disease, high blood pressure, or diabetes. These conditions are also part of the internist's specialty, and it may be especially comforting, if you have a complex health history, to take all your ills to one physician. At the very least, a lone practitioner should be able to avoid prescribing drugs that act against each other, as cortisone and barbiturates do, or act together to wreak havoc on your body, as aspirin and diabetes drugs do. (See Appendix C on drug interactions.)

There are upward of five thousand internists in current practice who have been certified by the American Board of Internal Medicine. This means that they took another three years of graduate medical education after finishing medical school, mostly hands-on experience in a hospital, and that they also passed certain exams. (Rheumatologists have the same background, plus another two years expressly devoted to rheumatology.)

Internists may successfully treat arthritis in much the same way as rheumatologists do, but when they fail to help, they fail for different reasons.

Improper diagnosis. Internists may not diagnose arthritis, or may not be able to pin down the type of arthritis a person has. Rheumatologists, on the other hand, are always looking for arthritis, and they are thus highly likely to find it. Although many people claim to have diagnosed their own arthritis on the basis of pain or swelling, a real medical assessment can be quite challenging. To help, the American College of Rheumatology has spelled out all the signs and symptoms that typify rheumatoid arthritis, and they have put these in a list that is used by doctors the world over. Even so, test results and physical examinations are not always definitive. What's more, there are *no* commonly accepted guidelines for diagnosing osteoarthritis, although the College is trying to develop such guidelines.

Lack of knowledge. Since internists are not strictly arthritis specialists, people assume they know less about the ailment than rheumatologists. In some cases, this is pure snobbery, in others, it's the sad truth. "My condition did not improve under the internist's care," reports a thirty-five-year-old librarian from West Virginia. "I have several deformed fingers because he did not prescribe correct treatment, nor did he refer me to a specialist. Since I went to the rheumatologist, his program of medication, rest, and exercise has enabled me to function on a nearly normal level, and I can work once again."

Poor attitude about arthritis. "My internist told me that everyone has aches and pains as they get older," writes a retired school superintendent from Massachusetts. Some internists just don't take arthritis seriously. This same school administrator went on to see a rheumatologist who gave him three prescriptions for anti-inflammatory drugs—and a chiropractor who put him on an exercise program. A retired travel agent from New York reports that his internist called arthritis "a natural ailment of old age with no cure," and suggested no treatment for *eight years,* then sent him to an orthopedic surgeon who wanted to perform two total knee replacements *immediately.* Our participant has found a new orthopedist on his own, however, who thinks surgery can be postponed or avoided with anti-inflammatory drugs and physical therapy.

To find an internist, check with your county medical society or look in your telephone directory under the "Physicians" listed in the Yellow Pages. Look for the heading "Internal Medicine." Some internists note right in their listing that they specialize in a certain area of internal medicine, which should help guide your choice.

General Practitioners and Family Doctors

- When these doctors know you well, they often know best how to care for your arthritis.

- GPs can work effectively with rheumatologists to take over your continuing care, even if you require specialized treatments.

If you have a good relationship with a nonspecialist who cares for "the whole you," consider yourself truly fortunate. "My GP has known me and my medical history for thirty-four years," writes a forty-one-year-old homemaker from New York. "He sent me to a rheumatologist, and I went for the tests, but I didn't think that doctor was taking my other ailments into consideration. I have diabetes, glaucoma, anemia, and asthma. So I'm sticking with my GP. He read the rheumatologist's report, and prescribed medications and treatments that fit me, the total person, in terms of what I can afford, what I can manage with my other conditions, my lifestyle, and my emotional needs."

Many of our participants enjoy the best of both practitioners. Having seen a rheumatologist one or more times for an expert assessment of their state, they go regularly to their family doctor for medical treatment—such as periodic gold injections, if necessary—and moral support. Arthritis, after all, is a chronic condition that waxes and wanes. There are times that it demands the ultimate from modern medicine, whether in the form of a bold drug combination, a high-tech diagnostic procedure, or a feat of surgical derring-do. There are also times when nothing is more important than the sympathetic ear of a doctor who knows you well.

General practitioners or family doctors often work very effectively *with* the specialists their patients have consulted. The rheumatologist who is too far away or too busy to take you on as a patient, may be only too happy to suggest a plan of action for your regular doctor to pursue with you. "My family doctor always treats me when I have a bad flare-up," says a plant engineer from Iowa, "since the rheumatologist is at the university, quite a ways away from here."

As the ratings from our survey participants show, general practitioners and family doctors have a slight edge over internists (about 5 percentage points) in providing dramatic long-term help.

Total number of **GPs** and **family doctors** seen	418	
Number rated by participants	397	(95%)
Outcome of treatment:		
Dramatic long-term relief	117	(29%)
Moderate long-term relief	99	(25%)
Temporary relief	121	(30%)
No relief (ineffective)	46	(12%)
Made participant feel worse	14	(4%)

As we interpret these numbers and the comments from participants, the advantage these practitioners have over internists is due partly to the long-standing nature of the doctor-patient relationship in many cases, and partly to plain old-fashioned good appropriate care. "My family doctor has treated me from the beginning, and I credit him for my not being laid up permanently at this stage of my life," writes a fifty-four-year-old Pennsylvania salesman who has had rheumatoid arthritis since age thirty-two. "I have been on gold for many years, plus anti-inflammatory drugs, exercise, good nutrition, and vitamins and minerals." Other survey participants rave about the practical advice they got from their family doctor, or the diet that launched their successful weight loss efforts.

A fifty-three-year-old office manager from California tells this story: "When I first went to a rheumatologist, he gave me no relief, but just kept saying, 'Wait and see.' I also saw a chiropractor, a physical therapist, and a Yoga instructor, who were helpful so long as I wasn't in intense pain. My family doctor is the *only* one who started me on various anti-inflammatory drugs, and we experimented until I found the right combinations. He also had me using splints to rest my hands, and when I could no longer walk, I had wonderful results from arthroscopic surgery done on both knees by an orthopedic surgeon he recommended."

Participants who are *dis*pleased with their general practitioners or family doctors make some of the same complaints we heard about internists. To wit: "Most GPs just don't have knowledge about arthritis," says a banker from New Hampshire. "They really don't seem to care about how one feels fighting stiffness, pain, and the inability to get around and do things."

At their worst, general and family practitioners may prescribe the wrong drugs. "My regular doctor," notes a beautician from Alaska, "was the one who just gave me codeine. I kept telling him that there must be a better answer, and he said that was all he could do. That's when I decided to go to an orthopedic surgeon—someone who knew about joints and could tell me what to do for my problem without turning me into a drug addict." The orthopedist switched her from painkillers to anti-inflammatory agents, gave her exercises to do, and taught her how to combine ice and heat for her knee pain.

Word of mouth may be your best guide to a good GP or family doctor, if you don't already have one. But if trusted friends or family members can't recommend anyone, turn to your county medical society for a referral.

Orthopedists (also called Orthopedic Surgeons)

- Their surgery, when needed, may greatly improve the quality of life.

- Orthopedists can give nonsurgical advice that equals that of any other practitioner.

Earlier in this chapter, we called these doctors heroes. They enter their specialty as the veterans of five years of post–medical school training in diseases and injuries that affect the bones and joints, as well as the muscles, ligaments, tendons, and the nerves that power them. Orthopedists do some of their most glorious battle in the operating room, where they have transformed a ravaged painful knee, for example, into a smoothly functioning joint that can bend readily, straighten painlessly, and do its part in helping you walk well without a crutch or a cane.

Surgery, when it works, works wonders. (See Chapter 7 for a detailed examination of surgery for arthritis.) "My orthopedic surgeon has helped me more than anyone," writes a retired teacher from Kansas. "He has performed eight operations on me—replaced both my knees, several joints in both hands, my left shoulder, and my right elbow—and the surgery has kept me out of a wheelchair. He has prescribed physical therapy and exercise as follow-up care, and he watches me carefully with periodic checkups."

Outside the operating room, orthopedists can and do provide many other kinds of treatment for arthritis, from prescription drugs and cortisone shots to braces and exercise advice. "The orthopedist took X rays and told me I was not ready for surgery," says a Wisconsin homemaker. "Instead, he talked to me about the right way to bend and sit, and how to make hot packs out of towels."

"My orthopedist prescribed a TENS unit [see Chapter 8] for me to use at home," a Florida pharmacist reports, "and it really helped."

A forty-nine-year-old secretary from Missouri, who has seen just one doctor in the twenty years she's had osteoarthritis, says of her orthopedist, "He is very sympathetic and encouraging. He's willing to listen to me, and he adjusts my medication for the most benefit to me." In short, there's nothing to stop an accomplished surgeon from being a good doctor in the best sense of the term.

Total number of **orthopedists** seen	350	
Number rated by participants	334	(95%)
Outcome of treatment:		
Dramatic long-term relief	160	(48%)
Moderate long-term relief	57	(17%)
Temporary relief	68	(20%)
No relief (ineffective)	30	(9%)
Made participant feel worse	19	(6%)

Orthopedists' ratings equal those of rheumatologists for providing dramatic and moderate long-term relief. The ratings match closely in the other categories too, except that orthopedists are twice as likely (6 percent versus 3 percent) to make their patients feel worse after treatment—because of the wrong advice, a poor surgery outcome, or a bad attitude. Here are some examples:

The wrong advice. "My orthopedic surgeon caused me the most harm by advising me to rest, instead of exercise," says a forty-three-year-old tennis instructor from New York.

Poor surgery outcome. "It's probably my own fault for going to the local hospital in the small town where I live," concedes a retired factory worker from Michigan, "but the orthopedic surgeon was incompetent and he hurt me. I walked with a cane before my foot surgery. Now I have to use crutches."

Bad attitude. A thirty-five-year-old vocational counselor from Texas reports that her orthopedist used scare tactics, actually "threatening" surgery if she didn't do her exercises. In California, a thirty-seven-year-old home health aide found an orthopedist who told her, "There's nothing you can do for it, and it's just going to get worse as years go on." "I believed him," she recalls, "but I found out through trial and error that exercise relieves my arthritis pain. The experience with the doctor led me to seek my own solutions—since he presented none."

With approximately 17,000 orthopedists in practice throughout the country, you have a good chance of finding a competent one—and another competent one in case you need a second opinion on questions about surgery. Your family physician should be able to help you make your selection, but if not, look to your county medical society or the Yellow Pages of your local telephone directory. Another route, since orthopedists spend so much time in the hospital, is to call the Department of Orthopedic Surgery at a hospital near you. If there's more than one hospital, pick the one that does the greatest number of arthritis-related operations, so you can be sure the doctors have the most experience. The American Academy of Orthopaedic Surgeons in Chicago does not offer any type of referral assistance.

Osteopaths (also called Doctors of Osteopathy, or D.O.s)

- Most osteopaths are in general practice—and may be indistinguishable from M.D.s.

- Osteopaths combine some of the best features of orthodox medicine and chiropractic care.

Technically, osteopaths are not doctors of medicine but doctors of osteopathy—a wholly different enterprise with its own philosophy and separate history. Osteopaths believe in the value of spinal manipulation, as chiropractors do, but they also prescribe drugs and perform surgery, just as medical doctors do. Indeed, the courses taught in colleges of osteopathy are so similar to those in medical schools that graduates have about the same degree of medical savvy, and that is why we are discussing osteopaths in the chapter on medical doctors.

Some osteopaths also go on for specialized graduate training in the same fields as medical doctors—including rheumatology—and sometimes in the very same training programs, but more than 85 percent of them are in general practice. Many people never notice that their family physician's or orthopedist's shingle says D.O. instead of M.D. And there may be nothing that happens *inside* the office to set the D.O. apart from other physicians.

Our survey ratings attest to the similarity in effectiveness shared by osteopaths and general or family practitioners.

Total number of **osteopaths** seen	192	
Number rated by participants	184	(96%)
Outcome of treatment:		
Dramatic long-term relief	53	(29%)
Moderate long-term relief	44	(24%)
Temporary relief	47	(26%)
No relief (ineffective)	30	(16%)
Made participant feel worse	10	(5%)

The ratings are similar to those of GPs, and some of the treatments identical (anti-inflammatories and painkillers, diathermy, gold shots, cortisone injections), but osteopaths helped several of our participants by their use of osteopathic manipulation. "The osteopath's manipulation helped no end," says a North Carolina housewife. "I would seek more treatment now, but we've moved and there is no osteopath near us." A few participants, who've had manipulation from both chiropractors and osteopaths, say they prefer the osteopath's brand of it.

Manipulation, however, no matter who performs it, rarely brings more than temporary relief, according to our survey, and also accounts for most of the "made me feel worse" reports from participants who are *dis*satisfied with their osteopath. "He tried manipulation on my back, but it only increased the pain," writes a clerk from Texas.

Osteopaths, much to their credit, give a great deal of helpful exercise advice, with lasting results. In fact, we heard more comments from participants praising exercises suggested by osteopaths than by any other doctors except physiatrists (see pages 37–39). "The only doctor who really helped me was an osteopath who told me how to exercise," says a retired gardener from Ohio. "Excellent" was the word a Tennessee psychologist used to describe the exercise program his osteopath devised.

The emphasis on exercise fits in well with osteopaths' reputation for being more "holistic" than M.D.s—more aware and more respectful of the nonmedical factors that can contribute to health. They are more likely to discuss nutrition as it relates to general well-being, for example, and to recommend fitness as preventive medicine. "The internist I saw was so insistent on surgery that I stopped going to him," writes a twenty-three-year-old receptionist from Washington. "But the osteopath was understanding and sympathetic. He encouraged me to keep trying with heat and physical therapy. He reviewed my vitamin regimen and advised me tenderly—almost as a friend."

Not surprisingly, several participants say they enjoy long-standing relationships with their osteopaths. "He is a very dedicated doctor who is interested in patients," observes a retired store owner from Florida, after seeing the same osteopath for forty years. "He diagnosed my condition and followed through with treatments and medication that won my complete trust and cooperation."

Of the 27,000 osteopaths in current practice, more than half can be found in small towns and rural areas where people need a family doctor. If you'd like more information about them, write to The American Osteopathic Association, 142 East Ontario St., Chicago, IL 60611.

Physiatrists (Doctors of Physical Medicine and Rehabilitation)

- Physiatrists (*not* psychiatrists) are experts on exercise.

- Long-term care of chronic conditions is the norm for these doctors.

"Why would I want to see a physiatrist?" one of our participants asked indignantly. "Arthritis is not a mental illness!"

Physiatry (pronounced *fizz-EYE-a-tree*) is one of the least-known medical specialties, and people seeing the word for the first time invariably mistake it for psychiatry, the mental-health profession. Regardless of this identity crisis, the physiatrist is probably the ultimate authority on exercise and rehabilitation following injury or surgery. A physiatrist's education now includes four years of graduate-level training after medical school. (As for psychiatrists, their role in helping participants control stress and improve their self-image is covered in Chapter 4.)

"The physiatrist is the best," writes a college professor

from San Juan, Puerto Rico. "He recommended exercises, plus physical therapy, changes in my diet, and aspirin."

"The physiatrist taught me exercises to strengthen my arm and shoulder," says a California sculptor, "and helped me to learn to use my left hand more for carving, so I can continue to work." He also gave her cortisone injections during periods of intense pain.

Relatively few physiatrists were consulted by our survey participants, however, and they did not achieve as much dramatic success as the other kinds of doctors we've considered.

Total number of **physiatrists** seen	34	
Number rated by participants	33	(97%)
Outcome of treatment:		
Dramatic long-term relief	7	(21%)*
Moderate long-term relief	9	(27%)
Temporary relief	11	(33%)
No relief (ineffective)	6	(18%)
Made participant feel worse	0	———

*These percentages have been rounded to the nearest whole number, with the result that ratings for some practitioners do not total 100%.

Physiatrists are the only physicians who maintained a perfect record for never leaving a participant in worse shape as a result of any word or deed, which is impressive. Their tailor-made exercises are safe and effective. Inappropriate or over-zealous exercise, on the other hand, can be quite dangerous (see Chapter 8), as it injured 174 of our participants, or 16 percent of the survey group.

While many doctors make the writing of a prescription their first order of business, the physiatrist tends to view it as a last resort. In routinely ministering to people who have been disabled by cancer, stroke, or spinal-cord injury, physiatrists like to offer the healing potential of nondrug alternatives such as water, ice, heat, movement, sound, and electrical stimulation. Another treatment they employ, although none of our participants experienced it, is to identify painful areas of damaged muscle, called "triggerpoints," which may accompany arthritis, and to inject these with either a local painkiller or a salt solution.

Physiatrists are not unreasonably averse to drugs—and they do prescribe anti-inflammatories for our survey participants. It's just that they've seen too many cases of medicine abuse. "The physiatrist took my pain seriously," writes a registered nurse from California. "He also understood my fear of becoming addicted to prescription pain meds, as so many of my R.N. friends are."

The worst criticism of a physiatrist in our survey comes from a Georgia office manager: "The physiatrist made a few good suggestions about posture and exercise, but her conversation was so optimistic, quoting so many platitudes, that I could not form a real doctor-patient relationship that came close to addressing my needs."

The best place to look for one of the approximately two thousand practicing physiatrists is in a large hospital, in the Department of Physical Medicine and Rehabilitation, where they often treat people with arthritis on an outpatient basis. For the names of physiatrists near you, call your county medical society or write to The American Academy of Physical Medicine and Rehabilitation, 30 North Michigan Ave., Chicago, IL 60602.

Neurologists

- Neurologists may be called in to assess nerve damage caused by arthritis.

- In some cases, they may also treat arthritis successfully.

Several of our participants took diagnostic tests for nerve damage from these specialists in diseases and injuries of the nervous system. But only three actually saw dramatic long-term improvement under a neurologist's care. "The neurologist has helped more than the internist or the chiropractors I saw," writes one of them, a real estate agent from Mississippi, "because he has a better understanding of muscles, joints, and nerves, and was able to treat it better from that perspective." The chances of getting dramatic long-term help from a neurologist, according to our survey results, unfortunately don't exceed the chances of being hurt by one.

Total number of **neurologists** seen	31	
Number rated by participants	23	(74%)
Outcome of treatment:		
Dramatic long-term relief	3	(13%)
Moderate long-term relief	4	(17%)
Temporary relief	7	(30%)
No relief (ineffective)	6	(26%)
Made participant feel worse	3	(13%)

Neurosurgeons

- Neurosurgeons may be able to provide dramatic relief if you need surgery on your back or neck.

- If you don't need surgery, you may receive no help at all.

While an orthopedic surgeon is usually willing to treat people with arthritis *whether or not* they require surgery, a neurosurgeon is strictly a surgeon who operates on the brain, the spinal cord, and the other nerves. If your problem requires their special expertise, you're likely to get relief. But if not, don't expect other help to be forthcoming. This situation accounts for the very high percentage of neurosurgeons rated as ineffective in our survey.

Total number of **neurosurgeons** seen	22	
Number rated by participants	22	(100%)
Outcome of treatment:		
Dramatic long-term relief	8	(36%)
Moderate long-term relief	2	(9%)
Temporary relief	2	(9%)
No relief (ineffective)	9	(41%)
Made participant feel worse	1	(5%)

"The neurosurgeon operated on my neck," writes a retired public relations man from Ohio, "because of bone spurs pinching a nerve and causing paralysis in my right arm. Now I can use the arm again, I can move my neck freely, which I couldn't do before, and I've had a major reduction in pain."

An insurance agent from Louisiana consulted a neurosurgeon about the osteoarthritis in her spine, but, she says, "He candidly tells me at this time there is no surgery that would help. He evaluates me every year or so in the event there has been a change in surgical options for me." Meanwhile, she gets her ongoing care from a rheumatologist who answers all her questions, prescribes drugs, and gives exercise advice.

If you have pain in your neck or back that hasn't responded to anyone else's care, consider discussing the problem with a neurosurgeon. If your doctor can't make such a referral, or you don't want to ask for one, check with your county medical society or with the hospitals in your area.

Other Practitioners

- Allergists and clinical ecologists may resolve arthritis pain with allergy tests and advice on avoiding certain substances.

- Doctors at pain clinics either get dramatic results or leave participants feeling worse off than before.

Our survey participants saw many different kinds of physicians in addition to the ones already discussed, but they saw some of them too infrequently for us to rate them. We felt we needed participants' comments on at least twenty practitioners in any given specialty to be able to rate that field. The list of doctors who were seen too infrequently to be rated includes allergists and clinical ecologists, anesthesiologists, cardiologists, dermatologists, emergency-room doctors, endocrinologists, gastroenterologists, general surgeons, hematologists, obstetrician/gynecologists, oncologists, ophthalmologists, otolaryngologists, pediatricians, plastic surgeons, radiologists, and urologists. (Acupuncturists, both M.D. and non-M.D., are covered in Chapter 4, and psychiatrists are considered together with other mental-health practitioners, also in Chapter 4.)

Although it would be misleading to try to assign ratings on the basis of five or ten practitioners in a given specialty, we would like to point out a few interesting observations.

- Twelve participants saw **allergists** or **clinical ecologists**, who tested them and found them sensitive to certain foods, bacteria, or molds. Treatment for the allergies was a combination of desensitizing injections and, in the case of foods, not eating the problem items. Of the ten participants who rated these practitioners, seven said they'd been dramatically helped. (At some large hospitals, in fact, allergy and immunology are *part* of the Department of Rheumatology, so you may be able to find all these specialists in one place.)

- Four of our participants whose joint pains started in childhood or adolescence, including a fifteen-year-old high school student from Nebraska, had received arthritis treatment from a **pediatrician**. And all four of them said they had benefited from these doctors' care.

- Physicians at **pain clinics** seem to offer an all-or-*less*-than-nothing proposition, judging from the experience of five participants who were treated by them. Three got dramatic long-term help, and two were left feeling worse off than before.

- A retired merchant seaman from Texas and a disabled veteran from Illinois who are treated at Veterans Administration (VA) hospitals report that most of their care, including surgery, has come from medical students who were not quite up to the task.

How to Get the Most out of Any Doctor Visit

"When my family doctor first diagnosed rheumatoid arthritis," a forty-seven-year-old Florida housewife writes, "he told me to go home, take aspirin until my ears ring, and come back next year. When you feel frightened and awful, that's not very comforting."

Surely *any* doctor has the responsibility to touch you gently, to treat you with respect, to explain your diagnosis, as well as the effects and side effects of various treatments, and to make suggestions of ways that you can further help yourself through exercise, for example, by taking warm baths or showers, and by protecting your joints. In the reality of a busy practice, however, there's a lot that never gets said. Often it is you, the patient, who—despite your pain, your fears, your personal problems, your money worries—still must take responsibility for getting the information you need. Here are some tips from survey participants on how you can do this.

Find a good doctor to begin with

If you don't yet have a doctor with whom you feel comfortable, use the ratings, comments, and access information in this chapter to help you find one. If you choose a specialist, remember that some physicians who call themselves specialists don't really have the credentials to use the word. *U.S. News & World Report* estimates that 30 percent of "specialists" fall into this category. A doctor who has gone through the formal specialty training and passed the necessary exams is a "board certified" specialist, or a "diplomate" of, for example, the American Board of Internal Medicine. Other so-called specialists may have as much experience or expertise, but have not met the requirements of the specialty-board examiners.

Credentials aren't everything. A good referral from someone you trust, whether it's your current doctor or a friend or relative, means a lot. What's more, it often happens that the very famous or very sought-after doctors are the ones who have the least time and energy to devote to you, which drastically reduces the quality of care you can expect to receive.

Most important of all is your take on the doctor. You have to feel that the two of you can work together as a team.

Communicate with your doctor

"I feel I have developed good communication skills over the years," says a twenty-nine-year-old participant from Indiana who has had arthritis since she was fourteen. "Communication is the key! It is the basis for choosing together what medication, exercises, and so on to try for your particular problems. Both the doctor and the patient have to work at this system. Communication is not always easy, but I'm sure it has been of benefit to me, *and* to the doctors and therapists who have worked with me." You can do your half this way.

- Think about what you want to tell the doctor ahead of time, so you'll be prepared for the visit.

- If writing down your symptoms or questions helps you, then write them, but remember that many doctors react badly to the sight of a long list of items. It may be better to leave the list home altogether, but if you use it, try to refer to it, and *communicate,* instead of just reading aloud.

- Be as brief as possible, out of respect for the doctor's schedule, but don't be cowed into thinking he or she doesn't have time to listen to you.

- Make your descriptions of symptoms or reactions to medications as specific as you can.

- Ask questions about anything that isn't perfectly clear to you. Then tell the doctor, in your own words, what you think he or she said.

- If you get home and realize you still have questions, or new questions are forming in your mind, call up and ask them now. If the doctor can't come to the phone, tell your questions to the person who answers the phone so the doctor can consider them before calling you back.

- Follow your doctor's advice, or explain why you don't want to.

Keep your perspective on the doctor-patient relationship

"I have often found that doctors lose interest and rapport after a few treatments," says a retired economist from California. "I believe this happens because many practitioners become irritated with their aging patients when they fail to deliver relief—and when the doctors realize that, in the course of time, they may find themselves in similar straits." Doctors, no matter how knowledgeable, are only human. And they can get as frustrated and as frightened as the rest of us. Some of them have never gotten over their embarrassment at talking about sexual matters, for example, while others are dangerously impaired—either because of incompetence or addiction to drugs or alcohol. By striving to communicate with your doctor, you have the best chance of knowing whether he or she is just having a bad day, or whether it's time for you to find a new doctor.

Summary of M.D. Practitioners

Highly recommended for diagnosis and ongoing care

Rheumatologists
Orthopedists

Recommended for continuing care of arthritis

General or family practitioners
Osteopaths
Internists

Recommended for special types of care

For most types of joint surgery: Orthopedists
For neck or back surgery: Neurosurgeons
For exercise advice: Physiatrists or Osteopaths
For rheumatoid arthritis: Rheumatologists

Not recommended

Neurologists

4

NON-M.D. PRACTITIONERS:
Which Ones Get the Best Results

■ What to learn from a physical therapist ■ What to fear from a chiropractor ■ What to look for in an acupuncturist ■ The virtues of exercise instructors and mental health practitioners

Some of the most successful programs for arthritis care use a team approach, with several kinds of professionals working together for a common goal— your well-being. Such a team might consist of (1) a **physician** who examines you, makes a diagnosis, prescribes drugs, and supervises your care; (2) a **physical therapist** who gives you wax or heat treatments, for example, and works out an exercise routine for you to follow at home; (3) an **occupational therapist** who shows you how to protect your joints and go about your daily activities with the help of special aids or smart tips on body mechanics; (4) a **psychologist** or counselor who might teach you a self-hypnosis technique for pain control, and help you work through any emotional difficulties arthritis could be causing; and (5) a **nutritionist** who talks to you about your diet and weight, with specific suggestions about how you can improve your eating habits.

Few of our 1,051 Arthritis Survey participants received this ideal level of attention, but many of them successfully assembled their own "teams" over the years and enjoy the advantages of receiving several—totally different—kinds of care. Thanks to their efforts, we can give you the information you need to find your own "players." We've already examined the physician members of the team (in Chapter 3). Now let's look at the non-M.D.s who have the most to offer, starting with the ones most frequently seen.

Our participants rated each kind of practitioner on the basis of the amount of help they received from his or her care, whether it was dramatic long-term relief, moderate long-term relief, or temporary relief. They judged a practitioner ineffective if they got no relief, and found a few non-M.D.s who left them feeling worse off than before. Of the two most popular non-M.D. practitioners seen in our survey, physical therapists have the edge over chiropractors.

Physical Therapists

- Physical therapists perform a wide variety of hands-on treatments that usually bring temporary relief.

- Their exercise advice can be the ticket to long-term improvement.

Most survey participants thoroughly enjoy the whirlpool treatments they get from the physical therapist; likewise the massage, the wax dips, the hot packs, the cold packs, the ultrasound, the diathermy, and the electrical stimulation. The variety is great, and sometimes the relief is, too.

"The hot packs were heaven," writes an investor from Idaho.

"The physical therapist used heat and massage, plus traction for sciatica pain that was brought on by arthritis," says a retired optometrist from Colorado. "I feel the traction definitely helped, and I've not had sciatica since I took those treatments in 1979."

"With a combination of cold pads, massage, and electrical stimulation," reports an Ontario travel agent, "I began to feel results in about three weeks. After five weeks, the pain in my knee was gone."

Some people feel that exercise instruction from the physical therapist has far greater value than any of the hands-on treatments—no matter how good these may feel at the time. A thirty-seven-year-old mother of two from South Dakota writes: "The physical therapist was fantastic for me—a lifesaver. After four years of severe rheumatoid arthritis and inactivity, I've experienced little, if any, loss of range of motion. I attribute that to the exercises I was taught. The exercises were painful at times, but very beneficial in the long run. The whirlpool, heat packs, and massages, on the other hand, were a great relief, but all very short-lived."

Exercise advice, in fact, accounts for most of the long-term relief that physical therapists are credited with providing.

Total number of **physical therapists** seen	440	
Number rated by participants	427*	(97%)
Outcome of care:		
Dramatic long-term relief	112	(26%)
Moderate long-term relief	77	(18%)
Temporary relief	183	(43%)
No relief (ineffective)	30	(7%)
Made participant feel worse	25	(6%)

*Occasionally, participants did not rate one or another practitioner because they had not yet had time to form a judgment. For each type of practitioner, we state the total number seen by our participants, but we used the number who were *rated* as the base for calculating the outcome of care.

Physical therapists typically use a combination of treatments, sometimes including splints or braces that participants wear on their hands or wrists, for example, to help prevent deformity. "Physical therapy was a godsend to me," says a Texas teacher. "It made me feel so much relief and helped me to regain some of the range of motion I had temporarily lost in my arms. The splints kept my wrists stable at night, so I could sleep."

If your particular regimen calls for physical therapy every week, or as often as seven days a week right after surgery, you'll probably spend more time with your therapist than with any other practitioner. This can be an emotional uplift, if you find someone who dispenses tender, loving care—or an educational bonanza, if you fill the time with talk as well as treatment. Moreover, a good physical therapist is long on practical demonstrations. "I had daily physical therapy to strengthen my muscles after knee surgery," writes a retired teacher from South Carolina. "The therapist also showed me how to use a paraffin bath for my hands, and gave me several gadgets for turning a doorknob, buttoning and unbuttoning my clothes, removing jar tops, and things like that."

The extremely high scores for temporary relief (43 percent) result from the hands-on treatments that *do* ease pain—but only for a few hours, or less. "The massage helped for a little while," says a waitress from Nevada, "but by the time I finished my work shift, the pain had returned." A salesman from California describes the brief relief situation this way: "It's like driving your car. You're going like sixty when you're driving it, but when you stop, that's it."

Physical therapists *rarely* fail to help the people in their care. In fact, no physician rated in our survey can match the physical therapists' extremely low *in*effectiveness rate of only 7 percent. Another 6 percent, however, caused harm by being incompetent, insensitive, or both. "The therapists I saw," notes an electronics technician from Oregon, "all seemed to possess a sadistic streak. The treatment was only so much torture for me, and any relief was brought about when they *stopped.*" An administrative aide from Rhode Island writes, "Physical therapy made my knee more painful to the point where I quit going after several appointments."

While sound exercise instruction may serve you well for the rest of your life, the advice of an incompetent therapist can be disastrous. For example, a New York policewoman says that five weeks of performing prescribed exercises and going to the physical therapist's office for treatments left her with debilitating low back pain—which she *did not have* in the first place.

How to find a good physical therapist

If you need a physical therapist, your doctor should be able to suggest one. Most orthopedists and rheumatologists have their favorites and may give special instructions to the therapist about how to proceed in your particular case. If your doctor does *not* recommend a physical therapist but you want to see one, you will probably have to ask your doctor for a *prescription* for physical therapy, since laws in most states forbid physical therapists to treat anyone without a doctor's permission.* Your doctor needn't know the first thing about physical therapy to prescribe it, however. Just the words *physical therapy* scrawled on a prescription pad will do nicely. Ideally, your physician will also write down the name of a competent therapist. If not, call the local division of your state chapter of the American Physical Therapy Association for a referral. (Their number should be available from your county medical society, even though county medical societies *don't* keep tabs on individual therapists.) Also, you can check the Yellow Pages of your telephone directory or go by word-of-mouth advice from other people with arthritis. Cybex, the internationally known manufacturer of several kinds of physical-therapy equipment, also runs a referral service for physical therapists who use Cybex machines. That number is 1–800–222–3245.

There are about 65,000 licensed physical therapists in hospital or private practice, all of whom have at least a college degree in physical therapy, and many who have an extra year's education and a master's degree to show for it. Some of them may specialize in certain areas of rehabilitation, such as physical therapy for cancer, heart conditions, or orthopedic problems. Before you take any treatment from a physical therapist you've found on your own, call and ask whether he or she has experience working with people who have arthritis. If not, ask to be referred to another one who does.

"The therapist I saw was not well versed in arthritis," laments a retired teacher from New York. "He never supervised me in the exercises he suggested, so I overdid them and further injured my elbows."

Only a few participants complained about the expense of physical therapy, and they solved the problem by learning

*The fourteen states that allow "direct access" to physical therapists *without* a physician's referral are Alaska, Arizona, California, Idaho, Kentucky, Maryland, Massachusetts, Montana, Nebraska, Nevada, North Carolina, South Dakota, Utah, and West Virginia. But even in these states, most people seek out physical therapy because a doctor suggests it. Illinois will probably soon become the fifteenth state on this list.

from the professionals how to use *some* of the treatments safely at home, on their own. You can do this, too. (See the tips on wax dips, heat, ice, and other self-help strategies in Chapter 17.)

Chiropractors

- Chiropractors' nonmedical approach is particularly appealing to some participants who can't take drugs.

- Chiropractors often provide good temporary relief, but their rate of making participants feel *worse* is higher than that of any other widely seen practitioner.

There are basically two kinds of non-M.D. practitioners—those who work with or for physicians, as most nurses and physical therapists do, and those who work independently of medical doctors on the basis of different healing philosophies, the way chiropractors tend to do. M.D.s, however, have long scoffed at chiropractors' heavy emphasis on spinal manipulation, and until recently, the Arthritis Foundation advised people with arthritis to "be suspicious of" chiropractic care in its pamphlet on *Arthritis Quackery and Unproven Remedies*. (The latest version of this pamphlet, called *Arthritis Unproven Remedies*, makes no mention of chiropractic.)

"I had chiropractic manipulation when my arthritis began three years ago," writes a forty-five-year-old locksmith from New Jersey, "but when I went to an orthopedist, I was told I had taken a big risk by letting the chiropractor touch my back, and that in the future, only a medical specialist could treat me." This antichiropractor bias may be changing, though, partly because of a lengthy legal battle that began in 1977, when chiropractors charged that the American Medical Association, the American College of Surgeons, and several other bastions of orthodox medicine had conspired to ruin the chiropractic profession. After ten years, a U.S. District Judge ruled in favor of the chiropractors, portraying them as the victims of "systematic, long-term wrongdoing." Recently, more than a dozen hospitals around the country have allowed chiropractors to join their staffs, or at least to treat some patients while they are in the hospital.

There are indeed good things to be said for chiropractic care. In addition to spinal manipulation, the thirty thousand-plus licensed chiropractors in the United States may use heat, ultrasound, electrical stimulation, traction, massage, and give exercise and practical advice. Before they enter private practice, they have to have at least six years of college study and clinic internship, including studies in anatomy, nutrition, X ray, and physical therapeutics. They can be caring, and they can be good listeners, our participants avow. What's more, some people seek them out expressly *because* of their non-medical philosophy.

"Since I can't tolerate any of the arthritis drugs with my ulcer," writes a retired advertising director from Illinois, "the chiropractor's gentle massage and heat gave marvelous, if temporary, relief."

"The chiropractor was better than the medical doctor," says a forty-one-year-old postal-service worker from Tennessee. "The chiropractor tried to help the problem, not mask the symptoms with drugs."

"I had a synovectomy on my right knee in 1981," reports a thirty-nine-year-old Wisconsin housewife. "My knee became even more stiff and painful after the operation. The chiropractor helped me get to walk again. I still go twice a week for relief."

"In my particular experience," opines a fifty-four-year-old factory foreman from Pennsylvania, "chiropractors are the only effective doctors to see. They know the muscular and skeletal systems of the body, plus they believe in proper nutrition, vitamin and mineral supplementation, and exercise. They will also admit it if they can do nothing, and send you to someone else for treatment—as opposed to the medical types, who will admit to no limitations of knowledge or experience."

Some participants said good things about manipulation, too, but *overall,* chiropractors had the lowest ratings of all widely seen practitioners—M.D. or non-M.D.

Total number of **chiropractors** seen	349	
Number rated by participants	345	(99%)
Outcome of care:		
Dramatic long-term relief	75	(22%)
Moderate long-term relief	53	(15%)
Temporary relief	118	(34%)
No relief (ineffective)	50	(15%)
Made participant feel worse	49	(14%)

As the ratings show, chiropractors deliver most of their help in the form of temporary relief. Although some participants feel improved for as long as three weeks after a chiropractic treatment, others find the effects disappear within a few days or a few hours. "I see a chiropractor because of arthritis in my neck and back," writes a fifty-four-year-old former truck driver, now disabled, from Illinois. "I get relief for about three hours after each treatment." A seventy-one-year-old Nebraska homemaker says, "The chiropractor helped for some time, but it got to the place where I would feel good after the treatment, and then the next day I would be right back where I started from." She eventually resolved her back pain with surgery and physical therapy.

Chiropractors' record for making their patients feel worse—14 percent—is the highest for any practitioner rated in our survey. And most of the harm comes from manipulation. "I went to a chiropractor first," says a retired glass worker from West Virginia, "and that was my big mistake, because I did not get better. I got worse. After a few adjustments, I could not sit down to eat or watch TV, but had to lie on the floor for relaxation, and it was painful to force myself to sit in a car long enough to go for my treatment. When I quit going, I got so I could sit again."

"The manipulation made me feel like a cripple," asserts a sixty-nine-year-old Florida woman. "The chiropractor told me I would feel worse before getting better, but that never happened. I had to go back to my internist and get a shot of cortisone and medication to help me feel better."

Nurses

- These professionals fill a variety of roles in several different settings, from hospitals to private homes.

- Nurses' positive attitude of caring and concern helps survey participants both physically and emotionally.

Nursing is called the caring profession, and the nurses who minister to our survey participants care for them in many different ways—as attending nurses in hospitals where participants have had surgery, as assistants in doctors' offices where they go for regular exams, as visiting or practical nurses who come to their homes, as nurse practitioners who provide some form of treatment, and as instructors in courses aimed at helping them remain independent. No matter which role the nurses fill, they seem to help most by sharing a personal warmth and an attitude of real concern. Here are the statistics.

Total number of **nurses** seen	108	
Number rated by participants	100	(93%)
Outcome of care:		
Dramatic long-term relief	22	(22%)
Moderate long-term relief	24	(24%)
Temporary relief	39	(39%)
No relief (ineffective)	10	(10%)
Made participant feel worse	5	(5%)

Nurses are often the ones who take the time to give small bits of advice that make large differences in the quality of a participant's life. "The nurse at my family doctor's office gives me moral support and a little praise," says a forty-two-year-old homemaker from Montana. "She gives me practical suggestions, too. Thanks to her I wear insulated mittens instead of gloves, insulated socks, and boys' shoes, usually, because they come with wider, rounder toes that keep my feet more comfortable."

An escapee from city life, who now lives quietly in the

woods of Wisconsin, gets reflexology treatments, or foot massages aimed at resolving pain elsewhere in her body, from a
nurse: "The treatments bring relief for twelve to twenty-four
hours. The nurse also taught me some stretching exercises and
gave me a relaxation tape. When I exercise and use the tape,
I get eight to twelve hours of relief. She has also recommended
a diet/vitamin/mineral program that seems to be keeping my
arthritis in check."

Exercise Instructors

- Many kinds of exercise instructors help survey participants find long-term relief.

- A safe, sane approach to exercise is the deciding factor in
  their success—not the type of exercise they teach.

Exercise instructors come in all guises, from health-spa owners
and track coaches to judo experts and Yoga teachers. In fact,
more participants mentioned Yoga instructors than any other
type of exercise teacher. Of the fifty-eight exercise instructors
seen, twenty-seven were Yoga teachers, and thirteen of these
(48 percent) helped their students find *lasting* relief.
    Whether exercise instructors teach people individually or
in groups, their record of success with our survey participants
is impressive.

Total number of **exercise instructors** seen	58	
Number rated by participants	55	(95%)
Outcome of instruction:		
Dramatic long-term relief	18	(33%)
Moderate long-term relief	12	(22%)
Temporary relief	18	(33%)
No relief (ineffective)	4	(7%)
Made participant feel worse	3	(5%)

One of the safest places to look for an exercise instructor is in
a water-exercise class at a local pool. A gentle workout in water

appears to be both pleasurable and possible, even for people who have a great deal of joint damage. It could be dangerous, however, to join an exercise class at a health club unless you tell the instructor that you have arthritis and may need some special modifications in the program. Many exercise instructors are experienced at working with people who have some kind of disability, and they are only too happy to oblige. "I go to a workout studio where the owner takes time with each student to set up a special individual program," says a writer from Missouri. "He was crippled himself for ten years, and is truly an inspiration to all of us who learn from him."

If your instructor is not sympathetic or knowledgeable about arthritis, proceed with caution, and let your body be your guide. A safe program starts out slowly and increases gradually. Many participants acknowledge that exercise may hurt a little before it brings relief. But movements that cause a lot of pain are not going to help you and may make matters worse. The slogan "No pain, no gain" does *not* apply to people who are already in pain and are exercising to banish it!

Mental-Health Practitioners*

- These practitioners teach valuable techniques for controlling pain with mental energy.

- Their "talk therapy" gets results, too, by helping participants accept themselves—and accept arthritis.

Psychiatrists, psychologists, and counselors are able to achieve more enduring pain relief for our participants than any other non-M.D. practitioner rated here. The secret of their success lies in the techniques they teach for exercising the mind's power over the body, including self-hypnosis, imagery, biofeedback, and relaxation. All of these mental tools improve with use, and participants continue to control pain effectively with them years after their last visit to a mental-health practitioner.

*All types of mental-health practitioners seen by our participants, including psychiatrists (who are M.D.s), are considered together in this section.

Total number of **mental-health professionals** seen	46	
Number rated by participants	45	(98%)
Outcome of care:		
Dramatic long-term relief	18	(40%)
Moderate long-term relief	12	(27%)
Temporary relief	7	(15.5%)
No relief (ineffective)	7	(15.5%)
Made participant feel worse	1	(2%)

The success of these practitioners does not imply that their patients' pain was "all in their heads," or milder than the norm. Participants who praise mental-health practitioners include those with rheumatoid arthritis and those with osteoarthritis, old and young, with pain ranging from moderate to severe. Indeed, most participants who believe in the "mind over matter" approach use it *along with* other kinds of treatment— medication, exercise, physical therapy—but reap a special bonus for trying to will themselves well. "I saw a psychiatrist who taught me how to use biofeedback," says a forty-year-old housewife from Ohio. "I can relax more and handle stress better because of it. I can also raise the temperature in various parts of my body, to decrease the pain there."

Psychologists and psychiatrists are also frequently consulted for psychotherapy, or the attempt to solve emotional problems by talking about them to a qualified practitioner. Several participants find psychotherapy to be an effective part of their treatment, as arthritis pain is frequently aggravated by stress. Also, some of them have been plagued by problems of denial, depression, and loss of self-esteem that followed in the wake of their arthritis diagnosis. "I had only one session with the psychologist," says a retired receptionist from Arizona, "but it helped change my self-image so that I was better able to deal with pain, and I became determined to help myself."

A twenty-two-year-old California student writes: "I've had rheumatoid arthritis since I was fifteen. I don't want to have to live with it, but I have to learn to do it anyway. The psychiatrist has helped me cope with the fact of arthritis, and given me ways to relieve pain."

There are so many kinds of mental-health professionals practicing so many different forms of psychotherapy or behavior modification that we could not even list all the types here. The best places to go for a referral are your doctor, a trusted friend or family member, or your county mental-health association. Knowing the type of help you want—self-hypnosis instruction, for example, or the chance to talk about your feelings—will speed the referral process along. If psychotherapy is your desire, a good recommendation is only the beginning, as *you* must determine, face-to-face, whether the therapist is the type of person who invites your trust and confidence. "I saw a psychiatrist for a period of six months," writes an artist from Colorado, "and she only made me feel worse. A psychiatrist who adds to the stress of an arthritis patient simply aggravates the problem."

Acupuncturists

- Many kinds of practitioners offer acupuncture, but training separates the effective from the less so.

- Acupuncturists often achieve lasting results for those who seek their help.

As with mental health practitioners, the acupuncturists in our survey are a mixed group of M.D.s and non-M.D.s. (Some chiropractors give acupuncture treatments, too, but ratings for all chiropractors are listed earlier in this chapter.) The treatment they offer, shrouded in history and mystery, has been used for thousands of years to assuage every imaginable symptom of illness, especially pain, and also to promote well-being in healthy individuals. More than half of the acupuncturists who treated our survey participants helped them find enduring results.

Total number of **acupuncturists** seen	37	
Number rated by participants	37	(100%)
Outcome of care:		
Dramatic long-term relief	12	(32%)
Moderate long-term relief	7	(19%)
Temporary relief	8	(22%)
No relief (ineffective)	8	(22%)
Made participant feel worse	2	(5%)

"The acupuncturist was the only one who knew what he was doing," swears a retired claims examiner from New York City. "In fact, the pain in my knee subsided after the first treatment. I am still visiting this gentle, knowledgeable Oriental medical doctor. I found the internist I consulted to be handicapped by his attitude on arthritis—'You'll have to live with it.' No comments on the chiropractor I saw, except to say that his knowledge and know-how were limited."

A doctor doesn't have to be Oriental to use acupuncture, of course, but teachers of acupuncture agree that the best practitioners are the ones educated in the *entire theory and use* of this ancient healing art. A GP or orthopedist, who has taken a weekend seminar in the placement of acupuncture needles for pain relief, for example, is not likely to be as successful as another practitioner—M.D. or non-M.D.—who has had several hundred hours of training in acupuncture's full scope and technique.

Ineffective acupuncturists are fairly common, our survey shows. So if you decide to try acupuncture, make sure you get the most out of the venture by choosing an experienced practitioner who is either state-licensed or certified by the National Commission for the Certification of Acupuncturists in Washington, D. C.

You'll probably need to try several treatments before you can judge whether the acupuncturist is helping you. At the same time, no responsible acupuncturist would tell you to stop taking your arthritis drugs as a prerequisite for receiving treatment. Like any other approach, acupuncture for arthritis is one element in a comprehensive program.

Although the risks of acupuncture appear vanishingly small, practitioners do leave some people feeling worse than before. "The acupuncturist did not help me," writes a thirty-five-year-old housing security officer from California, "as I could not stand the needles and the treatment caused me a lot of stress." Another participant reported negative results with one acupuncturist but then got a great deal of help when he went to a different practitioner.

Podiatrists

- These specialists can help solve arthritis-related foot problems.

- Orthotics (shoe inserts) prescribed by a podiatrist can make walking considerably more comfortable.

Although they are limited to treating the joints in the feet, podiatrists often get good results, and several of our participants thank them for providing far-reaching help. A podiatrist's surgery, for example, helped a California housewife walk again.

"The podiatrist was the only one who would listen to me at first," writes a telephone operator from Arizona. "He gave me physical therapy on my feet and ankles, had orthotics made for my shoes, which helped a lot, and he insisted that my internist check me for osteoarthritis and osteoporosis. It turns out I have both."

Total number of **podiatrists** seen	21	
Number rated by participants	21	(100%)
Outcome of care:		
Dramatic long-term relief	7	(33%)
Moderate long-term relief	4	(19%)
Temporary relief	7	(33%)
No relief (ineffective)	2	(10%)
Made participant feel worse	1	(5%)

The sole participant to blame a podiatrist for making him feel worse is a licensed practical nurse from Ohio who underwent an unnecessary and damaging operation on his foot. "Podiatrists can provide orthotics," he says, "which provide some relief. But in some communities, sporting-goods stores provide the same service—from people who are just as capable and certainly much less expensive!" Indeed, "over-the-counter" arch supports are a familiar sight in pharmacies and variety stores, too.

Podiatrists sometimes prescribe drugs, such as **Naprosyn**

or other anti-inflammatory agents. If you see a podiatrist who gives you a prescription, find out how it will mesh with the other medications you are taking.

Other Non-M.D. Practitioners

- Occupational therapists dramatically improve participants' ability to remain active and independent.

- Nutritionists and dietitians help most participants who seek and follow their advice.

Many other kinds of non-M.D. practitioners figure in our survey, including, in alphabetical order, aromatherapists, body workers, dentists, dietitians, herbologists, massage therapists, naturopaths, nutritionists, occupational therapists, and spiritual healers. Although we hesitate to rate any type of practitioner on the basis of fewer than twenty reports, we would like to share a few interesting trends and observations on these other health professionals.

- A massage from a physical therapist or a chiropractor may bring temporary relief, as we've seen, but a massage from a **masseur** or **massage therapist** may be a different story. Two participants out of nineteen found massage from this source to be useless, and another four participants say they were injured in the process. On the positive side, two participants ascribe dramatic long-term relief to their massage therapists, five get moderate long-term relief, and six get short-term benefits. You can probably tip the massage odds in your favor by seeking out a well-trained, *licensed* massage therapist who practices "medical massage."
- **Occupational therapists** gave advice and practical tips that thirteen out of seventeen participants found extremely or moderately useful over the long run. The suggestions had to do with performing tasks more easily, both at home and at work, and with ways to protect the joints from further injury. Another two got temporary help from occupational therapists. At their worst, these practitioners were ineffective or failed to tell

our participants anything they didn't already know—but they did not hurt anyone in our survey.

■ **Nutritionists and dietitians** helped thirteen out of fourteen participants who sought their advice. "The nutritionist changed my diet and told me to take vitamins E and C," writes a retired aluminum welder for Union Carbide. "This eased the pain and made me feel much better. After three months, I found I could cut down on the aspirin."

■ Two of the six **dentists** our participants saw were able to provide dramatic relief for jaw pain with a plastic mouthpiece to wear during sleep. Two others, however, removed all of the participants' mercury/silver fillings on the grounds that these were arthritis-aggravating. "I did not notice any improvement," an audiologist from Ohio says of this approach, "but I did not get any worse, either."

Summary of Non-M.D. Practitioners

Most highly recommended

> Physical therapist
> Exercise instructor

Also highly recommended

> Nurse
> Mental health practitioner
> Occupational therapist
> Nutritionist or dietitian

Worth a try

> Acupuncturist
> Podiatrist

Not recommended

> Chiropractor
> Massage therapist

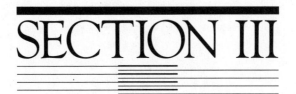

SECTION III

THE VALUE
OF ORTHODOX
TREATMENTS
FOR ARTHRITIS

All substances are poisons; there is none which is not a poison. The right dose differentiates a poison from a remedy.

—Philippus Aureolus Paracelsus (1493–1541)

An orthopedic surgeon who fell asleep in 1947 and awoke in 1987 could not comprehend the vast advancements. . . . Management of joint diseases in the adult by total joint replacement is possibly the most significant development in orthopedics in the past 40 years.

—Paul P. Griffin, M.D., from a retrospective in
Postgraduate Medicine, July 1987

So far I have spent about $25,000 over 35 years with different doctors, medicines, etc. The rheumatologist finally told me that aspirin was the best medicine he could prescribe.

—Survey Participant #1050, a retired teacher from
Virginia

5

RATING AND COMPARING THE MAJOR PRESCRIPTION DRUGS:
The First Across-the-Board Evaluation of Arthritis Medications

■ Personal preferences in anti-inflammatory drugs ■ Breaking the steroid habit ■ Going for the gold ■ The special uses of antirheumatic and cytotoxic drugs

All the major prescription drugs for arthritis—some twenty products that we'll discuss in this chapter—fall into just two broad categories, called, simply, the first line and the second line.

The first-line drugs are used to control pain and inflammation in both osteoarthritis and rheumatoid arthritis. They include the nonsteroidal anti-inflammatory drugs (NSAIDs), such as **Feldene** and **Motrin**, and the steroids, such as prednisone in pill form and cortisone injections into particularly troublesome joints. Aspirin, which is probably the most widely used and perhaps the most effective drug for arthritis, is also part of the first line. (However, since aspirin is an over-the-counter medication, not a prescription drug, it is covered in Chapter 6.)

The second-line treatments behave in mysterious ways that may slow the underlying disease process in rheumatoid arthritis: gold, in pills or shots; hydroxychloroquine, which is a malaria treatment that may slow down the destruction of the joints; penicillamine, a very different-acting relative of the famous antibiotic; and the cytotoxic drugs, originally developed for treating cancer. Some doctors relegate the cytotoxic drugs to a separate category—the so-called third line—to emphasize the fact that they are newcomers to arthritis care, and should be used with extreme caution.

Reports from the 1,051 participants in our nationwide Arthritis Survey allow us to rate and compare all these medications, both in terms of their positive effects on arthritis symptoms *and* their noisome side effects. At the end of this chapter, you'll find tips on buying and taking prescription drugs, including important questions for your doctor and inexpensive mail-order drug sources.

THE FIRST LINE:

Nonsteroidal Anti-Inflammatory Drugs (NSAIDs)

As we've said before, the lowly aspirin is generally recognized as the most effective arthritis medication. In high doses of about ten or twelve 5-grain tablets a day, it can work to control both pain and inflammation, and it's cheap, too. The trouble with aspirin, though, is that it irritates the stomach more than many people can bear. The threat of gastrointestinal bleeding and full-blown ulcers is very real to those who take arthritis-strength doses of aspirin. Indeed, aspirin's often intolerable side effects created the market for today's NSAIDs, all of which aim to be easier on the gut but none of which substantially improves on the original.

Though these drugs all have to prove themselves against aspirin's benchmark, they take their class name from the other arthritis "wonder drugs"—the steroids, including cortisone and prednisone. When cortisone was first isolated in the 1940s, it was hailed by some as the cure for rheumatoid arthritis because it banished inflammation so quickly and completely.

It didn't really cure the disease, however, it only masked the symptoms. And as time passed, the ugly side effects of long-term use became all too obvious—cataracts, bone fractures, and thin fragile skin, to name a few. Today steroids are given more sparingly and cautiously. The NSAIDs do not approach their power for reducing inflammation, but their side effects are considered far less toxic.

The first widely used anti-inflammatory drug other than aspirin that was *not* a steroid was phenylbutazone (**Butazolidin**). It's considered part of the NSAID family today, but when it first came out in 1949, steroids were scarcely used, so it wasn't called "nonsteroidal."

The first anti-inflammatory agent to appear in the wake of the wonders wrought (and havoc wreaked) by steroid drugs was indomethacin, known by its trade name, **Indocin**, and introduced by Merck Sharp & Dohme in 1963. It is still widely used, although it now competes with about a dozen newcomers on the American market, including two more drugs manufactured by the same company: sulindac (**Clinoril**) and diflunisal (**Dolobid**). Upjohn unveiled its candidate, ibuprofen (**Motrin**), in 1974, although the drug was originally developed by Boots, in England, where it is called **Rufen**. Today ibuprofen is also available in generic form, since its patent period has ended, as well as in nonprescription-strength tablets from several manufacturers.

If you read, as we've been reading, what doctors counsel other doctors about these drugs, you learn that there are no significant differences among them. And yet, one person with arthritis will thrive on **Indocin**, while the next person taking it will feel nothing but angry and nauseated until he tries **Motrin**, which works perfectly for him, even though it did nothing for the first person. No one can account for the wide variation in the way people react to these medicines, and, unfortunately, no one can predict which one is most likely to work for you. This means that you are in for a trial-and-error period that may be tough in many respects. But it also means that if the first drug doesn't bring relief, you're likely to hit on one that will.

Our survey participants have experience with all the NSAIDs, and their ratings allow us to compare them. The drug that offered them the highest rate of long-term relief and the lowest rate of unpleasant reactions was fenoprofen (**Nalfon**), produced by Dista since 1976. As you'll see, however, only thirty-eight participants took and rated **Nalfon**, while we had hundreds of reports on the more popular drugs such as **Motrin**, **Indocin**, **Naprosyn**, and **Feldene**.

The six most popular NSAIDs used by our survey participants are, in alphabetical order: **Clinoril**, **Feldene**, **Indocin**, **Motrin**, **Naprosyn**, and **Tolectin**. Let's compare these on several features, beginning with popularity. Here's how they stack up.

1. **Motrin** (ibuprofen)—554 participants
2. **Indocin** (indomethacin)—352
3. **Naprosyn** (naproxen)—335
4. **Feldene** (piroxicam)—326
5. **Tolectin** (tolmetin)—142
6. **Clinoril** (sulindac)—120

The above listing actually reflects the drugs' popularity among *doctors*, since our participants can't take an NSAID unless their doctors prescribe it. To figure the drugs' relative popularity among our *participants*, we'll use the rating scale that appeared on the questionnaire (Appendix A). The following list puts the drugs in order of the greatest percentage of top ratings—"plus 3," or "dramatic long-term relief."

1. **Clinoril** (sulindac)—26% of those taking it
2. **Feldene** (piroxicam)—23%
3. **Motrin** (ibuprofen)—19%
4. **Naprosyn** (naproxen)—19%
5. **Indocin** (indomethacin)—15%
6. **Tolectin** (tolmetin)—13%

If we pool *all* the positive ratings for each of the drugs—"plus 3" (dramatic long-term relief), "plus 2" (moderate long-term relief), *and* "plus 1" (temporary or minor relief)—the lineup takes this shape.

1. **Clinoril** (sulindac)—65% of those taking it
2. **Motrin** (ibuprofen)—64%
3. **Naprosyn** (naproxen)—64%
4. **Indocin** (indomethacin)—60%
5. **Feldene** (piroxicam)—59%
6. **Tolectin** (tolmetin)—55%

Yes, you guessed it. Turning the above list upside down puts the drugs in order of the highest percentage of "0" ratings from people who found them no help at all.

As for side effects, **Motrin** and **Naprosyn** caused the fewest, overall. Here's a list that shows the percentage of people taking each drug who reported *no* adverse reactions.

1. **Motrin** (ibuprofen)—38% of those taking it
2. **Naprosyn** (naproxen)—38%
3. **Tolectin** (tolmetin)—35%
4. **Feldene** (piroxicam)—34%
5. **Clinoril** (sulindac)—33%
6. **Indocin** (indomethacin)—30%

These comparisons are interesting, but as we said earlier, they don't predict the way the drugs will behave for you. It's more instructive to consider each one's record individually, in the light of what is known about the NSAIDs as a group. We'll also look at half a dozen other drugs in the nonsteroidal anti-inflammatory family in addition to these "top six." The following products are listed according to their frequency of use, beginning with those taken by the greatest number of survey participants.

Motrin
(ibuprofen, Upjohn)

Number of participants taking **Motrin**	554	
Outcome:		
Dramatic relief	106	(19%)
Moderate relief	96	(17%)
Temporary or minor relief only	155	(28%)
No relief (ineffective)	143	(26%)
No rating*	54	(10%)
Most common drug reactions:†		
No unpleasant side effects	210	(38%)
Stomach upset, pain, or indigestion	89	(16%)
Nausea and/or vomiting	72	(13%)
Dizziness or drowsiness	53	(10%)

*Participants did not rate a drug they had just started taking, or one to which they reacted badly and stopped taking before they could judge its effectiveness.
†Side effects listed in these ratings were reported by at least 10% of the participants on a given drug.

Like all NSAIDs, **Motrin** is both a pain reliever and an anti-inflammatory drug. It may work on your pain in a hurry, perhaps within a short time after you take your very first dose; but you may have to wait at least a week before you can tell how well it controls your inflammation. The same is true of the other drugs in this class. This is why your doctor will encourage you to stay with **Motrin**, for example, even if the first few weeks don't seem so promising. One strategy doctors use with NSAIDs is to prescribe them for two weeks, then, if there's no significant change, increase the dosage for another few weeks, and then, if there's still no improvement, try a different NSAID.

"While taking **Indocin** I suffered from nausea and abdominal pain," says a North Carolina homemaker. "**Nalfon** made me dizzy and caused a peptic ulcer. **Motrin** has helped more than the others, and with fewer side effects."

Indocin
(indomethacin, Merck Sharp & Dohme)

Number of participants taking **Indocin**	352	
Outcome:		
Dramatic relief	52	(15%)
Moderate relief	61	(17%)
Temporary or minor relief only	97	(28%)
No relief (ineffective)	102	(29%)
No rating	40	(11%)
Most common drug reactions:		
No unpleasant side effects	105	(30%)
Nausea and/or vomiting	65	(18%)
Stomach upset, pain, or indigestion	48	(14%)
Dizziness or drowsiness	44	(13%)

The side effects from most NSAIDs center on the gut, otherwise known as the gastrointestinal or GI tract. As you'll see from the ratings, nausea, vomiting, and stomach upset or pain are the most frequently mentioned side effects for the drugs in this class. And, as far as anyone can tell, the reason they cause so much grief is the *same* reason they bring so much relief. Aspirin and other NSAIDs apparently reduce inflammation and pain by blocking the body's production of substances called prostaglandins. There are *some* prostaglandins, however, that work to protect the stomach lining. The NSAIDs' shotgun destruction of them may leave the stomach open to injury.

What's more, since the NSAIDs are swallowed and spend some time inside the stomach, they get a chance to cause a little direct irritation while they're there. This is why your doctor has probably told you to take your medication with food or milk, so that you buffer the drug and hasten it along its way. Your chance of developing an ulcer if you have arthritis is at least one in five, due to these drugs. In fact, some of our survey participants listed a prescription ulcer drug—**Tagamet** (cimetidine), **Zantac** (ranitidine), or **Carafate** (sucralfate)—right under their arthritis medications.

The makers of **Indocin** tried hard to get around the stomach-irritation problem with a rectal suppository version of the drug, but no one in our survey was taking **Indocin** in that way.

"Of all the anti-inflammatories, **Indocin** is the most power-ful," writes a thirty-six-year-old househusband and father with rheumatoid arthritis, who has taken **Anaprox, Clinoril, Fel-dene, Meclomen, Motrin, Naprosyn, Oraflex, Orudis,** and **To-lectin. Indocin** has helped him as much as **Plaquenil** and prednisone, he says. "Sometimes I have to back off a little when I start getting dizzy and nauseous with it. Sometimes I get a little jumpy, too."

Naprosyn
(naproxen, Syntex)

Number of participants taking **Naprosyn**	335	
Outcome:		
Dramatic relief	62	(19%)
Moderate relief	61	(18%)
Temporary or minor relief only	90	(27%)
No relief (ineffective)	88	(26%)
No rating	34	(10%)
Most common drug reactions:		
No unpleasant side effects	128	(38%)
Stomach upset, pain, or indigestion	55	(16%)
Nausea and/or vomiting	45	(13%)

No medical researchers, whether they work independently or for a drug manufacturer, have attempted to compare all the NSAIDs in terms of their effectiveness and their side effects.* Much is known about both subjects, however, from the limited comparisons that have been done, and from doctors' long ex-perience in giving certain drugs to their patients and then hearing how they fared. This is how **Indocin** got its reputation for being more likely to bring on headaches and psychological effects, such as anger or confusion, and how **Meclomen** be-came known for causing diarrhea. These tendencies showed up in our survey data, too. Fully 15 percent of those partici-pants taking **Meclomen** said that it caused diarrhea, while only

---

*Admittedly, these drugs come and go pretty regularly, as we'll see, which makes it hard to pin down the entire group.

1 percent of those on **Motrin** and 3 percent of those on **Indocin** were troubled with diarrhea. As for causing headaches and psychological changes, **Indocin**, at 6 percent of those taking it, was more aggravating to our survey participants than **Motrin** (2 percent), **Naprosyn** (4 percent), and **Feldene** (2 percent). Other unfortunate associations reported by the drug manufacturers include **Tolectin** with allergic reactions and **Nalfon** with kidney damage. On the positive side, **Clinoril** is reputed to be kindest to the kidneys, although not completely benign, while **Meclomen** and **Feldene** are said to be easiest on the liver.

"I've been using **Naprosyn** since the summer of 1985," reports an electric-meter reader from California. "The pain was reduced immediately, and the pills have never bothered me. Even if I take them on an empty stomach, I get only very slight nausea."

Feldene

(piroxicam, Pfizer)

Number of participants taking **Feldene**	326	
Outcome:		
Dramatic relief	76	(23%)*
Moderate relief	46	(14%)
Temporary or minor relief only	73	(22%)
No relief (ineffective)	91	(28%)
No rating	40	(12%)
Most common drug reactions:		
No unpleasant side effects	110	(34%)
Stomach upset, pain, or indigestion	62	(19%)
Nausea and/or vomiting	44	(13%)

*Rather than carry out the percentages to decimal places, we round off, with the result that ratings for some drugs total 99 or 101%.

Feldene, although it is similar to other NSAIDs in most respects, has one advantage in that it's easy to swallow, or rather, you only have to swallow it once a day. Other NSAIDs have to be taken at least twice a day, or as often as four times a day, while aspirin users may need to down three or four tablets together at each dosage time. Some physicians—not to mention Pfizer Laboratories, the manufacturer of **Feldene**—believe that making an arthritis drug easier to take makes it more likely that people will remember to take it, and therefore get the most benefit from it.

Not long after **Feldene** was introduced in 1982, however, the Public Citizen Health Research Group began warning that **Feldene** was unsafe for older people. The high-dose regimen contained in a single capsule of **Feldene**, charged Dr. Sidney Wolfe, posed a special danger to individuals age sixty or over, whose bodies overreact to many drugs. Dr. Wolfe's group eventually petitioned the Food and Drug Administration to require a special warning label for **Feldene**, but the petition was rejected in 1986. Dr. Otis Bowen, then Secretary of Health and Human Services, said that **Feldene** was no more likely than other NSAIDs to cause serious gastrointestinal problems for the elderly.

Indeed, if you are over sixty-five, you may be more susceptible to any of the side effects from any of these drugs, and your doctor will have to prescribe them cautiously and watch you carefully.

"I've been taking **Feldene** for four and a half years," says a sixty-six-year-old educator from Delaware who gave the drug high marks. "Once I learned to take it in the morning with breakfast, I had no trouble with it. Last summer I had a complete upper and lower GI series, and the doctor said I was fine."

Tolectin
(tolmetin sodium, McNeil Pharmaceutical)

Number of participants taking **Tolectin**	142	
Outcome:		
Dramatic relief	18	(13%)
Moderate relief	17	(12%)
Temporary or minor relief only	43	(30%)
No relief (ineffective)	47	(33%)
No rating	17	(12%)
Most common drug reactions:		
No unpleasant side effects	49	(35%)
Stomach upset, pain, or indigestion	15	(11%)
Nausea and/or vomiting	14	(10%)

Being fancier updates of aspirin, all the NSAIDs have appreciably higher price tags. Some of them cost more than one dollar per pill. "I nearly fainted when I found out how much **Feldene** costs," says an audiologist from Indiana, "but I have no nausea and I feel much better."

If comparing the cost of **Tolectin**, for example, with aspirin makes you feel faint, remember that the cost of the pill is not the only expense of taking the drug. Writing recently in *The Journal of Musculoskeletal Medicine,* rheumatologists Daniel O. Clegg, M.D., and John R. Ward, M.D., point out: "If the cost of treatment for peptic ulcer disease and of hospitalization for GI hemorrhage is included, aspirin indeed may not be the least expensive anti-inflammatory medication." In other words, the more expensive drugs *may* save you from other medical expenses later. After all, attempting to *minimize* side effects is the NSAIDs' whole reason for being. In general, they are thought to cause less bleeding and fewer ulcers than aspirin. Some of them, like aspirin, can make your ears ring. Others may change your appetite or your blood pressure. Most of them have the potential, like aspirin, to cause a rash, itching, or hives. "After a few days of taking **Tolectin**," writes a Florida teacher, "I developed hives all over my chest and a rash on my abdomen and thighs. I phoned the doctor, but he did not appear at all concerned. Anyway, the hives and rash were gone after a day, never occurred again, and there have been no other side effects in over three years of taking **Tolectin**."

Clinoril
(sulindac, Merck Sharp & Dohme)

Number of participants taking **Clinoril**	120	
Outcome:		
Dramatic relief	31	(26%)
Moderate relief	25	(21%)
Temporary or minor relief only	22	(18%)
No relief (ineffective)	33	(28%)
No rating	9	(7%)
Most common drug reactions:		
No unpleasant side effects	40	(33%)
Dizziness or drowsiness	19	(16%)
Nausea and/or vomiting	15	(13%)
Stomach upset, pain, or indigestion	12	(10%)

For all the help they provide, the NSAIDs do not cure arthritis. Some laboratory studies with animals or individual cells have shown that one or another of these drugs appears to reverse the joint damage already done by arthritis, but this has yet to be proven in any group of humans.

Since they do not cure, NSAIDs are long-term therapy. And yet, as you may have noticed, their effects can wear off with time. "I used **Motrin** successfully for fourteen years," says a Weight Watchers lecturer from Delaware, "and then it finally quit working." A manager of a car dealership in Vermont writes, "I was on **Clinoril** for nine years and got a great deal of relief, but I apparently built up a resistance and by the end of that time it did very little for me."

Dolobid
(diflunisal, Merck Sharp & Dohme)

Number of participants taking **Dolobid**	84	
Outcome:		
Dramatic relief	9	(11%)
Moderate relief	11	(13%)
Temporary or minor relief only	21	(25%)
No relief (ineffective)	27	(32%)
No rating	16	(19%)
Most common drug reactions:		
No unpleasant side effects	24	(28%)
Nausea and/or vomiting	12	(14%)
Stomach upset, pain, or indigestion	12	(14%)
Dizziness or drowsiness	9	(11%)

NSAIDs may be prescribed for osteoarthritis or rheumatoid arthritis, to good effect, but the drugs play different roles in the two ailments. Rheumatoid arthritis is by definition an inflammatory disease, and NSAIDs are a mainstay of treatment. Even if you require one of the second-line drugs for rheumatoid arthritis, such as gold or penicillamine, your doctor will no doubt tell you to continue taking one of the NSAIDs.

The role of inflammation in osteoarthritis, on the other hand, is much foggier. Inflammation may be present *some* of the time, as opposed to most of the time, or it may be present in such a slight degree that only the most sensitive diagnostic measures can prove it's there. However, since the process of inflammation is thought to damage the joints, controlling it with NSAIDs when necessary makes sense—and, of course, the NSAIDs *also* act as painkillers. If you have osteoarthritis, your doctor will probably strive for the lowest dose possible, and he or she may suggest that you drop the NSAID from time to time, to see how you fare without it. This cautionary move is to avoid the risk of GI side effects. There is *no* danger of becoming addicted to any of the NSAIDs, as there is with narcotic painkillers.

"A few months ago, I stopped taking the **Dolobid** for about a week at my doctor's suggestion," writes a retired nurse from New Jersey who has had osteoarthritis for ten years. "But the pain in my hips and knees was much worse and more continuous then, so I went back on it." **Dolobid** works better for her, she finds, than the others she has tried: **Feldene, Motrin, Naprosyn,** and **Tolectin.**

Meclomen
(meclofenamate sodium, Parke-Davis)

Number of participants taking **Meclomen**	39	
Outcome:		
Dramatic relief	8	(21%)*
Moderate relief	8	(21%)
Temporary or minor relief only	8	(21%)
No relief (ineffective)	11	(28%)
No rating	4	(10%)
Most common drug reactions:		
No unpleasant side effects	13	(33%)
Diarrhea	6	(15%)
Nausea and/or vomiting	4	(10%)

*Rather than carry out the percentages to decimal places, we round off, with the result that ratings for some drugs total 99 or 101%.

"When I need to lift my spirits," writes a retired legal secretary from Wisconsin, "I think back to how bad it was before I started taking **Meclomen.** I had to stop using it twice because of extreme diarrhea, but I've had no further trouble with it in the three years since that time."

We've said that NSAIDs serve two functions: reducing

inflammation and relieving pain. For most of them, a relatively small dose is all that's needed to unleash their full pain-relieving power. Higher doses bring on the anti-inflammatory effect. As a general rule, then, if the drug controls your inflammation, it is doing all it can do to relieve your pain. But what happens if you are getting good control of your inflammation with the drug you're taking and yet you still have pain from time to time? Should you take more of the drug?

Most experts say no. An extra measure of the same medicine will not only fail to help you but it will raise your chances of suffering some adverse side effect; nor can you call in another NSAID to boost the power of the one you're taking. Since the NSAIDs are so similar to each other, using two together multiplies the risks of all side effects. Remember, too, that over-the-counter drugs such as aspirin and ibuprofen (**Nuprin, Advil**, and **Medipren**, for example) are also anti-inflammatory agents. Check with your doctor before you mix any of these with your prescription pills. Acetaminophen (**Tylenol** or **Datril**, for example), since it's *not* an anti-inflammatory, is a safer bet for added pain relief. Or your doctor may recommend a prescription painkiller for you to use from time to time.

Nalfon
(fenoprofen calcium, Dista)

Number of participants taking **Nalfon**	38	
Outcome:		
Dramatic relief	15	(40%)
Moderate relief	9	(24%)
Temporary or minor relief only	2	(5%)
No relief (ineffective)	5	(13%)
No rating	7	(18%)
Most common drug reactions:		
No unpleasant side effects	16	(42%)
Dizziness or drowsiness	4	(11%)

As we mentioned earlier, **Nalfon** brought the highest rate of dramatic relief of all the NSAIDs rated in our survey—40 percent, as compared to 26 percent for **Clinoril**, the next highest, and 19 percent for **Motrin**, the most widely used drug in our survey. As for side effects, **Nalfon** users were the least likely to suffer from them—42 percent reported no unpleasant drug reactions. **Motrin** and **Naprosyn** came the closest to matching this impressive record, as 38 percent of the participants taking each of these drugs said they had no troublesome side effects. The percentage of **Nalfon**-induced stomach upset was too low to be listed in the ratings—only 3 percent, which means that only one survey participant made such a complaint. Another 8 percent (three more participants) blamed **Nalfon** for their nausea.

One special category of drug fallout has not been mentioned yet, and that is the effect of the NSAIDs when used by pregnant or nursing women. In fact, none of the NSAIDs has been adequately tested for safety during pregnancy or nursing. If you are planning to have a baby, you'll want to discuss your medication with your obstetrician and make any necessary adjustments. If you have rheumatoid arthritis, you may find that your joint pain and inflammation all but vanish during pregnancy, anyway, perhaps because of the natural changes in hormone levels and the immune system that keep your body from rejecting the half-foreign cells of your baby.

Orudis
(ketoprofen, Wyeth)

Number of participants taking **Orudis**	38	
Outcome:		
Dramatic relief	2	(5%)
Moderate relief	9	(24%)
Temporary or minor relief only	12	(32%)
No relief (ineffective)	8	(21%)
No rating	7	(18%)
Most common drug reactions:		
No unpleasant side effects	9	(24%)
Stomach upset, pain, or indigestion	7	(18%)
Nausea and/or vomiting	4	(11%)

Although the NSAIDs make up a group, or family, of drugs, some of them are more closely related than others. For example, **Indocin**, **Clinoril**, and **Tolectin** make up one chemical

class, called indoles, while **Dolobid, Disalcid, Monogesic,** and
aspirin are part of another, called salicylates. Your doctor may
use these class lists in trying to find the right NSAID for you.
As the theory goes, if **Indocin** fails to help you, you probably
wouldn't find much comfort in either of its classmates, **Clinoril**
or **Tolectin.** That's the theory. In practice, however, the drugs
continue to defy anybody's predictions. Often enough, the
person who gets no comfort from **Indocin** goes on to have
great success with **Clinoril.**

"My internist prescribed **Orudis,** which has been the best
medicine I ever used," writes a retired salesman from Illinois.
Motrin, however, had no effect on him, he reports, although it
belongs to the same class as **Orudis. Naprosyn,** another member of this class (called propionic acid derivatives) gave him
stomach problems, but he's had no side effects from **Orudis.**

Butazolidin
(phenylbutazone, Ciba-Geigy)

Number of participants taking **Butazolidin**	33	
Outcome:		
Dramatic relief	10	(30%)*
Moderate relief	3	(9%)
Temporary or minor relief only	11	(33%)
No relief (ineffective)	7	(21%)
No rating	2	(6%)
Most common drug reactions:		
No unpleasant side effects	10	(30%)
Stomach upset, pain, or indigestion	4	(12%)

*These percentages have been rounded to the nearest whole number, with the
result that ratings for some drugs do not total 100%.

Of the six chemical classes of NSAIDs we mentioned above,
one has fallen far behind the others in popularity. This is the
class containing phenylbutazone (**Butazolidin**) and oxyphen-
butazone (**Tandearil**). Ciba-Geigy took **Tandearil** off the market in 1985, and put new restrictions on the use of **Butazolidin**
at that time. **Butazolidin** is no longer recommended as an early
choice, but only as a last resort if other NSAIDs fail, and it is
not to be used on a long-term basis. In addition to the usual

risks, **Butazolidin** has the potential to block the bone marrow's life-sustaining production of new blood cells.

Disalcid and Monogesic
(salsalate, Riker [**Disalcid**] and Central Pharmaceuticals [**Monogesic**])

Number of participants taking **salsalate**	25	
Outcome:		
Dramatic relief	6	(24%)
Moderate relief	5	(20%)
Temporary or minor relief only	4	(16%)
No relief (ineffective)	4	(16%)
No rating	6	(24%)
Most common drug reactions:		
No unpleasant side effects	9	(36%)

Before a drug company can market a new drug, it must run trials in which large numbers of volunteers (healthy ones first, then people who have the target disease) take the drug. Through this process, the company proves to the Food and Drug Administration that the new product is safe, and that it indeed works as it is intended to. Once the company wins FDA approval for the drug, salespeople introduce it to physicians, who then prescribe it for their patients. And that's when another trial, of sorts, begins. Because some new drugs go to market looking fine, only to fall flat later when thousands of people begin taking them in earnest. This is what happened to the now defunct benoxaprofen (**Oraflex**), introduced by Eli Lilly in early 1982 and pulled off the market by summer's end, after allegedly causing some sixty deaths in the United States and England. During the time it was available, fifty-nine of our participants tried **Oraflex**, with poor results overall.

Oraflex
(benoxaprofen, Eli Lilly)

Number of participants who tried **Oraflex**	59	
Outcome:		
Dramatic relief	4	(7%)
Moderate relief	4	(7%)
Temporary or minor relief only	14	(23%)
No relief (ineffective)	30	(51%)
No rating	7	(12%)
Most common drug reactions:		
No unpleasant side effects	15	(25%)
Stomach upset, pain, or indigestion	9	(15%)
Nausea and/or vomiting	7	(12%)

In 1987, McNeil Pharmaceutical recalled its new drug, suprofen (**Suprol**), after an untoward number of people suffered flank pain and kidney damage while taking it. Only two of our survey participants had tried **Suprol**, and neither one encountered this problem. Nine participants had used another McNeil drug that disappeared in 1983, zomepirac (**Zomax**), and six of them sorely missed it.

"Several years ago, when I first noticed arthritis pain," writes a Minnesota homemaker, "**Zomax** was the first thing prescribed for me. It was wonderful, and I got complete relief. A short time later it was taken off the market, supposedly to be returned in six months. I am still waiting for its return. Nothing else—**Indocin, Feldene, Motrin, Naprosyn**, or **Tolectin**—works as well."

As we've seen, the cast of NSAID characters is a changing one, with new drugs entering frequently, and both old and new drugs making a command exit on occasion. Carol A. Warfield, M.D., director of the Pain Management Center at Boston's Beth Israel Hospital and assistant professor at Harvard Medical School, advised recently in *Hospital Practice* that doctors "refrain from using newer NSAIDs until a track record of safety is established."

Three new NSAIDs have come *on* the market in the short time since we completed our survey. These are diclofenac (**Voltaren**, Ciba-Geigy), which was ushered in with a testimonial from baseball hero Mickey Mantle, carprofen (**Rimadyl**, Roche), and flurbiprofen (**Ansaid**, Upjohn).

Though new to the United States, **Voltaren** has been marketed in Canada and abroad for more than ten years, and three of our survey participants were already taking it, two of whom live in Canada. A fifty-year-old psychologist from Saskatchewan, for example, just started taking **Voltaren** when **Naprosyn** became ineffective after seven years of giving her great relief. She can't yet rate the new drug, she says, and she is warding off its possible side effects with tricks she's learned over the years: "All these drugs upset my stomach, so I take them after milk and use **Tagamet**."

A sixty-four-year-old school custodian from Ontario says that two 50-milligram **Voltaren** tablets per day make him feel "very good," and cause no side effects of any kind. The one American, a forty-three-year-old New Hampshire real estate agent, heard about **Voltaren** from his Canadian mother-in-law, and he began traveling north to see a rheumatologist in Canada, where he buys his prescribed **Voltaren** in six-month supplies. "It's easier on the stomach than the other drugs I've tried," he says, "and its effects seem to last longer."

According to a report in *Drug Therapy* (September 1988), **Voltaren** is rapidly eliminated from the bloodstream, which may make it safer for elderly people, but it does stay inside the joints for a long time. It is the first of a new class of NSAIDs called phenylacetic acids. As for **Rimadyl**, the FDA is thus far recommending that it be given only to people who have not responded to, or cannot tolerate, other drugs.

Steroids

The drugs in this group, though also part of the first line, are no longer offered first. Their impressive power is held in reserve until other first-line measures have been tried. And while it was once common practice to prescribe large doses of steroids for long periods of time, most doctors today use low doses for safety's sake, and frequently set up an every-other-day dosage regimen to further minimize drug side effects. You may be offered a short course of steroids to get you through an arthritis flare-up, or to tide you over a period of switching from one slow-acting drug to another, but your doctor will probably move to reduce the dose fairly quickly or get you off the drug altogether. From time to time, you may also have steroids injected directly into a severely affected joint. This technique gets the drug right to the site where it's needed most.

The steroid family drugs are synthetic copies of hormones that our bodies normally produce. Other names for them are corticosteroids, glucocorticoids, and adrenocortical steroids. The drugs themselves include dexamethasone (**Decadron** is one example), hydrocortisone or cortisol (**Cortef**, for one), methylprednisolone (**Medrol**), prednisolone (such as **Delta-Cortef**), and prednisone (**Deltasone** and others).

All of the steroids date from the 1940s and 1950s, and they all have a history of use in the treatment of many conditions other than arthritis, from asthma to cancer. Indeed, a few of our participants got their first taste of prednisone for a totally unrelated problem, and found arthritis pain relief to be the chief side effect of the drug. "Two years ago I had bypass surgery, after which I developed pericarditis [inflammation of the membrane around the heart]," writes a sixty-two-year-old homemaker from North Carolina. "I was treated with prednisone for five months, from August through December, and I had no pain from arthritis during that time."

Prednisone and other pills

Compared to the NSAIDs, the steroids are far more effective at relieving pain and reducing inflammation. As the ratings show, 52 percent of our survey participants taking steroid pills get dramatic relief, and another 33 percent report moderate or temporary relief. No NSAID comes close to that score. Steroids works so well, in fact, that many participants willingly put up with any number of troublesome side effects in exchange for the relief they get. "I have taken prednisone continuously for about eight years," writes a forty-four-year-old Texas police officer, "and I guess the side effects have come from it. My kidneys hurt, I have blurred vision because of cataracts, growth of excessive hair, and lots of water retention, causing me to swell up at the face." Puffed-out cheeks or "moonface" is a common side effect of these drugs. Less obvious but more insidious is the high blood pressure that can also come with fluid retention.

Number of participants taking **oral steroids**	133*	
Outcome:		
Dramatic relief	69	(52%)
Moderate relief	25	(19%)
Temporary or minor relief only	19	(14%)
No relief (ineffective)	5	(4%)
No rating	15	(11%)
Most common drug reactions:		
No unpleasant side effects	33	(25%)
Fluid retention, with hypertension or moon-face	22	(17%)
Thin fragile skin, bones, muscles, or tendons	15	(11%)

*"Steroids" include prednisone (110 participants), cortisone acetate (9 participants), methylprednisolone (7 participants), dexamethasone (3 participants), prednisolone (3 participants), and triamcinolone (1 participant).

Conspicuous by its absence in the list of side effects here is any mention of gastrointestinal distress, which is so common with the NSAIDs. Only five participants taking steroids complained of nausea (4 percent), three of stomach upset or cramps (2 percent), and one of diarrhea (less than 1 percent). The more serious side effects of steroid use, in addition to the ones listed in the ratings, include the risk of eye damage, diabetes, and increased susceptibility to infection. Some people have reportedly developed ulcers, too, from steroid use, although no one in our survey complained of ulcers from this source. Depression, anxiety, and other psychological fallout from steroids is well documented in clinical studies, and was reported by nine of our participants (7 percent).

"I hate prednisone," writes a homemaker from Connecticut. "Yes, it did help me through the bad flare-ups, but it made me jumpy and edgy, snapping at people for no real reason. I had trouble sleeping, too."

Steroids are also known to create a kind of drug habit called functional dependence. Because they are so similar to the natural hormones produced by the adrenal glands, steroid drugs may shut down the body's own production of those hormones. This means that if you've been taking prednisone for a while, you can't suddenly stop, lest you leave yourself virtually defenseless against infection, and find your arthritis symptoms much, much worse. Instead, you must be "weaned" off slowly, under close medical supervision.

"I took prednisolone for almost four years," writes a fifty-five-year-old farm wife from Ohio. "It made me feel wonderful at first. I could do things I couldn't do before. But the doctor didn't tell me it could cause diabetes, which I now have, or that it was dangerous to go off the medicine suddenly. At one time, I decided to quit taking it because of some of the changes that were occurring with me. I became miserable with pain and high fever, and I was practically crippled. It took me a while to realize the connection between stopping the medicine and the horrible way I felt."

Today, prednisone is used along with other treatments, including NSAIDs. "The internist I saw after I took rheumatoid arthritis twenty-six years ago," writes a coal miner from West Virginia, "told me to take aspirin, twenty-four a day, but they didn't do anything at all toward controlling the disease. I went directly from aspirin to prednisone. Since then, I have been tried on new medicines, first **Indocin**, then **Motrin**, but staying in the meantime with prednisone. By taking **Feldene** now, which works well for me, I am able to take a lesser dose of prednisone."

Getting down to the lowest dose possible, experts agree, should be the goal for anyone taking prednisone or other steroids.

Cortisone and related injections

Steroids can also be given as a shot in the arm—or the knee, the hip, the wrist, whichever part hurts most. For a joint that has been immobilized by pain or stiffness, steroid injections can bring dramatic relief that typically lasts anywhere from a few days to a few months. "Cortisone shots gave me instant relief," says a retired telephone operator from Louisiana, "and the relief lasted from a week to six months. Once I remember I couldn't even lift my arm, and as soon as I received the injection in my shoulder, my arm was free from pain and I could raise it." The best practitioners capitalize on this startling degree of relief by coupling the injections with physical therapy and safe exercises that are likely to bring about long-term improvement. They will also warn you that overuse of a suddenly pain-free joint may cause more damage in the long run.

Steroid shots promise only temporary help, but a few of our participants find themselves enjoying extremely lasting benefits from shots they took years ago. "I had a cortisone injection in my knee on May 1, 1983," reports a Florida homemaker. "The doctor said it would last for four or five months, but I have been very fortunate in that the knee has not given me any great pain that can't be helped with **Ascriptin** [aspirin] tablets." A retired social agency director from Seattle writes: "I find the shots are a blessing to me, and last several years. They say it's dangerous to take them, but as far as I'm concerned, it's better than crying all the time with pain or being in a wheelchair. I don't see how it's hurt me."

By the same token, "temporary help" from steroid shots can be relatively long-lived, compared to other treatments. A nurse from Illinois, for example, says she gets "temporary relief" lasting from three to six months after an injection of cortisone. Keep this in mind as you look at the ratings for "temporary" help.

Number of reports on **steroid shots**	485*	
Outcome:		
Dramatic relief	183	(38%)
Moderate relief	103	(21%)
Temporary or minor relief only	95	(20%)
No relief (ineffective)	57	(12%)
Participant felt worse after injection	27	(5%)
No rating	20	(4%)

*For at least twenty-three of our participants, results from steroid shots differed so greatly from one injection to the next that they listed two or more separate ratings for this treatment.

Because of the way steroid shots are given—in different joints at different times, and spread out over intervals of months or years—the experience and the amount of relief may vary greatly for some people. "I got some pain relief from cortisone in my knee," recalls a retired postal clerk from Wisconsin, "and the first time I had a shot in my hip it gave me relief for months. But the second injection in my hip six months later brought no relief at all. The pain even seemed to get worse."

"I've had many, many injections in all the affected joints during bad flare-ups over the years," writes a thirty-four-year-old homemaker from Maryland. "The injections help after several hours, although the spot where the needle goes in always hurts for a day or two. Cortisone will usually settle my hips, knees, ankles, and elbows, but it has no effect on my back, shoulders, and neck." Cortisone definitely helps some joints more than others for several participants who have tried shots in various painful places. And while the places vary from one person to the next, we had more reports of *ineffectiveness* for cortisone shots to the joints of the back and neck than to any other part of the body. This is apparently true because the joint spaces of the spine are not accessible by injection, and getting the drug into the surrounding tissue does little good, if any, according to the manufacturers.

Another, perhaps obvious point is that the effectiveness of any steroid injection depends to a large extent on the skill of the person giving the shot. Since the needle must be properly positioned inside the joint space, the practitioner must be ultrafamiliar with the anatomy of the joint.

Cortisone shots, as we've said before, are not a cure. Even if they work for you, they will likely have to be repeated someday. "Cortisone shots help me a lot for about two months," says a Texas carpenter, "then I need another one." There is a limit to the number of times any one joint can be injected, however, before the procedure poses a threat of damage to the cartilage or bone there, or both. And, although steroids that are specially prepared for injection into the joints are considered safer than pills or intramuscular shots that spread steroids through the bloodstream, the drug still builds up in the body, and its effects are cumulative. In other words, the more you take, the greater your risk of long-term difficulties, which include osteoporosis and cataracts. "I was taking shots of **Depo-Medrol** every two months in each thumb," writes a retired salesman from Florida. "It was the most effective medication I've ever had, but after a couple of years, I was advised by another doctor that it might be destroying my bones."

Aside from the dangers of long-term use, a few of our participants note that steroid shots eventually lose their effectiveness anyway. "The cortisone injections gave instant relief," writes a nun from Missouri, "but in time the effects lasted only a day or two, instead of weeks." A joint that is crying out for repeated injections is probably a candidate for surgery. "I had three cortisone shots in my left knee before my total joint replacement," says a thirty-six-year-old New York freelance writer with rheumatoid arthritis. "The first was a miracle, the second great, and the third so-so, as the disease progressed."

Steroid injections rarely fail to bring relief, but some people do find them useless, and others actually feel worse after having one. "The cortisone injection I had did not help the pain," recalls a restaurant owner from Staten Island, "and I couldn't move my arm at all for almost two weeks." Here's another negative report from an Idaho homemaker: "Cortisone in my knee made it get black and blue and more painful. The only relief I had came when the bruised area healed." And an Ohio teacher tells us that she has lost the use of the joint where cortisone was injected.

THE SECOND LINE

The drugs that make up the second line are reserved almost exclusively for the treatment of rheumatoid arthritis. They are also called remittive, or disease-modifying antirheumatic drugs, because they may bring about a remission by countering the disease process itself, although no one can say just how they do so. Another name for them is slow-acting, and they do take a long time—weeks or months—to take effect. The oldest and most popular among them is the injection of gold salts. This treatment has become the standard against which all other second-line drugs are judged.

Gold: The Gold Standard

Gold was first used to treat rheumatoid arthritis for the wrong reasons. That was in the 1920s, when the disease was thought to be a chronic infection in the joints. Renowned German bacteriologist Robert Koch had shown that gold and other heavy metals, such as arsenic and mercury, could fight the tuberculosis germ in the test tube, and it was only natural to try the novel therapy on other infectious diseases. Gold looked promising against rheumatoid arthritis, and doctors quickly built up evidence to support its use. But by the mid-1940s, when gold had proven itself effective, most scientists had abandoned the belief that arthritis was an infectious disease. So gold was then *rejected* by doctors because it didn't fit the prevailing theory of the day. A few diehards continued to use it anyway, however, and a couple of decades later, gold resurfaced in the 1960s as a standard treatment. No theory yet explains its effectiveness, but that doesn't stop anyone from using it, since gold works, after all, and since the cause of rheumatoid arthritis remains a mystery.

Gold injections

"After three or four months on gold injections," writes a retired teacher from New York, "the miracle started and I was a new person. I now take one injection a month, and in general I feel well with very occasional bouts of pain."

Although gold is the standard, it does not stand alone. If used, it is but one element in a regimen including, for example, exercise, physical therapy, and other medications. "I have been on gold almost from the onset of the arthritis twenty-two years ago," says a salesman from Pennsylvania, who stretches and walks regularly—on his doctor's advice—to keep limber. "I credit the gold, plus a combination of **Indocin** or **Feldene** and some other medications, for keeping me as well as can be."

Gold injections carry weighty risks, and your doctor will no doubt talk to you about these before you start the therapy. You'll be seeing a lot of your doctor if you take gold injections, most likely going to the office for a shot every week during the first few months. You'll also be tested at each visit for any of the toxic side effects the gold may cause. These include kidney problems and bone-marrow suppression. Much more common side effects, which you will see for yourself if they develop, are itchy skin rashes and sores in the mouth. "I had gold shots for six months," writes a housewife from Iowa, "and they did wonders for me. But after six months I broke out all over my body and the rash itched something terrible. That was a year and a half ago, and I still have some of the spots." A credit analyst from New York says, "Gold injections seemed to put the rheumatoid arthritis into remission. Then, after thirteen injections, I broke out in a rash, and the doctor stopped the treatment." Even if you can tolerate the itching, the rash signifies that the drug is causing a toxic reaction, and it will do worse damage unless you stop taking it.

Several researchers have shown that gold controls pain and inflammation, and prevents further deformity, for as many as two-thirds of those who try it. It is such a well-liked therapy that you may be encouraged to take a series of gold *again* if an earlier trial failed to help you. Several of our participants reported two or even three experiences with gold injections. "I tried gold three times in different cities, with different doctors, but it was no help," writes a librarian from Missouri. A retired tax representative from California recalls, "Gold gave me so much help that I discontinued treatment. I had to resume the injections at a later date, and they had absolutely no effect then. I often wonder if further damage could have been prevented had I not stopped gold in the first place."

Number of participant trials of **gold shots***	146	
Outcome:		
Dramatic relief	50	(34%)
Moderate relief	25	(17%)
Minor or temporary relief only	15	(10%)
No relief (ineffective)	35	(24%)
No rating	21	(14%)
Most common drug reactions:		
No unpleasant side effects reported	62	(42%)
Allergic reaction, including rash, itching, or sores in the mouth	34	(23%)

*The product used is either gold sodium thiomalate (**Myochrysine,** Merck Sharp & Dohme) or aurothioglucose (**Solganal,** Schering Corporation).

A small minority of practitioners today believe in the value of gold treatments for osteoarthritis, but only eleven of our participants with osteoarthritis got the chance to try gold injections, and just one of them got any lasting help. Gold may also fail to help people with rheumatoid arthritis, and it makes some of them feel worse. The following account comes from a retired specialized clerk for the armed forces: "I had three gold injections, and each time I could not move my body the next day because all of my joints hurt too much. In those three weeks, I missed three days of work because of the shots."

Several of our participants used gold successfully for long periods of time—ten, twenty, or even thirty years—before it finally lost its effectiveness for them. They never developed any side effects, they just woke up one day to find that the treatment didn't work anymore, and it was time to try something else. Others got good results for several years before a toxic reaction ended the therapy. "Gold did the best," claims a housewife from Michigan, "but I developed a rash and ulcers in my mouth. Now I'm on oral gold."

Gold in pill form

This relatively new treatment won FDA approval in 1985. Auranofin, or **Ridaura**, as it was named by its manufacturer, Smith Kline & French, means the end of the bothersome rear-end injections for many people with rheumatoid arthritis. It's thought to be a little safer than the shots but also a little less effective, and some doctors don't trust it because they like the chance to see and evaluate their patients before each dose of gold. If you take the capsules, you simply swallow them yourself, twice a day, although you still need to see your doctor every month for blood and urine tests. **Ridaura** carries the same dangers as injectable gold, and already it has a reputation for being a more frequent cause of diarrhea.

Number of participants taking **Ridaura**	41	
Outcome:		
Dramatic relief	8	(20%)
Moderate relief	7	(17%)
Minor or temporary relief only	6	(15%)
No relief (ineffective)	14	(34%)
No rating	6	(15%)
Most common drug reactions:		
No unpleasant side effects	11	(27%)
Diarrhea	8	(20%)
Rash, itching, or mouth sores	6	(15%)
Nausea	4	(10%)

Plaquenil: The Antimalarial Drug

The primary use for hydroxychloroquine (**Plaquenil Sulfate,** Winthrop-Breon) is in the treatment of malaria, but it can also tackle rheumatoid arthritis, for reasons no one really understands. Like gold, **Plaquenil** is slow-acting and may take as long as four to six months to make any appreciable difference in the way you feel. Doctors consider it to be less effective than gold or penicillamine, but then, it's quite a bit safer. The major threat from **Plaquenil** is to the retina of the eye because the drug winds up in that tissue, where it can disturb your vision. Three survey participants taking **Plaquenil** (8 percent) mentioned this problem. Indeed, it's so possible, and so reversible, that a prescription for **Plaquenil** typically comes with a referral to an ophthalmologist.

"Before I started on **Plaquenil**," writes a retired Canadian research chemist, "all the prescription drugs I took made my white blood cell count too low. I get good relief from **Plaquenil**, with no noticeable side effects. But, since the drug may damage the retina, I see an ophthalmologist twice a year who tests my eyes for color vision and visual field." A social worker from Indiana, after four years on **Plaquenil** and regular eye exams every four to six months, says she is doing well on both counts.

Number of participants taking **Plaquenil**	39	
Outcome:		
Dramatic relief	11	(28%)
Moderate relief	6	(15%)
Minor or temporary relief	2	(5%)
No relief (ineffective)	8	(21%)
No rating	12	(31%)
Most common drug reactions:		
No unpleasant side effects	16	(41%)
Nausea	4	(10%)

Another comparatively safe disease-modifying drug favored by some rheumatologists is sulfasalazine, which is an anti-inflammatory agent approved by the FDA for the treatment of ulcerative colitis, and used sporadically for forty years to treat rheumatoid arthritis. Only three of our participants had experience with sulfasalazine, however, and the reports were mixed: One got dramatic relief, one got moderate long-term relief, and the other one couldn't say.

Penicillamine and the Copper Connection

If you've ever thought about wearing a copper bracelet, you know that the copper leaching into your skin from the jewelry is rumored to have healing powers. This is *just* a rumor, though, and our survey participants' experience shows the copper bracelet for what it is: a piece of jewelry. (See Chapter 9.) Penicillamine, on the other hand, *removes* copper from the body. This makes it the ideal treatment for people with the extremely rare illness called Wilson's disease, who build up too much copper in their body organs and then suffer brain damage, cirrhosis of the liver, kidney dysfunction, and other potentially fatal problems. What penicillamine does that makes it so effective in reducing the pain and inflammation of *arthritis,* however, is unknown. It appears to quiet the disease by influencing the immune system. Copper removal may have everything or nothing to do with the fact that penicillamine works.

"Before trying penicillamine," writes a sixty-one-year-old

accountant from New York, "I used a cane and was hardly able to walk. Now I am almost free of pain and swelling."

Number of participants taking **penicillamine***	36	
Outcome:		
Dramatic relief	13	(36%)
Moderate relief	8	(22%)
Minor or temporary relief	3	(8%)
No relief (ineffective)	8	(22%)
No rating	4	(11%)
Most common drug reactions:		
No unpleasant side effects	8	(22%)
Nausea and/or vomiting	5	(14%)

*Penicillamine is sold as capsules (**Cuprimine**, Merck Sharp & Dohme) or tablets (**Depen**, Wallace Laboratories).

Unlike the vast majority of arthritis drugs, penicillamine must be taken on an *empty* stomach—at least an hour before meals or after any other drug, food, or milk—for it to have maximum effect. Penicillamine is used *with* other drugs and treatments. "I have been taking the combination of **Feldene** and **Cuprimine** for nearly three years now," says a thirty-five-year-old librarian from West Virginia, "and am *very* pleased with the results. I have had no side effects other than some light-headedness and occasional nausea." For others, penicillamine's noxious side effects include kidney problems (8 percent of our participants), rashes (6 percent), muscle weakness (6 percent), as well as bone-marrow suppression and syndromes that resemble other diseases, including systemic lupus erythematosus, which is characterized by arthritis and other disorders.

It takes two or three months of treatment to tell whether penicillamine will work for you. This is the case with all the slow-acting agents, as we've seen. Aside from their long start-up time, these drugs pose a problem for doctors in deciding which one to try first. As a general rule, X ray evidence of serious joint damage is the signal to go for gold, but many doctors like to start with **Plaquenil** because, if it works, it offers the safest treatment. Penicillamine is probably the least popular of all, and is usually reserved for those who get no help from gold. Recent research at the Johns Hopkins Medical Institutions in Baltimore, however, suggests a way to identify, *in advance,* the people with rheumatoid arthritis who are most likely to benefit from penicillamine. By following the progress of a group of eighty-eight patients over the course of a year, the Hopkins doctors saw that the majority of those who got the most out of penicillamine shared a common genetic marker—a protein on their cell surfaces called HLA-DR2. Scientists have already identified certain genetic markers that tag some people as being more than likely to develop arthritis. The Hopkins research holds out the hope that these same genetic markers may one day point the way to the most effective treatment, as well.

Cytotoxic Drugs: Chemotherapy for Arthritis

The drugs in this group have been used to halt the uncontrolled cell growth that characterizes cancer, to help keep transplanted organs from being rejected by their new hosts, and, more recently, to slow the runaway inflammation of rheumatoid arthritis. They are praised for their demonstrated ability to bring relief when all else fails. And they are feared for their awesome side effects. Some of them can *cause* cancer, strangely enough, as well as bone-marrow suppression, sterility, or cirrhosis of the liver.

The cytotoxic drugs inlcude azathioprine (**Imuran,** Burroughs Wellcome), chlorambucil (**Leukeran,** Burroughs Wellcome), cyclophosphamide (**Cytoxan,** Bristol-Myers), and methotrexate (**Methotrexate** and **Rheumatrex,** Lederle). **Imuran** and **Rheumatrex** are the only ones that have been approved by the FDA for use in arthritis, and **Rheumatrex** just became available in January of 1989. Since methotrexate was used by our participants (with a high rate of success) while it was considered "experimental," we include a detailed account of it in Chapter 11, along with other experimental approaches.

Unfortunately, we cannot rate **Imuran,** since it was taken by only nine of our participants. Of the nine, two credited the drug with giving excellent relief, three said it helped somewhat, two found it of no use, and two reserved judgment. **Imuran** is also called an immunosuppressive drug, because it can damp the immune response. Since the destruction in rheumatoid arthritis is believed to be caused by an immunity to one's own body, it makes good theoretical sense to fight the arthritis by suppressing the immune system. As you might imagine, however, calling off the immune response can make a person more vulnerable to colds and other illnesses. Five of our survey participants taking these drugs complained of lowered disease resistance as a side effect.

"**Imuran** has definitely helped my arthritis," writes a forty-four-year-old retired teacher from Ohio, "but it has broken down my immunity badly. I've had pneumonia, diagnosed by X ray, five times in the last eight months."

Tips on Drug Safety and Purchase

The following suggestions are based on survey participants' comments and material from the National Council on Patient Information and Education.

At the doctor's office

- Learn the *name* of any drug your doctor prescribes for you, and ask what it is supposed to do for you.
- Make sure you understand how and when to take it (before meals, after meals, with milk, etc.).
- Determine how long you are supposed to stay on the drug—and what would happen if you stopped taking it for any reason on your own.
- Ask whether there are any foods or drinks that might interfere with the drug's action (milk, for example) or multiply its side effects (alcohol, perhaps). Also find out whether the drug makes it dangerous for you to drive.
- Get an idea of the possible side effects to look for, and what you should do if you experience any of them.
- Get your own copy of any written information that the doctor has available about the drug.
- Mention to the doctor the names of the medications you already take, whether they are prescription drugs or over-the-

counter staples in your medicine chest. It's also very important to mention any allergic reactions you've ever had to any drug.

At the pharmacy

- Read the prescription before you hand it over, and check the drug you get to make sure it's what the doctor ordered. Some pharmacists substitute generic drugs for brand names, and while these are usually less expensive, they may not be the equal of the original. If your prescription says "DAW," or "Dispense as Written," it means your doctor does not want you to take the generic version.
- If your pharmacist is accessible, repeat your questions about the drug and any precautions about taking it. The pharmacist may tell you something the doctor overlooked.
- If your drugs are paid for by an insurance plan, it probably makes no cost difference to you where you buy them. But if you are paying for them out of your own pocket, you may do well to shop around, comparing prices, or to order some arthritis drugs through the mail. The American Association of Retired Persons operates twelve such mail-order pharmacies, and you can learn of the one nearest you by writing to Retired Persons Services, Inc., 1 Prince St., Alexandria, VA 22314. Or try the Arthritis Foundation Pharmacy Service, P.O. Box 10490, Des Moines, IA 50306–0490.

At home

- Take the drugs as directed.
- If you forget some of your doctor's directions, call and ask for a reminder.
- If you develop problems while taking the drug, report them to your doctor immediately.

Summary of Prescription Drug Treatments for Arthritis

The First Line

NSAIDs—Good control of pain and inflammation, although finding the best one for you may take some time.
Steroids: Oral—Great relief, but dangerous as high-dose or long-term therapy.
Intra-articular injections—Excellent spot relief for painful joints.
Intramuscular injections—Effective for control of severe arthritis flares or during start-up period of second-line drugs.

The Second Line

Gold: Injections—Time-honored treatment for advanced rheumatoid arthritis.
Pills—Easier to take but not quite as effective.
Antimalarial—The safest of the second-line drugs, provided it can do the job for you.
Penicillamine—The standard treatment for rheumatoid arthritis when gold fails to help.
Cytotoxic Drugs—Gold's newer rivals, some of them only recently approved, though used successfully.

WARNING: All drug treatments carry the risk of side effects, and not one of them constitutes a cure in itself. Whatever you take, take it along with exercise, proper diet, rest, physical therapy, and all necessary precautions.

6

OVER-THE-COUNTER DRUGS:
From the Miraculous to the Preposterous

■ Aspirin ■ Acetaminophen ■ Ibuprofen ■
Combinations ■ Rub-on balms

The most widely used and most highly regarded treatment for arthritis is an over-the-counter drug. Its name, of course, is aspirin, and more than half of our 1,051 survey participants rely on it every single day. Many of them give aspirin a "plus-3" rating—the highest on our scale.

Most participants are thrilled that they can buy aspirin without a prescription because it means their favorite drug stays cheap and readily available. But they also curse the fact that "plain old aspirin" is the best medicine for arthritis. And they hate the myth, spawned by some aspirin advertisements, that arthritis is nothing more than "minor aches and pains"— easily managed by the same pills everyone else uses to chase a headache or a fever.

Separating the facts from the myths, the misleading claims of manufacturers, and the well-meaning advice of friends who swear by some nonprescription treatment, whether it's **Tylenol** or **Tiger Balm**, is what this chapter is all about. In it, we'll give you the benefit of our participants' experience with over-the-counter drugs, from tablets and tonics to creams, lotions, and sprays. We'll back their testimony with reports from the medical literature, and give you tips on how to buy and use these products with savvy and safety.

Aspirin

Perhaps the most important thing to say about aspirin, simply, is that it works, and works well. No prescription drug for arthritis really matches aspirin's proven effectiveness. Here's how the original wonder drug fared statistically in our survey.

Number of participants using **aspirin***	598	
Outcome:		
Dramatic relief	121	(20%)
Moderate relief	239	(40%)
Minor or temporary relief only	210	(35%)
No relief (ineffective)	19	(3%)
No rating (too soon to tell, etc.)	9	(2%)

*This number includes 543 participants currently taking aspirin and 55 who no longer take it but who rated it in comparison to other treatments.

Totaling the positive ratings reveals that aspirin gives at least some relief to 95 percent of those who use it—and perhaps to as many as 97 percent. Most of the prescription anti-inflammatory drugs for arthritis, by comparison, help between 60 and 80 percent of the participants who take them. "I have tried several arthritis drugs prescribed by my doctor," writes a retired businessman from California, "but aspirin seems as good as anything." Even prednisone, the miraculous steroid, at 85-percent overall effectiveness, lags behind "plain old" aspirin. (See Chapter 5 for a full discussion of prescription medications for arthritis, plus individual ratings.)

Aspirin is not only good medicine. It's cheap. The brand you choose and the place you shop may drive the expense up or down, but not by much when you compare aspirin prices to the cost of other anti-inflammatory drugs, some of which sell for more than one dollar *per pill.*

Although it is used for every imaginable pain, from toothache to cancer, and although thousands of Americans take aspirin regularly to ward off heart attacks, aspirin remains uniquely suited to the treatment of arthritis. All three of aspirin's major actions are called into play in arthritis. It acts as: (1) an analgesic to ease pain, the hallmark of the disease; (2) an anti-inflammatory to control inflammation, the culprit responsible for much joint damage; and (3) an antipyretic to reduce fever, which frequently plagues people with rheumatoid arthritis.

The amount of aspirin you take probably depends on the type of arthritis you have. For osteoarthritis, for example, aspirin is mostly a pain reliever, and you use it as often as your pain demands. But to treat rheumatoid arthritis, aspirin levels have to build up in your body, and you may be urged to take as many as a dozen or even two dozen a day to get the full anti-inflammatory effect.

You'd almost think aspirin had been tailor-made for arthritis, but it came about as a failed attempt to create a man-made substitute for quinine. In the 1800s, when malaria was rampant and supplies of natural quinine couldn't fill the need, German chemists set out to synthesize quinine in the laboratory. They did not succeed. None of their concoctions cured malaria. But one of them, acetylsalicylic acid, the drug we now call aspirin (or A.S.A. in Canada), did prove to quell fever and pain.

Although acetylsalicylic acid was synthesized in 1853, it did not become commercially available until decades later, in 1899, when the Bayer Pharmaceutical Co. introduced it and coined the trade name "aspirin." Another half a century passed before scientists learned through animal experiments in the mid-1950s that aspirin could also control inflammation. And it has been only fifteen years since medical researchers began to fathom *how* aspirin works its various wonders—apparently by blocking the body's production of substances called prostaglandins, some of which cause pain and inflammation.

Aspirin's most common side effect . . . and what to do about it

The dark side of aspirin therapy lurks in the stomach, where even one tablet can cause a little bleeding, and where prolonged heavy use has lead to ulcers. If you depend on large quantities of aspirin for controlling your arthritis, then the chance of your developing an ulcer is probably somewhere between one in four and one in five. In hospitals where doctors have studied the effects of long-term aspirin use, as many as 25 percent of their patients with rheumatoid arthritis have ulcers from the treatment.

The 598 participants who rated aspirin in our survey have osteoarthritis or rheumatoid arthritis or both, and they take anywhere from one to thirty-six tablets a day. Of these, 151 (25 percent) complained of some kind of gastric distress, whether it was upset stomach, heartburn, or ulcers.

Aspirin manufacturers have tried to protect their customers' stomachs with several strategies, but each one has its shortcomings. *Buffering* the aspirin with an antacid, for instance, may keep you from feeling that you have an upset stomach but doesn't seem to ward off ulcers in the long run. Some examples of buffered aspirin are **Bufferin** (including **Arthritis Strength Bufferin**), **Ascriptin**, and **Arthritis Pain Formula**. The very *highly buffered* aspirin products that must be dissolved in water, such as **Alka-Seltzer**, *do* succeed in sparing and even *protecting* the stomach. There's a catch, though. They contain so much sodium that no one on a low-salt diet can use them, and no one should use them on a regular long-term basis. They also cost more than plain aspirin.

Coated aspirin keeps itself under wraps as long as it stays in the stomach. The protective coating around **Ecotrin**, for example, does not dissolve until *after* the pill leaves your stomach. This makes it a poor bet for fast pain relief but fine for many people taking large daily doses of aspirin. A thirty-four-year-old Florida homemaker rates **Ecotrin** higher than any of the twenty prescription drugs she's taken for rheumatoid arthritis, saying it eases the pain and doesn't bother her stomach. For some people, though, the coating and delayed dissolving can cut down the amount of aspirin that actually gets into the bloodstream.

Aspirin *suppositories* only switch the irritation from the stomach to the rectum, and what's more, they don't deliver the drug reliably.

So what else *can* you do to protect yourself? Here are a few suggestions, based on a combination of survey participants', doctors', and pharmacists' advice:

- *Drink a full glass of liquid* with your aspirin, to dilute its irritating effect. Water and milk are the best choices. Anything alcoholic is the worst because it doubles the damage that can be dealt to your stomach. Never mix aspirin with alcohol.

- *Eat something* to act as a buffer. Be aware, though, that a big meal can slow down the aspirin's entry into your bloodstream. This shouldn't matter at all if you are taking large doses regularly to build up a high level of aspirin in your body. However, if you're swallowing two tablets in the hope of quick pain relief, don't eat more than a small snack.

- *Take an additional drug to protect your stomach,* such as **Maalox** or **Mylanta**, which are also sold over the counter, or **Tagamet** or **Carafate**, which are anti-ulcer medications your doctor may prescribe. Another approach, just recently approved by the Food and Drug Administration, is to take aspirin with misoprostol (**Cytotec**), a drug that apparently undoes the stomach damage aspirin causes but without blocking its good effects. (See Chapter 11.)

Less common side effects

Another unpleasant aspirin side effect is the ringing, clicking, or humming sound that you may hear as an accompaniment to aspirin therapy. The noise is a signal that you've had too much, and you must try to use less. It often turns out, however, that the people who are the most susceptible to tinnitus, or ringing in the ears, are also the ones who get the greatest benefit from aspirin. Among the 598 survey participants who use aspirin, 57 (nearly 10 percent) complain that their ears ring.

A few participants notice that they bruise easily, apparently because of aspirin's blood-thinning effect, and that the bruises tend to last a long time. (See Chapter 15 for information on how vitamin C may counteract this effect.) Others find themselves growing drowsy after they take aspirin, but they don't necessarily object to the feeling. Indeed, for every participant who complains of daytime drowsiness, there's another who counts on aspirin for help with relaxing and getting to sleep at night.

According to the Aspirin Foundation, about one person in five hundred is truly allergic to the drug and suffers an attack of asthma or hives upon taking it. In our group of 1,051 survey participants, however, 8 individuals (about 4 in 500) say they do not use aspirin because they are allergic to it.

Aspirin by other names, in other forms . . . and even by prescription

Aspirin is aspirin, whether it's **Norwich** or **Bayer** or any other brand. Name brands cost more than generic, or so-called "house" brands, but the price difference reflects each product's packaging and marketing, not its content. Most drug companies, in fact, get their raw material—acetylsalicylic acid—from the same supplier, mix it with starch and other inactive ingredients, and then shape the mixture into aspirin tablets etched with their own company name. As long as the product you buy is labeled "USP aspirin,"* you can be sure it measures up to the government's quality standards. Aspirin is *not* just aspirin, however, when it's **Anacin**, **Excedrin**, or **Vanquish**, all of which count caffeine among their ingredients.

Typical aspirin tablets give you 325 milligrams (mg), or 5

---

*USP stands for United States Pharmacopeia, the agency that sets the drug standards enforced by the Food and Drug Administration.

grains of the drug. Most "extra strength" formulas contain 500 milligrams, or about half again as much aspirin per pill.

After all we've said about aspirin's being an over-the-counter drug, we have to mention the exceptions to this rule. Several survey participants take one of the high-dose formulations sold only by prescription: **Easprin**, a coated aspirin that is the equivalent of three ordinary tablets (975 milligrams, or 15 grains), and **Zorprin**, which contains 800 milligrams of aspirin in another kind of stomach-sparing coat. Convenience is a major advantage of prescription-strength aspirin, especially for those participants who would otherwise have to swallow three or more pills every few hours. Another advantage is the fact that they can have their drug costs reimbursed by medical insurance.

Aspirin and other drugs

Aspirin doesn't mix well with several other drugs in general, and with a number of arthritis drugs in particular. If you take medication for diabetes or a heart condition, don't take aspirin unless you clear it with your doctor. The same goes for anticoagulants (blood thinners), diuretics, and drugs that lower blood pressure.

I can't take aspirin because I take Clinoril, some participants say, or *because I take Naprosyn,* or some other prescription product in the NSAID (nonsteroidal anti-inflammatory drug) family. And they're right. These drugs are so closely related to aspirin that taking them both together does little good, if any—and dangerously increases the likelihood of suffering the bad side effects of each. All of the NSAIDs, as aspirin itself, are designed to relieve pain *and* control inflammation, so take one *or* the other, and discuss the decision with your doctor.

Over-the-counter products made of ibuprofen, such as **Nuprin** or **Advil**, behave just like their prescription-strength parents, the NSAIDs **Rufen** and **Motrin**. Mixed with aspirin, they may produce double-whammy side effects.

Methotrexate (**Methotrexate, Rheumatrex**), used by forty-eight of our participants to control severe rheumatoid arthritis, can have toxic side effects all by itself. Aspirin may aggravate them.

The steroid drugs, including prednisone, may undermine the effect of aspirin, so there's no point in taking both. And if you combine aspirin with gout medications such as **Benemid** or **Anturane**, then the aspirin can wipe out the good effects of those drugs—and make your gout feel worse.

Also, if you plan to have surgery, whether for arthritis or any other condition, talk to your surgeon about cutting back on aspirin as a pre-op precaution. This could save you from a serious loss of blood during your operation.

Acetaminophen: The "Aspirin Substitute"

Most people know the name **Tylenol** better than the name of **Tylenol**'s key ingredient—the nonaspirin painkiller acetaminophen. More of our participants use **Tylenol** than any other over-the-counter aspirin substitute, although some of them like **Anacin-3, Panadol, Datril,** and various other brands of acetaminophen.

Acetaminophen has been available in the United States since 1955. It is definitely effective against arthritis pain, our participants report. The fact that it has little or no power to combat inflammation simply doesn't bother many of them.

Number of participants taking **acetamino- phen**	201	
Outcome:		
Find it moderately to dramatically helpful	177	(88%)
Find it of no use (ineffective)	14	(7%)
No rating	10	(5%)

Acetaminophen has very few side effects. It rarely upsets anyone's stomach and it doesn't cause ulcers. This makes it the treatment of choice for many participants who have been burned by aspirin or other anti-inflammatory drugs. "I tried **Naprosyn** and **Indocin**," writes a housewife from North Carolina, "but I was nauseated all the time. **Tylenol** is helpful for me." A gardener from New York says, "**Tylenol** has the same effect on my pain as aspirin, and it doesn't seem to retard blood clotting the way aspirin does." Overuse of acetaminophen over long periods of time, however, can do serious, perhaps even fatal damage to your liver. And a one-shot overdose may be just as dangerous.

Tablet for tablet, acetaminophen works at the same dosage level as aspirin—325 milligrams in a regular-strength tablet and 500 milligrams in most extra-strength products.

Some of our participants take acetaminophen because it is so *un*likely to interfere with the drugs they must take for their other health problems. Indeed, acetaminophen is hardly ever to blame for intensifying the side effects of another drug. Exceptions are **Dolobid**, a nonsteroidal anti-inflammatory, and members of the anticoagulant family, including medications such as **Coumadin**. If you take one of these blood-thinning drugs, check with your doctor before using acetaminophen.

"I take **Tylenol Extra Strength**," writes a retired teacher from Louisiana, "and I get just as much relief as I did from **Indocin, Motrin**, and **Naprosyn**—without the internal bleeding. My only complaint is that six to eight pills per day can get expensive." Other participants lower the expense by using generic brands of acetaminophen, which may sell for half the price of nationally advertised names. Regular-strength tablets of any brand cost less than "extra strength" formulas, so it also makes sense to try taking two of the regular strength before deciding to buy the larger-dose pills.

Ibuprofen: The Latest Aspirin Rival

Anything aspirin can do, ibuprofen can, too, including fight inflammation, relieve pain, reduce fever, and upset the stomach.

Ibuprofen was first marketed as a prescription drug in Europe by Boots, under the name **Rufen**, before Upjohn introduced it to the United States in 1974 as **Motrin**. Within a decade, however, ibuprofen found its way around the prescription pad and over the counter, where some of our participants buy it in packages labeled **Advil, Medipren**, and **Nuprin**. Some of them consider it the best arthritis drug of all: "Ibuprofen has given me a period of freedom from all pain," writes a sixty-one-year-old secretary from Washington, who had switched from aspirin to ibuprofen five months before joining our survey. "There were a couple of days when it didn't seem to help, and then suddenly I realized my hands weren't hurting for the first time in ten years."

Number of participants taking **ibuprofen***	120	
Outcome:		
Find it moderately to dramatically helpful	93	(77%)
Find it of no use (ineffective)	13	(11%)
No rating	14	(12%)

*This is the number of participants who take over-the-counter ibuprofen in the form of **Advil, Medipren, Nuprin,** or other brands.

The over-the-counter brands of ibuprofen rated here *coexist* in the marketplace with the original prescription products, **Motrin** and **Rufen,** which remain among the all-time most popular drugs for arthritis. Indeed, more than half of our survey participants filled at least one prescription for **Motrin.** (See Chapter 5 for more information about **Motrin,** plus ratings.) What separates the prescription drug from the nonprescription is the amount of ibuprofen in each tablet. Over-the-counter brands contain 200 milligrams of ibuprofen per pill, while **Motrin** has 400, 600, or 800 milligrams, depending on which strength your doctor prescribes. But obviously, you can take enough 200-milligram tablets to give yourself a prescription-strength dose of ibuprofen.

As a rule, it is best to take just enough of an anti-inflammatory drug to get the most help with the least trouble. Taking a lot does not necessarily produce added relief, but it *does* leave you more vulnerable to side effects. The advice to "Take two aspirin and call me in the morning" has been repeated so often that most people think one aspirin is only half a dose. But 325 milligrams of aspirin or acetaminophen, or 200 milligrams of ibuprofen—the amount in one regular-strength tablet of these drugs—may be all you need at any one time.

Just as ibuprofen mimics aspirin's pain-relieving and anti-inflammatory effects, it often produces the same unwanted side effects: upset stomach (with the potential to cause ulcers) and ringing in the ears. "**Medipren** is great for me," says a twenty-two-year-old housewife and mother from Kansas. "It doesn't cost as much as my other medicine. But it bothers my stomach." If your stomach is sensitive to ibuprofen, you can try to ward off an upset with the same steps that apply to aspirin, such as taking the pill with food or milk.

Other Pills: Combos and Come-ons

Two over-the-counter pills mentioned in our survey were not used widely enough to rate them comparatively, and they don't quite fit in the categories we've mentioned so far. **Excedrin**, for example, is aspirin *and* acetaminophen, 325 milligrams of each, with about half a mug of coffee's worth of caffeine added to the mix. Of the twelve participants who mentioned **Excedrin** by name, eleven found it helpful and one judged it ineffective.

Doan's Pills, touted as special medicine for back pain, contain a close relative of aspirin called magnesium salicylate. (Aspirin, once again, is acetylsalicylic acid. Both these drugs belong to the same drug family, called salicylates. Other family members include the prescription drugs diflunisal [**Dolobid**] and salsalate [**Disalcid** and **Monogesic**].) The ten survey participants who mentioned **Doan's Pills** were split up the middle about them. Five said the pills did something for them and five felt they did nothing. According to the Public Citizen Health Research Group in Washington, D.C., magnesium salicylate has no special advantage over aspirin for treating back pain, although **Doan's Pills** are considerably more expensive than aspirin.

Rub-on Balms

More than 70 percent of our participants have sought pain relief by rubbing some kind of lotion, liniment, cream, oil, or gel on a painful part. Fully 742 of the 1,051 participants in our survey say that they have used a rub-on balm. According to most of them, the rest of the group is missing out on something good.

The Arthritis Foundation lumps all "topical creams" together with various forms of "harmless" baloney (including copper bracelets and uranium mines) in its brochure on *Arthritis Unproven Remedies.* And indeed, there is no scientific proof that any of these home remedies provides any substantive help. But there is a measure of relief to be had here, our participants say, even if it's only temporary, and there's no serious harm in trying.

Many of these products are counterirritants. That is, they try to make you forget about pain by irritating your skin to make it feel hot. The heat, in turn, may soothe some soreness and stiffness. Survey participants who understand this relationship still enjoy the sensation: "I don't think **Ben·Gay** does any real good," says a retired teacher from Indiana, "but the warmth it produces makes you feel better." Several participants share a different theory about how and why such liniments help: "You rub on the **Aspercreme**," a Colorado homemaker explains, "and the *massage* is the truly effective part."

Balms and liniments are the particular favorites of participants who don't get any help from drug treatments. "No drug has ever helped me," says a housewife from Florida. "I find the best remedy for temporary relief that works for me is **Absorbine Jr.** I carry it at all times." Other participants find rubs to be of special help at certain times, such as immediately before or after exercising, or at bedtime: "**Ben·Gay** and **Sloan's Liniment** are wonderful for me," writes a shipping clerk from California. "If I take a scalding hot bath, cover my knees and ankles with liniment and wrap them in Ace bandages, I can sleep for a few hours with no discomfort."

Several of these products, including **Aspercreme** and **Myoflex**, contain salicylates. The implication is that aspirin, or other members of its drug family, could relieve pain in a certain area by being applied directly to the surface of the skin there. As we've seen, however, aspirin *irritates* the stomach if it's swallowed, or sometimes the rectum if it's used in suppository form. On the skin, too, it is irritating, not anesthetizing. Aspirin can relieve pain only by getting into the bloodstream. True, some aspirin may be absorbed through the skin and into the blood when applied this way, but mostly it just rubs the skin the wrong way. "At first I tried a lot of different liniments," writes a dry cleaner from Arizona, "but some of them felt like they would burn my skin off, so I stopped using them."

WARNING: If you are allergic to aspirin or other salicylates, then you must avoid using rubs that contain them, too.

In all, our participants tried about thirty brands of balms and got at least some temporary relief or sense of well-being from all of them. Here is a list of the most popular ones, arranged in order of their effectiveness.

Name of Product	Number of Participants Who Used It	Number Who Say It Helped	Percent Who Found It (Somewhat) Effective
Myoflex	32	26	81%
Mineral Ice	26	21	81%
Icy Hot	79	61	77%
Absorbine Jr.	27	20	74%
Ben • Gay	202	142	70%
Mentholatum	35	22	63%
Heet	51	31	61%
Aspercreme	126	72	57%

Two other popular brands, although they were used by too few participants for us to rate them comparatively, also deserve mention. **Banalg** is favored by twelve of the sixteen participants who tried it. "Massage with **Banalg** works best of all," maintains a nurse from Texas. And **Tiger Balm** pleased fourteen out of fifteen who used it, especially this librarian from Ohio: "**Aspercreme** helps by relaxing the joint, but **Tiger Balm** is the best. It warms, relaxes, and anesthetizes the areas where I have severe pain."

The differences in effectiveness among these products are not striking enough to serve as strong recommendations for one brand over another—especially when you consider the other differences among them, including cost and *smell*. A veterinary assistant from Florida insists, "If it doesn't smell strong, it doesn't help!" The aroma of wintergreen or menthol, however, really offends some participants who denounce the "smelly relief" offered in a rub. Take a whiff if you can, before you buy.

Summary of Over-the-Counter Treatments for Arthritis

Aspirin—Still the mainstay of treatment for people with arthritis, aspirin is an effective and inexpensive way to control pain and inflammation. Even though it is sold without a prescription, its potency calls for caution if you use a lot, or if you take it with other types of over-the-counter or prescription medicine.

Acetaminophen—One of the safest pain-relieving drugs available, acetaminophen is not effective for the inflammation that often accompanies arthritis. Its kindness to the stomach, however, may make it the best available drug for people who have arthritis and ulcers.

Ibuprofen—The newest of the top three nonprescription painkillers, ibuprofen works much the way aspirin does to relieve pain and inflammation. Some people find that it even surpasses aspirin, but, like aspirin, it can upset your stomach and sound bells in your ears.

Rub-on balms—Even though there is no scientific justification for finding relief in any of the lotions, liquids, creams, or gels sold for arthritis relief, these products do have a soothing effect on joint pain for most of the people who try them. Choose one in your price range that doesn't hurt your skin or offend your nose.

7

SURGERY FOR ARTHRITIS:
A Surprisingly Successful Solution

■ Dramatic results from joint replacement ■ Fusion ■ Arthroscopic surgery ■ Facts about procedures and risks ■ How to prepare yourself for surgery

To walk without a cane, or even a limp.

To move without pain for the first time in years.

These are the outcomes of surgery that our Arthritis Survey participants call "miraculous." And they are commonplace miracles. Indeed, success and satisfaction are by far the most common results reported by those participants who had one or more joints replaced or repaired. As most of them tell the story, the end result is well worth all the pre-op anxiety they suffered and all the post-op inconvenience.

"The outcome of my two operations—total left hip replacement in 1984 and total left knee replacement in 1986—has been a vast improvement in the quality of my life," says a freelance writer from New York. "A five-mile walk is no big deal to me now. Going from nearly being in a wheelchair to limpless walking is nothing short of miraculous."

If you are currently facing a decision about joint surgery, this chapter will tell you the encouraging truth about the level of improvement you can expect from various types of operations, and why some procedures get better results than others. You'll learn the risks involved, too, and the things *you* can do in preparation for surgery to assure yourself of the best possible outcome.

In all, 194 participants, or slightly more than 18 percent of the 1,051 members of our survey group, had joint surgery. Many of them had two or more operations because, for example, both their hips, both their knees, or all their knuckles had been badly damaged by arthritis. Others had their wrists fused, bone spurs removed, or tendons repaired. Most of the operations fall into one of these major categories, all of which are covered in this chapter:

arthroplasty—the replacement (partial or total) or resurfacing of damaged joints

arthrodesis—the fusing together of bones to make a joint more stable

arthroscopy—the technique for accomplishing surgical procedures through small incisions, using fiber optics and miniature tools

synovectomy—the removal of the joint lining

Arthroplasty

Total joint replacement is the flashiest, most dramatic achievement in arthritis treatment of the past several decades. Many people swear that the surgery gives unparalleled pain relief and a return to near-normal function. Yet, most surgeons still consider it the *last resort* for people with arthritis—an option to hold in reserve until all else fails. This is because an artificial joint, no matter how well it works, has a limited life span. If it is cemented in place, it can come unstuck. If it is pushed too hard through strenuous activity, it may break. In either case, it will have to be replaced, and the bones that support the replacement's replacement will have to be further cut—and further compromised.

The challenge of total joint replacement is to copy nature with materials that are not really the equal of bone and cartilage. Metal implants have been used to repair the living skeleton, historians say, for as long as humans have practiced surgery. But not until this century were the materials and techniques available to make replacement parts work well in the body's hostile environment. Most metals crack under the pressure, or corrode, or cause infection. Even stainless steel can *break* when it has to do the work of a person's shoulder.

Today, close to 200,000 total joint replacements are performed in the United States every year. Most of these are hips and knees made of metal alloys (cobalt chromium is one) and tough plastics, or finger joints fashioned from silicone rubber. Scores of specially engineered joints already compete in the marketplace, and new modifications are constantly being introduced, so that the replacements ever more closely approximate the form and function of the original (nature's) design. One of the early artificial knees, for example, created in the 1950s, was a hinge that replaced the worn-out surfaces of the joint and anchored itself with long metal shafts driven into the bones of the leg. A human knee, however, doesn't open and shut like a door on a hinge, but rolls, glides, and rotates in an extremely complex fashion. Current designs allow for this freer, more natural kind of movement.

Total knee replacement

At the knee, the bottom of the thigh bone (femur) meets the top of the shin bone (tibia), and the two move effortlessly in tandem, thanks to their caps of glistening cartilage. When arthritis destroys the cartilage, however, the bones are left to grind painfully against each other. A surgeon performing a total knee arthroplasty cuts away the damaged bone ends and replaces them with a matched set of implants that let the bones glide smoothly once again.

More people in our survey have undergone total knee replacement than any other form of arthroplasty. The overall results they report are excellent, and some of those who are the most satisfied with their surgery are walking around with no trouble on artificial knees that have been in place for ten or twelve years. "Surgery will not restore 100 percent natural movement," says a forty-two-year-old writer from Kentucky who had both her knees replaced in the 1970s, "but it will relieve pain drastically and restore a major portion of lost mobility. The psychological effect of all this for me has been a greater feeling of self-esteem and self-worth."

There are seventy-eight total knee replacements listed in the ratings below, representing the fifty-one survey participants who had this type of surgery on one or both knees. Five participants in the group needed repeat surgery because their first artificial joint worked loose or otherwise failed. Each procedure is rated separately.

Number of **total knee replacements**	78	
Outcome:		
Dramatic relief	52	(67%)
Moderate relief	12	(15%)
Minor or temporary relief	1	(1%)
No relief	3	(4%)
Made participant feel worse than before	4	(5%)
No rating (too soon to tell)	6	(8%)

Strictly speaking, we have to call the 67-percent figure for "dramatic relief" a "short-term" outcome, because some participants were rating the procedure just two or three years after surgery. And while this period of time could be considered extremely long-term relief for a new drug, surgery is such a major undertaking that its results must be measured in decades—and *two* decades is about as long as most artificial joints are expected to last.

As you can see, a few participants had been through total knee replacement so recently that they didn't try to evaluate it. The period immediately after surgery is quite painful for some people, and most of our participants say that full recovery takes three to six months. "I was very fortunate," writes a sixty-seven-year-old Iowa housewife who had one knee replaced in March and the other in April of 1986, "as my recovery was painless after the first eighteen hours each time. I had full use of both knees in about two and a half months."

What kind of replacement will I get? Several participants know the type of knee they received, such as the Zimmer or the Austin Moore (named for their designers), the Geometric or the Multiradius (named for their design features). Surgeons choose styles of knees from a wide array of models, some already approved for general use by the Food and Drug Administration and some so new that they are still considered experimental or investigational devices, to be used only by surgeons involved in clinical research. The choice of joint implant depends a lot on the type and degree of destruction in the original joint, not to mention the surgeon's personal preference. At some hospitals, in fact, surgeons work with bioengineers to help put their own ideas for new joint designs into production.

What happens after surgery? The implanting of the new joint is only the beginning of a successful replacement. Physical therapy is the next phase, and it covers everything from teaching you how to use crutches or a walker to demonstrating and supervising exercises that will strengthen the muscles that make your new knee go. (These muscles, including the quadriceps at the front of the thigh and hamstrings at the back, may be quite weak if pain has kept you inactive before surgery.) The exercises our participants describe include both *active* movements, such as extending the knee while wearing small weights around the ankle, and *passive* motion. "After my total knee replacement," writes a retired electrician from West Virginia, "my left leg was put in a motion machine that moved my leg as if I was riding a bicycle. I used this for several days and it kept my knee flexible. I was also given exercises and instructions as to what I should and shouldn't do with my new joint." Even after some participants left the hospital, they returned two or three times a week for physical therapy and then continued exercising regularly on their own, mostly by walking, swimming, or riding a bike or an exercycle.

What risks do I face? Total joint replacement is major surgery and patients face all the known risks of being put under general anesthesia or numbed with a spinal. Over the long run, the special risk of replacement is the possibility that the new joint will come loose and the pain return. Five of our participants had to have repeat surgery on their artificial knees within ten years of the original operation. "I was one of the first men to have two total knees and two total hips," says a thirty-five-year-old artist from Ohio. "Actually, I've had three total knees over the years, the first two in 1972 and 1973, and one redone in 1983."

Loosening is the most common risk with joint replacements, but infection is the most serious. It is quite rare today, thanks to the extreme precautions taken at most hospitals, including the astronaut-type helmets the doctors and attendants wear to keep their exhaled breath from contaminating the new joint—or you—during the long hours required for this surgery. Despite all the safeguards, infection can sometimes undermine the new joint by spreading to it from some other part of the body days or weeks after the operation. A fifty-six-year-old teacher from Massachusetts tells how her artificial knee was undone by a tooth:

"In June of 1982, I had a total knee replacement and an uneventful hospital stay that lasted eleven days. But five days later, at home, severe pain set in. I took a series of tests that revealed a strep infection in my knee. The doctors determined the source to be some dental work I'd had done, for which my dentist should have given me penicillin. I had to be treated with intravenous antibiotics for forty-nine days—yes, seven full weeks. Then I had another operation in October. The surgeon found then that the bone around the new joint had become soft, brittle, and jagged with multiple fractures. The cement had cracked and so the prosthesis was loosened. Ligaments, too, had been destroyed. The second joint replacement took seven and one-half hours, and I spent more than eight months on crutches. Physical therapy is *still* going on, because of the damage to the ligaments. But this experience is just a fluke. Most of the time a knee replacement gives a great deal of pain relief and greater mobility. It's like a new lease on life. I know because I had surgery on my other knee the year before all this happened, and that knee is fine."

Total hip replacement

The hip was the first joint to be successfully replaced on a wide-scale basis, thanks mostly to the brilliant efforts of British surgeon Sir John Charnley, who figured out the best combination of materials for creating an artificial joint and implanted a series of them in his patients in the early 1960s.

Previously, hip parts had been made of everything from wood and hand-carved ivory to Pyrex, Bakelite, and Teflon, as well as metals such as gold, silver, aluminum, lead, copper, iron, and zinc. But no combination was ideal. Even the best of the metal-on-metal designs, though precision-ground for a perfect fit of ball in socket, wore each other down and dumped metal debris into the joint space. They also squeaked. Dr. Charnley became "the father of modern total hip arthroplasty" by designing a hip that was part metal and part polyethylene, with virtually no friction between the moving parts.

Although Dr. Charnley's concept was readily applied to the knee and other joints, hip replacement remains the most successful of the arthroplasties. The reason lies in the anatomy of the hip. The bones there are large enough to accommodate prosthetic parts that hardly ever break. And the ball-and-socket action of the joint has proved easier to imitate than the complex workings of the wrist, for example, or the ankle. In total hip arthroplasty, the surgeon cuts away the top of the thighbone, with its ball-shaped knob, and replaces it with a metal one that has a long shank to fit inside the bone. The damaged socket (acetabulum) also gets cut out and a new cup is screwed or cemented into the pelvis.

Number of **total hip replacements***	58	
Outcome:		
Dramatic relief	46	(79%)
Moderate relief	8	(14%)
Minor or temporary relief	0	———
No relief	0	———
Made participant feel worse than before	0	———
No rating	4	(7%)

*This is the number of *procedures;* the number of *participants* who had one or both hips replaced is 45.

Dr. Charnley cemented his implants in place with an acrylic bone cement called polymethyl methacrylate, or PMMA, which added an element of solidity to the surgery. Instead of sinking the shaft of the hip ball into the thighbone, for example, and counting on a perfect fit to hold it there, surgeons could shoot some cement into the bone along with the implant. When it hardened, it would create a solid bond. Surgeons have found ever better ways over the years to improve PMMA's performance—mixing it in a vacuum chamber or whirling it in a centrifuge to get the air bubbles out, then applying it with a high-pressure caulking gun that drives it into all the nooks and crannies of the surrounding bone. Even so, some experts now claim that the *cement* eventually makes the replacement come *unstuck* by engendering a barrier between itself and the bone.

When surgeons set about performing rereplacement of implants that have loosened, they often discover that a membrane has grown all around the cement, resembling the synovial membrane that normally surrounds the joint. Inside the membrane they find tiny particles of PMMA cement—and evidence that the membrane is doing chemical battle with these particles, releasing substances that cause the bone around the cement to retreat, or resorb, and the implant to grow progressively looser.

Since the cement may be the weakest link in the joint-replacement process, new implant designs are trying to get around the problem.

What will hold my new joint in place? Several participants mentioned that the hips they received were of the new "cementless" variety, also called "bony ingrowth prostheses," which are the latest word in joint replacements. Instead of being fixed in place with bone cement, these implants rely on their porous surfaces, which invite living bone tissue to grow in and around them and forge a permanent fusion. Although the recovery period may be lengthier, waiting for the new joint to take hold, the cementless implant is expected to last longer—perhaps indefinitely. (We say "perhaps" because the new designs haven't been around long enough for *anyone* to evaluate their very-long-term success.) Bony-ingrowth joints should also stand up to the stresses and strains of a more active lifestyle, making them a more likely choice for younger people. Also, surgeons suspect that younger bone may be more capable than elderly bone of infiltrating and incorporating a cementless implant.

Which is better, cemented or cementless? Orthopedic surgeons haven't reached a conclusion on this yet. Indeed, some situations require them to implant "hybrid" hips and knees that are cemented on one side of the joint and cementless on the other.

Finger-joint replacement

What Dr. Charnley did for the hip, Dr. Alfred B. Swanson did for the joints of the fingers in the mid-1960s, and at least fifteen of our participants were able to fill out their survey questionnaires in longhand thanks to the implants that bear his name.

Dr. Swanson discovered early on that metal replacements wouldn't do for the fine bones of the hands or feet. His success, like Dr. Charnley's, depended partly on his own creativity, and partly on finding the right material for the job. This was a flexible and durable synthetic rubber called silicone (and later dubbed "Silastic"), created by the Dow-Corning Corporation, and made available to Dr. Swanson for his research. The revolutionary finger joints he devised turned out so well that Dr. Swanson went on to fashion some two dozen other kinds of replacements out of silicone, including toe joints, wrist bones, and parts of the elbow.

The Swanson finger joint is a one-piece design that roughly resembles a flower with two stems—one at the bottom and one growing out the top. If the implant replaces the knuckle of your index finger, for example, one of its stems will extend into the bone of that finger and the other into the adjoining bone of your hand, leaving the wider middle portion to cushion and hold the proper space between these bones. The middle part is also a flexible hinge, easily operated by your muscles and ligaments. Once implanted, it should not only restore pain-free motion but also stabilize the joint, keeping the bones properly aligned. Survey participants whose hands were deformed by rheumatoid arthritis, with their fingers skewed at an exaggerated tilt, were pleased with the change in their appearance after surgery.

The finger joints take no cement. In fact, the stems actually glide, just a fraction of an inch, inside the bones as they move, like pistons in cylinders. To fix the implants rigidly in place, Dr. Swanson explained, would put intolerable strain on them.

Number of **knuckles** replaced*	75	
Outcome:		
Dramatic relief	62	(83%)†
Moderate relief	1	(1%)
Minor or temporary relief	10	(13%)
No relief	1	(1%)
Made participant feel worse than before	1	(1%)

*Nineteen participants had from one to ten finger joints replaced, most often the large joints at the bases of the fingers.
†These percentages have been rounded to the nearest whole number, with the result that ratings for some procedures do not total 100%.

An eighty-one-year-old retired accountant from upstate New York described the exercises he did after receiving artificial joints in the thumb and fingers of both hands: "The physical therapist brought me a glove that had small lead weights attached to it. I would put on this glove and then raise and lower each finger ten or fifteen times. I did this twice a day for several weeks, then once a day for a fairly long time." This participant also spoke frankly about the difficulties of recuperating from his hand operations, which were done in the fall of 1984 and the spring of 1985: "I was sent home four days after the operation with my whole arm immobile and held straight up in a foam cushion. I had to have complete care, including washing, feeding, and bathroom, for weeks. It was very hard on me and on my wife."

Several people judge the recovery period, with all its disability and dependence, to be as much of a trial for their families as for themselves. "I was fortunate to have an understanding family," writes a fifty-five-year-old Michigan homemaker whose surgery entailed four operations within ten months: both wrists and all the fingers on both hands, including two tendon transplants to make her fingers functional. "After surgery there was very little I was able to do for myself, and I had to rely on family members. For a while, all I could manage was to squeeze a Nerf ball or therapeutic putty for exercise, and soak my hands in warm water. It's been a year now, and though I guess I'm still recovering, my hands get stronger with use. I can once again cook, do laundry, some limited gardening, shop, run errands, clean the house, and even crochet and do other handcrafts. I have about 60 percent function in my hands at this point. However, the *pain is gone!*"

For the accountant mentioned, unfortunately, the trying recovery period did not end so happily. "There was pain relief for about a year," he says. "After that, although my fingers *looked* better, the mobility was not helped. My wife is typing the answers on the questionnaire because I am unable to write or even hold a pen."

Other partial and total replacements

The hips, knees, and knuckles are far and away the most frequent sites for total joint replacement, and the results are usually excellent. Several other participants had some of the less commonly performed joint replacements, including the shoulder, elbow, wrist, and ankle. There were too few of these operations for us to rate them individually, but it's worth noting what happened with each type of joint.

- Five out of the six **total shoulder replacements** were successful, and the one that failed was redone to become one of the five successes. "Although my first right shoulder replacement did not work out," reports this wholesale paper dealer from Virginia, "the second time was perfect. I have almost complete relief, but limited use of the joint. I've also had total replacement of my right hip and knee, with complete relief of pain in both. My advice is: *Do not delay.* Have surgery performed *mit schnell, muy pronto,* after obtaining the best surgeons."

- A retired teacher from Kansas underwent **elbow replacement** twice, once in 1986 and then over again in 1987. "My orthopedic surgeon has helped me more than anyone," she says, after two total knee replacements, surgery on both hands, and left shoulder, in addition to the two elbow operations.

- "It does relieve the pain," reports a thirty-three-year-old nurse from Pennsylvania who had a **total wrist replacement**, "but I have very little mobility, and the joint feels fake. I'd think twice before having the other wrist done, whereas my artificial hip brought me total pain relief, much greater mobility, and generally made me feel like new."

- All four participants who had a **total ankle replacement** were extremely pleased with the outcome, although this procedure, like total wrist replacement, is still considered experimental.

- Nine survey participants had a **partial joint replacement** of the hip or knee, seven of whom reported dramatic relief. Partial replacements work well for people whose joint damage is not so extensive as to require total replacement. In the hip, for example, the ball part alone may be replaced. Or the joint can be **resurfaced** by scraping the ball part smooth and capping it with metal, and also cleaning the socket and putting in a new plastic lining. It is also possible to replace one side of the joint and resurface the other. Partial replacement leaves the door open, so to speak, for total replacement later, if the joint continues to deteriorate. Two of our participants did eventually trade in a partial hip for a total replacement.

"I had a partial hip replacement that made me feel fine for a year," writes a sixty-nine-year-old housewife from Wisconsin, "but then it came loose and had to be redone, so my partial hip replacement was followed eighteen months later by a total one. After the second surgery I gained weight, probably from inactivity, and my prosthesis has come loose again—this time after six years. I have much pain now and remain inactive. I doubt that I will have another operation because I have emphysema, and the prognosis is not good."

Overall, our survey shows that nine out of ten joint replacements provide at least some relief, and about three-quarters of these can be of dramatic help.

Number of **partial or total replacements***	247	
Outcome:		
Dramatic relief	184	(74%)
Moderate relief	26	(11%)
Minor or temporary relief	12	(5%)
No relief	8	(3%)
Made participant feel worse than before	5	(2%)
No rating	12	(5%)

*This number includes partial or total replacement of the hips, knees, fingers, shoulders, elbows, wrists, ankles, and toes, representing the combined experiences of 106 survey participants.

Although none of our survey participants underwent replacement arthroplasty with a **joint transplant**, some surgeons are attempting to apply the lessons learned from organ transplant to joint replacement. Only a few hundred such operations have been performed since 1975 in the United States and Canada. The joints have come from accident victims under the age of forty and free of disease. If their hip or knee is taken within twelve hours of death and transplanted in a day or two, it may give ten or twenty years of painless movement to the right recipient—a would-be active young person with the same body build. There is no tissue typing required, surgeons explain, and no need to fear transplant rejection or to take immunosuppressive drugs, but the new joint has to match the old one in *size*.

Resection

Resection arthroplasty is the removal of damaged bone and cartilage at the joint without replacing them. Before Dr. Swanson invented his Silastic hinges, many people's severely affected hand and finger joints were treated this way. Today, some of the joints in the feet are still relieved by resection arthroplasty, as this forty-seven-year-old Florida housewife explains: "In March of 1986 I had a Hoffman resection of both feet. My metatarsal bones were cut off where they were un-jointed and protruding on the bottom, and my toes realigned. I have about 80-percent pain relief now, and walk at least a mile a day, plus I can wear more normal shoes. It took almost a year to recover, during which time I was quite dependent and immobile, having had surgery on both feet, but I would do it again in a minute."

An equally enthusiastic photographer from Massachusetts, age sixty-nine, calls the outcome of her two 1975 metatarsal resections "a total miracle." "I had screaming pain upon walk-ing," she recalls. "The surgery gave me back my life."

Another successful use of resection is the cutting away of painful, disfiguring bunions from the base of the big toe. The following ratings combine the experiences of fifteen partici-pants, ten of whom had metatarsal resection on one or both feet, and five who had one or two bunions removed.

Number of **resections**	27	
Outcome:		
Dramatic relief	23	(85%)
Moderate relief	2	(7%)
Minor or temporary relief	1	(4%)
No relief	0	
Made participant feel worse than before	1	(4%)
No rating	0	

Arthrodesis

Before joint replacement became popular, surgery often re-lieved arthritis pain by fusing the bones at their meeting place. A fused joint lost natural motion, it's true, but it gained strength, and besides, the promised freedom from pain was worth the sacrifice for many people. Today, fusion, or arthrod-esis, is still regarded as the best surgical treatment for certain joints, especially the ankle and wrist, where several small bones come together, and where replacement is far from rou-tine. In the spine, where replacements are not even at-tempted, fusion of two or three vertebrae may bring relief of severe neck pain or lower back pain. "Cervical fusion brought me total pain relief," reports a Rhode Island secretary, "although I now have much less range of motion in my neck."

Arthrodesis is also preferred in certain *situations*. A person with recurrent infections, for example, who faces a greater-than-average risk of losing an artificial joint because of loosening after infection, might be better off with a fused shoulder than a new shoulder.

The participants in our survey who had one or more joints fused are extremely pleased with the results.

Number of **fusion** procedures*	35	
Outcome:		
Dramatic relief	30	(86%)
Moderate relief	3	(8%)
Minor or temporary relief	0	———
No relief	1	(3%)
Made participant feel worse than before	0	———
No rating	1	(3%)

*This number combines the wrist, ankle, finger, toe, and spinal (including cervical spine) fusions reported by 18 survey participants, most of whom also had joint replacement surgery on their hips or knees.

No glue or cement is used to make the bones of a fused joint stick together. Instead, the surgeon cuts away all the damaged cartilage and bone, shaping the joint so that the bones interlock in the ideal position. The joints closest to the fingertips, for example, may be fused, if need be, in a slight crook—a position that lets you use them to write, or button your coat, or pick up coins from a countertop. "Ten years ago I had the knuckles in my right hand replaced, and the joints of my fingers fused to make them bendable," writes a housewife from Tennessee. "Before the operation, they wouldn't bend and I couldn't hold anything in that hand at all. Now it works great."

Once the bones to be fused are positioned just so, they get fixed in place with a bit of wire. The wire stays in for several weeks until new bone has a chance to grow around the joint and form a natural seal. Often, small bone chips are also inserted at the fused joint, because they encourage new bone to grow. The bone graft may come from elsewhere in your own body—from the top of your pelvis, for example—or from a "bone bank," just as blood for transfusions comes from a blood bank.

New versions of arthrodesis in the wrist combine the best advantages of fusion and joint replacement. The joint between the arm bone and wrist can be fused, while other small bones of the wrist are resurfaced or replaced with silicone implants. This combination can relieve pain and shore up a weak wrist while leaving the natural motion of the hand intact. "I had a total fusion in my right wrist," says a Michigan homemaker, "and a partial fusion on the left with an artificial joint. This is a new surgical procedure that gives me some movement."

A fifty-three-year-old travel agent from Washington reports that the first twenty-four hours after her ankle fusion were extremely painful, and full recovery took about a year. Now, however, her exercise regimen includes low-impact aerobics three times a week, tennis once or twice a week, depending on the weather, and a daily walk.

Arthroscopy

The arthroscope is the device that has opened up the knee and selected other joints to lights, cameras, and surgical implements—and all without opening them very wide. Through an incision as small as a quarter of an inch, a surgeon can now get the best possible diagnostic picture of the inside of a joint, and, if necessary, perform surgery through another small hole with specially designed microtools.

The small scale of the procedure—the tiny incision, the short hospital stay—lead many people to believe that arthroscopy is a minor matter. But surgery via arthroscopy is still surgery and usually calls for general anesthesia. What's more, the recovery period may last just as long as recovery from other types of surgery, depending on what gets done with the arthroscope. If you hear of someone who is up and about the morning after, you can bet that person had little more than a diagnostic look-see with a local anesthetic.

Despite all the fanfare surrounding arthroscopy, however, especially the exciting stories of world-class athletes whose careers were saved by arthroscopic surgery, our participants had less success with it than with the other forms of surgery they rated. Some of the operations carried out with arthroscopy simply don't improve life as dramatically as a joint replacement, say, or a fusion procedure. Here are the things that surgeons can do with arthroscopy to help people with arthritis: remove debris from inside the joint, scrape off bone spurs, and take out the joint lining (synovium). A salesman from Illinois described his arthroscopy the way it felt to him, as "microsurgery of right knee to remove sand and gravel."

Number of **arthroscopic procedures***	22	
Outcome:		
Dramatic relief	8	(36%)
Moderate relief	5	(23%)
Minor or temporary relief	1	(5%)
No relief	5	(23%)
Made participant feel worse than before	1	(5%)
No rating	2	(9%)

*Although 80 participants reported they underwent arthroscopy as part of diagnostic testing, only 20 had surgery with this technique, and 2 of them had two procedures apiece. All these operations were performed on the knee.

Synovectomy

In rheumatoid arthritis, the main culprit responsible for pain and swelling is thought to be the paper-thin membrane that surrounds and lubricates the joint, called the synovium. Inflammation can spur this membrane on to wild overgrowth, until it becomes so thick and unwieldy that it fills the joint space, puffs out the surrounding skin, moves bones, and ruptures tendons. As inflammation rages, the synovium also secretes enzymes that eat up the cartilage. Little wonder, then, that surgeons thought to stem the destruction by *synovectomy*—removing the synovium. "I had a synovectomy on my right knee in 1962," writes a former coal miner from West Virginia. "All of the inflammation, swelling, and practically all of the severe pain left, and full mobility in the knee returned." An executive recruiter from Texas, who had a wrist synovectomy in 1978, says it relieved about 90 percent of his pain.

Number of **synovectomies***	25	
Outcome:		
Dramatic relief	11	(44%)
Moderate relief	5	(20%)
Minor or temporary relief	1	(4%)
No relief	6	(24%)
Made participant feel worse than before	1	(4%)
No rating	1	(4%)

*Sixteen participants had one or more synovectomies. The joints operated on were 11 knees, 4 hands, 3 wrists, 2 feet, 1 finger, and 1 that was not specified.

Synovectomy is not performed as frequently as it used to be, partly because doctors have found that the membrane often grows back. "I had greater mobility for a year after the synovectomy on my left knee in 1970," says a fifty-eight-year-old homemaker from Minnesota, "but then the diseased synovial membrane grew back, and there is very little mobility now."

Even if the membrane does not overgrow the joint space again, the joint destruction may continue to get worse after synovectomy. "I had synovectomy on one knee in 1967, and then the other knee the next year," reports a retired engineer from Tennessee. "After these operations I had less pain and I got around better for years, until my knees completely deteriorated and I had to have them both replaced, one in 1985 and the other in 1986. The replacements have given me total pain relief and good mobility."

Other Surgical Procedures

Our participants underwent several other kinds of surgery for arthritis, but not in large enough numbers for us to evaluate their relative effectiveness. **Osteotomy**, for one, was a popular way to relieve hip and knee pain in the late 1950s and early 1960s, but it got upstaged by joint replacement. Now, according to articles in the medical literature, it may be making a comeback, especially for people who are considered too young to receive an artificial joint.

Osteotomy entails cutting a bone to correct the alignment of the joint. At the knee, for example, if the thighbone and shin don't abut squarely, there may be too much stress on one part of the joint, and the cartilage and bone at the overloaded meeting place will wear unevenly. By cutting a wedge-shaped piece out of either bone, a surgeon may tip the balance, so to speak, and get the person's weight distributed evenly across the joint, the way it should be.

Two of our participants were relieved to have their **rheumatoid nodules removed**. These are lumps that form under the skin of some people with rheumatoid arthritis. They may appear on the fingers, or near the knees or elbows, and they may hurt anytime they are touched.

Other surgical procedures include attempts, most of them successful, to repair or release tendons and ligaments, and a couple of highly unusual procedures for rare complications of rheumatoid arthritis. A forty-three-year-old Washington real estate agent began losing his voice very soon after he developed rheumatoid arthritis. Surgery freed his vocal cords, he writes, restoring 75 percent of his voice. A thirty-five-year-old Pennsylvania lab technician needed surgery to remove inflamed tissue around her heart.

Survey Participants' Advice About Surgery

No matter what their operations entailed, most of the surgery veterans among our survey participants agree on certain points about joint surgery—including preparations and follow-up procedures that can increase the likelihood of a successful outcome. If you are considering surgery for arthritis, consider their suggestions.

1.   *Have it done!* This was the most frequently offered advice about surgery from the group of participants who'd been through it, and the most common comment was, *I'm glad I did it. It was definitely worthwhile.*

2.   *Give the whole process your most serious considera-tion.* Surgery for arthritis is *elective* surgery, which means that you must choose whether and when to go through with it. The pain and disability that bring you to this decision have likely

been worsening over a period of years, so there's no need to make snap judgments now.

3. *Get a second, and even a third opinion.* By all means get the opinion of at least one other doctor. A second surgeon's analysis is valuable, but so is the opinion of a physician who's used to dealing with joint problems *non*surgically, like a rheumatologist or a physiatrist (doctor of physical medicine and rehabilitation). The expert opinions should cover whether or not you need surgery, and if so, which type of procedure is likely to help most.

4. *Choose your surgeon carefully.* It's a simple case of practice making perfect. The more elbows that surgeons replace, the more proficient they become with the technique. Many orthopedic surgeons specialize in treating certain areas of the body, for this very reason, and you owe it to yourself to find one who is especially adept at doing whatever you need done. "Inquire long and carefully," says a retired carpenter from California. "Get the very best surgeon in the field. The very best costs no more than the mediocre."

5. *Pick the best available hospital.* The fact is that hospitals, like specialists, differ in their track records for safely accomplishing certain procedures.* Some of our participants chose the hospital first, for its fine reputation in joint surgery, secure in the assumption that any surgeon affiliated with that institution would be well qualified.

6. *Learn all you can about your surgery beforehand* by questioning your doctor(s), reading any available information, and talking to one or two people who have undergone the same type of operation. This will help you form a realistic picture of what's to be done, what the immediate aftermath may be like for you, how much time you may need to fully recover from surgery, and what long-term results you can expect.

7. *Get in shape for surgery.* If you are overweight and need surgery on your hips, knees, or feet, this is the time to try to shed extra pounds. A low-calorie but nutritious diet makes

---

*In 1986, the U.S. Health Care Financing Administration released a list of hospitals all over the country that had distressingly high death rates for nine types of surgery, including major joint procedures. The list demonstrates the importance of picking a hospital where the surgery you need is performed *frequently.*

the most sense, because you need to reduce the strain on your weight-bearing joints *and* keep up your general health to withstand the physical stress of surgery. A crash diet could leave you dangerously weakened. Also talk to your doctor about all the *medications* you take regularly, such as aspirin, as some may need to be cut back or stopped altogether in preparation for surgery. Ask about food supplements, too, such as adding vitamins A and C, as well as iron, to help speed your recovery, or cutting out fish oil because it might prolong bleeding.

8. *Prepare your family for the role they will play.* Although the goal of your operation may be to restore your physical independence, the immediate recovery period could call for more help from your family than you've ever needed before. Involve them in the planning stages, and help them find out what will be expected of them.

9. *Follow post-op directions.* Exercise the joint according to the instructions you receive from your doctor or physical therapist. Make sure you understand what you can and can't do during the recovery period and beyond, and, again, if it's a weight-bearing joint that's had surgery, don't give it any added weight to bear.

10. *Think positively.* There is every reason to believe that the surgery will turn out well, so try to keep that thought uppermost in your mind—before the operation and during the recovery period. A fifty-four-year-old housewife from Tennessee observes, "I would highly recommend these operations [she's had eight] for people who have a good attitude toward this sort of thing. The attitude is very important. It takes nerve to go through surgery. Confidence in your doctor helps, and the moral support of family and friends."

Summary of Arthritis Surgery

Arthroplasty—Total hip replacements are the most successful surgery in this category, followed closely by knee and knuckle replacement. Replacement of other joints, such as the shoulder, is performed less frequently but can also be quite successful. Where the joint damage is not too extensive, partial replacements or resurfacing may be all that's needed to relieve pain.

Arthrodesis—Wrist, ankle, or neck fusion may give pain relief and joint stability in exchange for full range of motion. Arthrodesis may also be favored over joint replacement for people with recurrent infections who would face a high risk of losing a replacement joint.

Arthroscopy—Microsurgery techniques enable surgeons to perform diagnostic exploratory surgery inside certain joints, and also to remove joint debris and scrape off bone spurs.

Synovectomy—Removing the grossly inflamed synovial lining of the joint may bring great relief, but the membrane sometimes grows back.

Osteotomy—Cutting the bones near the joint to correct misalignment may be better than joint replacement for younger people.

Other—Operations to remove rheumatoid nodules, to repair tendons and ligaments, free the vocal cords, and remove inflamed tissue around the heart were also successful for our participants.

8

ELEVEN EFFECTIVE EXTRA TREATMENTS FOR REDUCING ARTHRITIS PAIN

■ Exercise ■ Hydrotherapy ■ Heat/Cold ■ Ultrasound ■ Psychological Counseling ■ Wax ■ Massage ■ Traction ■ TENS ■ Splints ■ Biofeedback

The best of the current treatments for arthritis are combination plans—mixtures of methods that work *together* to bring pain relief, keep joints flexible, and slow the progress of the disease. The medicine prescribed or the surgery performed by your doctor, no matter how dramatically effective, does not stand alone. The truth is that the exercises you've learned to do at home for fifteen or twenty minutes a day are every bit as important. And exercise instruction is just one of a variety of other professional treatments, neither medicinal nor surgical, that help our Arthritis Survey participants to feel and function well. The list of these additional treatments includes many forms of physical therapy, such as diathermy, hydrotherapy, massage, and ultrasound, as well as psychological counseling and biofeedback. (See Chapter 10 for information about the unconventional extras—acupuncture, manipulation, and Yoga.)

Some of these extra treatments work better than others,

of course. A few bring at least some measure of relief to nearly everyone, while others work about half or three-quarters of the time. Our participants' comments allow us to rank the following topics in order of their *relative effectiveness,* beginning with the ones that produce the greatest degree of help for the 1,051 members of our survey group.

Treatment	Number of Participants Who Tried It	Number Helped by It
Exercise	836	794 (95%)
Hydrotherapy	83*	75 (90%)
Heat/Cold	123*	104 (85%)
Ultrasound	47*	38 (81%)
Psychological Counseling	46	37 (80%)
Wax	30	22 (73%)
Massage	298	211 (71%)
Traction	46	29 (63%)
TENS	30	18 (60%)
Splints	125	74 (59%)
Biofeedback	42	20 (48%)

*These numbers may be underestimates, as 371 of our participants who received physical therapy did not say what the treatments entailed. Hydrotherapy and heat were likely included in the sessions, and perhaps ultrasound as well.

Exercise

The overwhelming majority of our participants—836 individuals—say they exercise regularly because of arthritis, and the effort pays off for fully 95 percent of them. The chief benefits they get from exercise are increased flexibility of their affected joints and some measure of pain relief. Exercise also improves their general health, participants say, lifts their spirits, and keeps their weight down. A few even credit exercise with helping them fight stress, giving them more energy during the day, and helping them sleep better at night.

"Even though exercise is the last thing I feel like doing

when my arthritis is unbearable," writes a teacher from Illinois, "I always feel better later on after I force myself to get up and move around. Exercise doesn't aggravate the joint; it loosens up the stiffness." A retired physician from Mississippi says, "I believe that without the exercising I have done over the years I would now be in a wheelchair!" (See Chapter 18 for a rundown of the fitness exercises favored by our participants; Chapter 19 tells you how to perform stretching and strengthening exercises tailored to specific joints.)

Some 350 of our participants were taught exercise—or at least told to exercise—by their doctors. Almost as many others learned their exercise routines from physical therapists, nurses, or instructors at health clubs, gyms, pools, schools, and senior centers. Hundreds take the advice of books and magazine articles on the subject, and some are self-taught.

In general, activity is better than inactivity, but the wrong exercise can sometimes be as dangerous as the wrong medication. Out of 1,051 participants in our survey, 174 (17 percent) reported being harmed at least once by inappropriate or overzealous workouts. Getting and following expert exercise advice is a good way to help you avoid injury. But where do you go for suggestions?

You can expect the most helpful individual attention to come from a practitioner who knows about your medical history, about exercise in general, and about the particulars of exercise designed to preserve range of motion in joints threatened by arthritis. Here are a few of the best choices.

- **Your doctor**, especially if you're seeing a physiatrist, an osteopath, or a rheumatologist (see Chapter 3). These three specialists gave the most helpful exercise information to our participants. Doctors who are not exercise experts can at least advise you on safe limits and refer you to someone who knows how to teach the specifics, such as a physical therapist.*

---

*Some chiropractors are quite knowledgeable about exercise for arthritis, but on the whole, our participants did not fare well under chiropractic care. (See Chapter 4.)

- **A physical therapist** who has both interest and skill in helping people with arthritis. Sound exercise advice from these practitioners often led to long-term improvement for our survey participants. (See Chapter 4.)

- **The exercise instructor** at your local Y or fitness center. If you enroll in a general exercise class, make sure to tell the instructor that you have arthritis and that you may need to do some exercises differently or not at all. Many exercise instructors, including Yoga teachers, have the ability to provide such individualized help. (See Chapter 4.)

- **Group classes** specially designed for people with limited movement, such as aquatic exercise at a community pool. Classes may be offered near you from time to time by your local chapter of the Arthritis Foundation.

In recent years, videotapes that can be played on a home VCR unit have become popular substitutes for exercise classes. Survey participants mentioned several exercise tapes produced especially for people with arthritis and sold through the Arthritis Foundation (1314 Spring Street N.W., Atlanta, GA 30309).

The amount of time our participants devote to exercise varies from a few minutes to a few hours a day, depending on their family obligations, business demands, age, and physical fitness—including the degree of joint damage they have. "I spend fifteen minutes a day on range-of-motion exercises," writes a forty-year-old Iowa homemaker, "because I tend to get stiff and sore if I don't do them daily." A retired car dealer from Florida, age sixty, follows a much more ambitious routine: "I bicycle five miles per day, walk two miles per day, do stretching exercises in bed for half an hour every day, and type—to keep my fingers active—for about two hours a day."

There is no simple formula for determining an optimum amount of exercise time, but there are rules for safe exercise that seem to apply to just about everyone, whether your routine involves moving your fingers in warm water or walking miles at a time. Indeed, so many of our participants offered the same advice that we were able to create this list of exercise guidelines.

- *Don't overdo it.* "Know your limits," writes a store manager from Texas. A Georgia housewife adds: "Learn to pace yourself. You may have to change your daily routine on bad days."

- *Exercise regularly—every day if possible.* "A little bit daily, faithfully and regularly, is much more effective than more exercise done sporadically," explains an editor from New York.

- *Listen to your body.* "Don't push through pain," advises a retired purchasing agent from Maryland. "If you start to hurt, *stop!*"

- *Start any new exercise program slowly, and increase gradually.* "Set your own goals and don't be influenced by jocks or normal know-it-alls," says a freelance writer from New Mexico.

- *Choose exercises that are easy on the joints.* "And never try to exercise or force a joint when it is swollen," writes a factory worker from Virginia.

- *Learn to exercise properly, and follow the instructions you receive.* "Find a good person who is knowledgeable and can relate to your individual body problems," a New York psychotherapist suggests.

- *Get your doctor's OK before you embark on a new exercise regimen.*

- *Warm up before and cool down afterward.* "Always warm up thoroughly," says an insurance secretary from Texas. "Cool-down is also important, and should contain some easy stretching, just like the warm-up."

- *Don't give up.* "Exercise can get very discouraging when you are alone and have to do it," sympathizes a retired postal worker from New Jersey. "You seldom see immediate results, but sometimes you have to keep at it just to stay even. When you don't exercise, you tend to limit yourself more each day."

Among the 215 participants who do *not* exercise regularly, many find their jobs or other daily activities to be so physically taxing that they have neither the time nor the energy for a structured exercise period. "I just do all I can," writes a forty-nine-year-old teacher from Nebraska. "I recommend: Keep moving, keep living, don't stop!!!" Others say they are hoping or planning to start an exercise program soon. And a small minority say they find exercise too painful to pursue.

Hydrotherapy (Water)

Baths, spas, springs, tanks, and tubs that deliver the soothing powers of water all work well for our participants. Hydrotherapy ranks among the oldest forms of medical treatment and remains one of the best-loved. Even though its good effects are temporary, the sensation is so pleasant that immersion has become a daily ritual for many of our participants. When they are not receiving whirlpool or Hubbard tank* treatments from their physical therapists, they seek the hydrotherapy of their own bathtubs at home or the hot tub at a nearby health club.

Hydrotherapy can be considered a form of whole-body heat treatment—an extremely efficient way to warm up many painful joints at one time. Survey participants say the warmth relieves both pain and stiffness. (Inflammation, however, is better served by cold, as explained on page 143.) Participants also find that the buoyancy of the water takes the strain off their weight-bearing joints, while the whirlpool's churning action gives them a gentle, thorough massage. "I've had chiropractic, acupressure, massage, and physical therapy with diathermy and hydrotherapy," writes a retired proofreader from New York. "The whirlpool hydrotherapy is the only treatment that helps me significantly. In fact, it helps a great deal."

Some of our participants report that they do their exer-

*What separates the Hubbard tank from an ordinary whirlpool bath is the special apparatus that can lower you into the water and lift you out again.

cises in the whirlpool because the water makes movement easier. "This feels great while I'm doing it," reports an Indiana social worker, "and also gives me carryover mobility later in the day."

Most hydrotherapy makes do with ordinary tap water, but a few of our participants got the chance to bathe in renowned mineral springs. "Three years ago I spent four days at Hot Springs, Arkansas," writes a retired salesman from Illinois, "and had hot-bath treatments at the spa there. On the third day I had a full body massage that, along with the hot baths, did make me feel great. But as soon as I would cool off or get chilled, my muscles would tighten and my joints would again become sore and tender."

Thermotherapy (Heat)—and Cryotherapy (Cold)

Many survey participants find relief from pain and stiffness with thermotherapy, because heat increases the circulation where it is applied and helps the muscles relax. Professional methods for getting heat to affected joints include hot compresses, heat packs (sometimes called hydrocollators), heat lamps fitted with infrared bulbs, and devices that beam a comforting dose of warmth in the form of shortwave or microwave diathermy.

"An Army physical therapist taught me how to survive in an environment where I have to use aching joints," writes a forty-five-year-old commissioned infantry officer from Hawaii. "I find that direct heat on my shoulders and elbows, applied with a hot cloth, improves the mobility and gives temporary relief."

Most participants who enjoy professional heat treatments find that they can be helped just as much with the hot pads, hot-water bottles, or heat lamps they use at home. Heat is heat, after all, and it usually helps. An advantage of the professional thermotherapy is that it often comes complete with another form of treatment, such as massage or muscle stimulation. And a good practitioner, mindful of the real danger of burning you, may be more careful than you would be about where the heat source is placed and the length of time you are exposed to it.

For example, most professionals say you should never lie on a heating pad, but put it on top of the painful part, and never use heat on a joint that is already hot and swollen. They also advise stopping any heat treatment session at the twenty- or thirty-minute mark.

The opposite of thermotherapy is cryotherapy, which aims to put the freeze on pain. Many doctors and therapists believe that cold is actually *more effective* for pain relief than heat. Some of our survey participants strongly agree, although more of them use heat than use ice.

Cold treatments penetrate farther and last longer than most forms of heat, and cold has the added advantage of working to *reduce inflammation.* Professionals apply it much the way you would, with gel-filled, refreezable cold packs, or plastic bags filled with ice or a mixture of water and ice. They make sure to protect your skin from frostbite with a thin cloth and an eye on the clock—limiting cold treatments to twenty minutes every few hours. And they sometimes alternate heat and cold to maximize the benefits of both.

Ultrasound (Deep Heat)

The penetrating waves of ultrasound can heat small areas of the body so quickly that a treatment may go from start to finish in just *two* minutes, or ten at the most. Indeed, ultrasound is the only form of thermotherapy that has been shown to raise the temperature of tissues underneath the surface muscles. Heat pads, packs, and lamps, on the other hand, warm just the skin and surface muscles, letting the increased blood flow do the rest of the work.

Physical therapists and chiropractors were the most likely sources of ultrasound treatments for our participants, some of whom enjoyed relatively long-lasting benefits. "I found ultrasound the most beneficial of all therapeutic aids," writes a twenty-year-old college student with rheumatoid arthritis. "Ultrasound gave me relief from the pain in my hips for about twenty-four to thirty-six hours."

As any form of heat, however, ultrasound can *aggravate inflammation.* "The ultrasound was very painful for me because of my inflamed nerves," reports a former legal secretary from California who fares much better with ice and TENS (see pages 147–148).

Psychological Counseling

The medical literature is full of conflicting reports about the role of psychological counseling in the treatment of arthritis. Is it important, or is it just an added expense for people already strapped with high medical costs? In studies conducted at medical schools and hospitals, various types of psychological dishes have been added to the treatment menu—supportive group therapy, for example, or relaxation training—while doctors tried to see whether the treatments affected people with arthritis in ways that could be measured, such as their grip strength, pain level, and degree of inflammation. Some experts show objective proof that treating the mind helps the body, while others argue that the evidence is weak or wanting.

The nature of our survey research is fundamentally different from these studies, since we rely totally on our participants' accounts of what happened to them and not on laboratory results or the observations of clinic personnel. By their own reckoning, survey participants *do* find psychological intervention to be of value. It actually relieves pain for some of them and it helps others overcome emotional problems that have burgeoned around the fact of their arthritis, such as anxiety or depression.

Forms of psychological counseling that are directly aimed at pain control include relaxation training, guided imagery, and self-hypnosis. (Biofeedback is also a pain-control strategy taught by some psychologists, and is described separately on page 149.) All of these approaches require that you marshal your powers of concentration to alter your perception of pain or even to change the course of your illness. For example, you might be asked to picture yourself in some much-loved place as a way to take your mind off the pain you feel, or you might be encouraged to conjure up a healing image—the fire in your joints, perhaps, being doused by guardian cells traveling through your body. Some of our participants regularly practice such techniques of thought control and they know that their success does not mean their pain is minor or imaginary. "I use self-hypnosis taught to me by a psychologist," writes an insurance underwriter from Louisiana. "It works better than some medications I've tried for helping me deal with the pain."

Treatments that address arthritis-related psychological problems include behavior modification and the many forms of individual or group psychotherapy. These gave some of our participants the help they needed to regain a lost measure of self-assurance or self-esteem. "During one of my very worst struggles with rheumatoid arthritis," says a secretary and mother of four from Texas, "I was given the number of a psychologist who has rheumatoid arthritis and who had led groups for the Arthritis Foundation. I was too ill for an office session, so she agreed to counsel me on the telephone. From talking with this kind lady, I realized that I was not alone in my disease or in the emotional havoc it causes."

Wax (Heat)

Heat pads may be fine for the neck and back, and ultrasound ideal on an elbow, but some participants say there's nothing like a coating of wax to warm their hands and feet—over, under, and around every single joint of every finger or toe. Here's how it works: You dip your hands several times into the molten wax of the paraffin bath, then lift them out. The warm wax hardens immediately and you must hold the coated parts still, lest you crack the wax and let out the heat. The therapist then wraps your hands in plastic bags and heated towels, leaving you to enjoy the effect for about fifteen to twenty minutes. At the end of the treatment time, the wax peels off easily, since it is premixed with mineral oil.

Several participants found wax dips such a high point of physical therapy that they bought or learned how to make their own paraffin baths at home. (See Chapter 17 for full instructions.)

Wax treatments tend to be kinder to your skin than repeated soaking in hot water, although a laboratory technician from Pennsylvania reports that the paraffin occasionally causes a mild skin rash on her hands. The rash doesn't detract much from the pleasure, though, she adds.

Massage

Massage may work some of its good effects by the heat and increased circulation it generates. Some experts in pain control further believe that rubbing a painful area sends a different sort of message along nerves that travel to the brain. In other words, the "massage message" blots out, or at least interferes with, the "pain message."

"I had massage treatments for six months from a physical therapist," writes a homemaker from Oregon. "These began very gradually, massaging only my feet at first, and then the rest of my body after a few weeks. The treatment helped me a great deal." A former USDA inspector from Colorado adds, "I don't much like to get bent in the directions the physical therapist bends me in. It doesn't feel all that great, but the massage part feels great anytime, and is really relaxing."

Survey participants who praise massage say they like it because it feels good—soothing and relaxing—even when it does not relieve pain. From the wrong hands, however, massage can make pain more pronounced. Our participants preferred massages from physical therapists, chiropractors, and osteopaths to those given by massage therapists who didn't understand the sensitivity of arthritis-stressed joints. "Massage by a holistic massage therapist did me in," says a retail buyer from New York. "I've had trouble with my hernia ever since."

Traction

Whether it's performed with weights and pulleys or a motorized machine, traction is supposed to relieve pressure and pain by pulling apart joint spaces that have narrowed and by freeing nerves that may be pinched. The vertebrae in the back and neck are the most frequent sites targeted for traction, although one of our participants was greatly helped by traction treatments on her legs during a hospital stay. "In 1980 I became completely bedridden," the forty-six-year-old Wisconsin house-wife recalls. "My rheumatologist put me in the hospital for a six-week stay with drug treatments and physical therapy, including traction on my legs. I believe the traction is what helped me most to walk again."

A few participants who received and benefited from traction say that the treatments sometimes caused nausea, headache, or jaw pain. Others found their original problem made worse by traction: "I feel traction harmed me," writes a receptionist from Florida. "It's as though my neck has been stretched so far that there is no elasticity left." People with rheumatoid arthritis need to be cautious about traction, especially neck traction.

Two of the participants who were helped by traction received a form known as "inversion traction" or "gravity inversion," which involves lying for short periods of time in a head-down tilted position. With their feet up and heads down, they found that the ever-present tug of gravity became a therapeutic device.

TENS (Transcutaneous Electrical Nerve Stimulation)

The fact that electricity can ease or erase pain has been known for many centuries—ever since the times when electric fish or eels were used as physician's assistants. The compact ultramodern way to pit electricity against pain is with a device called a TENS unit, which has been around for only a few decades but has proven effective for some participants' arthritis pain. "TENS diminishes my pain considerably," says a college professor from Massachusetts.

The doctor or physical therapist who introduces you to TENS hooks you up to the device by taping its electrode-tipped wires to your skin at carefully selected points, depending on where you hurt. Turning on the battery-operated device delivers the electric current through your skin to the nerves. The relief you may feel within a few minutes is real, and it may last hours or days, although technology cannot

explain why. The current may somehow short-circuit your perception of pain, or it may precipitate a flood of endorphins—
your brain's own internally manufactured morphine.

"The TENS unit is the only thing that I've found effective," writes a housewife from Utah, "and it has no side effects." Actually, the gels and tapes used to secure the
electrodes may cause skin irritations, if you're susceptible to
them, and using the unit at the wrong setting can throw your
muscles into spasm. But if you receive good instruction, and
you respond to the treatment, you may want to purchase your
own TENS unit for home use. "I'm on my second one," says a
Michigan housewife. "I had the first for eight years until I just
wore it out." You need a prescription to get a TENS unit, not
to mention several hundred dollars to buy one, or a smaller
sum to lease the equipment.

Splints

A strap-on mechanical aid that rests a joint, or keeps it stable
while you work, or prevents deformity—or all three—is called
a splint. Some of our participants say that splints also give them
pain relief and protection from further injury. "I've had at
least four splints on my right hand," says a nutritionist from
South Carolina. "The orthopedist kept changing them as my
hand changed, and those splints saved me from surgery."

The function of a splint determines its form, and each one
can be fashioned from a variety of materials, such as a combination of plastic, cloth, and metal, with Velcro fasteners.

Splints are often used "as needed," while driving or dressing, for example, or at night to keep the joint in the safest, most
comfortable position. "The wrist splints help, but I hate them,"
writes a Pennsylvania piano teacher. "They aren't very roman-
tic to wear at night, and once I accidentally hit my husband on
the head with the metal plate in my sleep."

This may sound like a truism, but splints can't help you
unless you wear them. A California dental assistant reports
"immense" help from her splints, "particularly after I decided
to wear them religiously." In contrast, a Connecticut housewife gave them up, even though they helped, because they just

got in her way, especially when she was caring for her children.

A few participants leveled serious charges against splints for undermining the joint they were supposed to support. A retired tax assessor from Rhode Island says, "After four months of wearing a splint on my left wrist, I felt that my wrist was getting weaker, so I discontinued wearing it."

Biofeedback

A biofeedback device gives voice to the unseen, unheard vital processes that your body carries out without your conscious control. An ordinary thermometer is a biofeedback device—a meter that can show how your body temperature fluctuates over the course of a day. With practice, several of our participants have learned to use biofeedback devices to gain control over one or more of the body's automatic functions, and gain pain control as well.

One kind of hand-held biofeedback device gives a shrill whistle, for example, in response to a microscopic amount of perspiration on your palm. If, upon hearing the tone, you bend the powers of your mind to relaxation, you can stem the flow of sweat and make the machine hum quietly. More important, however, is the beneficial effect of relaxation on body tension and pain perception. "I have tried biofeedback for the arthritis pain in my jaw," writes a Colorado homemaker, "and I find it helps me a lot. I listen to the general relaxation tape the psychologist gave me, and work on relaxing my facial muscles, and this seems to relieve the tension and pain in my jaw."

It should be clear by now that the biofeedback device is a means to an end. It is simply a monitor, no matter how elaborate it may be. The real painkiller in biofeedback is the relaxation technique you master. This may take a lot of work. "Biofeedback does help," says a high school chaplain and counselor from Ohio, "but it takes an extreme investment of time and concentration." "It's useless at the workplace," adds a California electrician, "and also very expensive!"

Summary of Additional Orthodox Treatments

1. *Exercise* is the best, provided it's tailored to your needs. You may want to seek professional advice for instruction, while letting your own body be your guide to what exercise (and how much) you can do.

2. *Hydrotherapy* feels great while you're wet, and whirlpool treatments are especially helpful for reducing pain and increasing mobility, but the effects are temporary.

3. *Heat* is an effective treatment for pain and stiffness. *Cold* works even better than heat for some people's pain, and it also helps relieve inflammation.

4. *Ultrasound,* the most penetrating form of heat therapy, may achieve even better results in less time, with more lasting effects.

5. *Psychological Counseling* is a worthwhile adjunct to arthritis care, whether the therapist focuses on strategies for pain control or on the emotional problems arthritis can create.

6. *Wax* treatments in paraffin baths literally seal the hands (or feet) in warmth, and thereby provide a respite from pain.

7. *Massage* is at least soothing and relaxing, and may also relieve pain when it is performed by a knowledgeable practitioner.

8. *Traction* can relieve some kinds of pain by taking pressure off pinched nerves. In the wrong hands, this treatment can hurt as much as help.

9. *TENS,* the electrical painkiller, works by interfering with the brain's perception of pain.

10. *Splints* can relieve pain through physical support, while protecting a joint from injury and deformity.

11. *Biofeedback* requires your own finely honed powers of concentration to help you achieve relaxation and pain relief.

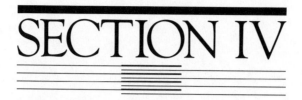

SECTION IV

WHAT YOU NEED TO KNOW ABOUT UNCONVENTIONAL TREATMENTS FOR ARTHRITIS

Be not the first by whom the new are tried,
Nor yet the last to lay the old aside.

> —Alexander Pope, from *An Essay on Criticism* (1711)

"I didn't say there was nothing better," *the king replied. "I said there was nothing* like *it."*

> —Lewis Carroll, from *Through the Looking Glass* (1872)

My experiences would indicate that what helps is often an individual thing, and each new treatment must be approached with cautious *enthusiasm.*

> —Survey Participant #388, a school cafeteria server from Colorado

9

AN UNCENSORED LOOK AT ARTHRITIS "QUACKERY" FROM COPPER BRACELETS TO STINGING BEES

■ *What is quackery, anyway?* ■ *The green wrist effect* ■ *The solvent solution* ■ *Folk medicine* ■ *The sting*

There has probably been more haranguing, more breast-beating, and more outrage expressed on the subject of quack remedies for arthritis than on any other aspect of the disease. Estimates of the number of people with arthritis who have tried foolish or dangerous remedies run higher than 90 percent. And estimates of the money wasted on these quests are routinely figured in the billions of dollars per year.* Physicians often depict quackery as a boogeyman that preys on people in pain, making them discard proven treatments in favor of overblown promises—a walk down the primrose (oil) path. Some physicians blame themselves for the quack crisis. Dr. James F. Fries, director of the Stanford Arthritis Clinic, has said: "The fact that patients try unorthodox treat-

*This amount of money would buy several hundred copper bracelets for every man, woman, and child in this country with any of the one hundred forms of arthritis.

ments and go to quacks is an indictment of medical care. It smacks of poor communication on the part of physicians, lack of results, and a failure to deliver hope to patients." Whatever the reason, the medical consensus is that quackery is pervasive and pernicious.

Our nationwide Arthritis Survey offers no support for these claims or fears. Our 1,051 survey participants avoided quackery, for the most part, despite self-assessed pain ratings of 10 (the highest on our scale) and disease duration of more than thirty years in some cases. Two-thirds of them never tried so much as an alfalfa tablet or a sip of cod liver oil. And of the one-third that did report using an unproven treatment, the majority had limited themselves to wearing a copper brace-let—on a lark, on the urging of a friend, or on the grounds that a five-dollar piece of junk jewelry couldn't hurt, so why not? Less than one-tenth of 1 percent of our participants actually went against medical advice in trying potentially dangerous unorthodox treatments, such as traveling to a clinic in another state or country for hormone/steroid shots, or trapping bees in a jar and then getting them angry enough to sting the affected joint.

We conclude that either the threat of quackery is a fabrication—a straw man set up to divert attention from other issues in arthritis—or the haranguing has had its desired effect. In any case, people from every level of income and education are appropriately suspicious of mail-order miracles.

What Is Quackery, Anyway?

The real reason that the Arthritis Foundation catches nine out of every ten people trying some quack cure is that its definition of quackery is broad enough to include *anything* that isn't written on a prescription pad. The list of suspects in the Foundation's pamphlet on *Arthritis Unproven Remedies* names acupuncture, spas, diets, vibrators, and topical creams, among others. This means that every time you purchase **Aspercreme** or **Myoflex**, you are flirting with quackery, because the preparations are home remedies that haven't been proven effective for arthritis in scientific studies.

You know full well, however, if you follow news of arthritis research, that one decade's quack cure may turn out to be the next decade's orthodox treatment. As we saw in Chapter 5, gold was first used for rheumatoid arthritis in the 1920s, proved to be effective, but was then rejected for many years because its use smacked of alchemy and mysticism. Pragmatism brought it back, however, and it is now a cornerstone of conventional care.

Sometimes the lines separating the orthodox from the unorthodox are thinly drawn, further confusing the meaning of quackery. For example, during the time that snake and bee venom were both denounced as suspicious hokum in the United States, a purified form of the venom from Bolivian stinging ants was under serious investigation by respected rheumatologists. And now, although snake venom is still considered a harmful way to gamble with arthritis, bee venom is coming under legitimate study.

Similarly, while most doctors frown on cod liver oil, many look favorably upon the capsules of fish oil containing omega-3 fatty acids. (See Chapter 11.)

The most useful definition of quackery hinges on the spirit in which a treatment is offered and the attitude with which it is tried. Anything that *promises* a cure is suspect, and anyone who ignores medical treatment while embracing such promises is asking for trouble; however, that leaves a lot of room for personal experimentation with a variety of products and plans that not only do no harm but may do a lot of good. A change in diet that actually improves the way you eat is a prime example. (See Chapters 13 and 14.)

Why I Decided (Not) to Try It

Participants' attitudes on quackery vary widely, from the few who are ever willing to try something new to the majority who reject unproven remedies out of hand.

"I've tried every concoction friends would tell me about," writes an Oregon woman disabled by rheumatoid arthritis, "from honey, vinegar, and iodine to gin-soaked raisins, with no results. The copper bracelet didn't help. The DMSO didn't

help either, and it makes you stink. But when you have RA—
and the pain and the emotional and physical problems it
causes—you're willing to try anything to be the old you again."

"Arthritis is enough of a problem without becoming a
guinea pig for quack medicine," says an adult-education instructor from New Mexico. "Take nothing unless it's approved
by the *New England Journal of Medicine.* If a cure is found,
I'll know it by the six-inch headlines in my daily newspaper."

The Most Popular Unproven Remedies

Copper bracelets

More people in our survey tried wearing a copper bracelet
than any other unorthodox or folk remedy. (Indeed, more people had experience with copper bracelets than with several of
the orthodox therapies, including gold salts and surgery.) A few
participants wore copper rings, too, copper earrings, or even
a copper insole in their shoes. But it was mostly for naught.
"The copper bracelet did nothing," reports an audiologist
from Indiana. "I also wore a copper insole in one shoe for one
day, and it was the worst day I'd had in months. On top of that,
it gave me a metallic taste in my mouth and caused a run in
my nylons." Rating copper bracelets on the basis of our participants' reports shows the jewelry to have *less* than a placebo
effect.

The term *placebo effect* comes from clinical research in
medicine. To test the value of a new drug, for example, doctors
gather a group of volunteers who have the illness the drug is
supposed to treat. Then they give the new treatment to half
the volunteers, while the other half get a placebo, or sugar
pill—something that's really nothing but that looks and tastes
just like the actual treatment. If the real drug is effective, then
the people getting it should improve, and the people getting
the placebo should feel no different from before. But a strange
thing happens in these studies, as years of research have revealed. That is, some number of volunteers taking the placebo
begin to feel better for reasons no one can explain. This is the
placebo effect. It is probably a mixture of hope, faith, and good

fortune. Thus, the bottom line in drug studies is that the new drug, to prove itself, must get whopping-good results compared to the placebo.

Even in studies where a new drug is *not* compared to a placebo, there can still be a placebo effect. That is, some number of people taking the drug may feel better by virtue of the placebo effect and not because the drug is really helping them. Scientists expect this to happen to as many as one-third of the volunteers involved.

In our survey, copper bracelets proved more useless than a sugar pill. We might have expected them to work by placebo effect alone for about 70 of the 211 participants who wore them. As it turned out, however, only 31 got any kind of help at all, whether it was pain relief or a boost for their morale. As they report, our participants were more likely to find that their skin had turned green or black than to notice any improvement in the way their joints felt.

Number of participants trying **copper jewelry**	211	
Outcome:		
"It helped."	13	(6%)
"It may help."	14	(7%)
"It helped my morale."	4	(2%)
"It did nothing."	180	(85%)
Most frequently mentioned side effects:		
"It turned my skin green [or black]."	34	(16%)
"It made me feel I'd wasted my money."	33	(16%)

Although the bracelets do no good, they do no real harm either. "I once got a copper bracelet for kicks," says a freelance writer from New York, "and kicks are all I got! It was an interesting piece of jewelry in which I invested a few bucks."

"I've used a copper bracelet for sentimental reasons," reports a childcare giver from South Dakota. "My pretty grandma always wore one. She was hopelessly handicapped with arthritis, however, and her hands were useless claws by her sixties, so I can't say I have much faith in the copper."

"Copper bracelets are really neat," quips a novelist from Florida. "They turn your arms green! They jingle and get caught on things, too. I wore them on each wrist for approximately two months, with no relief."

"Sure I've tried copper bracelets," writes an Arthritis Foundation Self-Help Course instructor from Indiana. "But other than 'psychological relief,' you only get green wrists. There's no harm in them, so if they make you 'feel better,' then it might be worth having green wrists!"

DMSO

DMSO (dimethyl sulfoxide) had its heyday in the 1960s and 1970s, when it was called an unproven remedy in the best sense of the term—that is, an experimental treatment under clinical investigation for a variety of problems ranging from athletic injuries to rheumatoid arthritis. After an exhaustive review of this research, however, a special committee of the National Academy of Sciences declared DMSO too iffy and too risky to become a prescription drug. The FDA has since *approved* it for treating the symptoms of one particular illness—a rare bladder disease called interstitial cystitis. But as far as arthritis is concerned, DMSO is considered more unproven than ever.

Prescription DMSO for cystitis is manufactured by Research Industries Corporation of Utah, and is sold under the name **Rimso-50.** It is a 50-percent solution, prepared to be instilled directly into the bladder. Most DMSO available in the United States is less pure and more strong, though, meant to be used either as a solvent (99-percent solution) or for veterinary treatment (90-percent gel) of bruises, sprains, and other ills that befall horses and dogs. That doesn't stop people from trying to see if it works to relieve arthritis pain though. About half of our survey participants who used it found that it did help, albeit temporarily.

Number of participants who tried **DMSO**	47	
Outcome:		
"It helped."	23	(49%)
"It did nothing."	24	(51%)
Most frequently mentioned side effects:		
Garlic/onion breath	7	(15%)

DMSO is colorless and odorless by itself, but once applied, it may make your breath reek within a few minutes, and the smell may persist for hours. A magazine editor from New Jersey said it made her smell like "ripe pizza," while several other participants complained of a strong garlic taste after use, or "onion breath." The odor foils the best efforts of researchers, since no placebo gives quite the characteristic flavor of real DMSO. Some studies have been done by giving DMSO to all of the volunteers and then tallying up the number who improve. But the results have not been convincing.

Our results are not convincing, either. At 49-percent effectiveness, DMSO certainly does *not* outperform standard arthritis treatments. For comparison, most of the prescription anti-inflammatory drugs help 60 to 80 percent of those taking them. (See Chapter 5.) We cannot recommend the use of DMSO, but if you are determined to test it on yourself anyway, please consider these warnings and tips from our survey participants.

- Try to find DMSO that has been formulated for human or veterinary use, and not as a commercial solvent, so as to avoid impurities.

- DMSO can cause skin rash. Researchers say that a 70-percent solution of DMSO (with 30 percent water) is the best compromise between effectiveness and irritation. People with fair complexions, however, may not be able to tolerate more than a 50-percent solution.

- Because DMSO carries anything *on* your skin *into* your bloodstream, make sure your hands and the area to be treated are very clean.

- The threat of DMSO is to the lens of the eye, although real damage has been shown only in animal tests. Even if you never touch the solution to your eyes, it may wind up there, and the long-term effects are unknown.

- Beware of foreign clinics offering DMSO injections, as some of these have been found to mix steroids and other drugs with the DMSO, and to give shots without medical supervision.*

Remember that even DMSO's most ardent promoters, including Dr. Stanley Jacob, who did the pioneering research at the University of Oregon Medical School in Portland, do not claim that DMSO is a cure for arthritis. At best, it can reduce pain and increase mobility for some people, but it does not affect the course of the disease. Nor can anyone explain how it works to achieve its good effects. In the authorized account of his work, *DMSO: The True Story of a Remarkable Pain-Killing Drug* by Barry Tarshis, Dr. Jacob said, "We've found that DMSO works better for arthritis above the waist than below the waist, and found that the most resistant part of the body to DMSO treatment is the hip." (More than one-third of our participants had arthritis in at least one hip, and well over half said their knees were affected.)

One of our participants, a fifty-six-year-old Oregon homemaker with osteoarthritis, received periodic DMSO injections from Dr. Jacob several years ago as part of an experiment. "The shots really helped me," she recalls. "I would limp in, and then be able to drive home myself. One shot lasted a couple of months, while the rub-on helped me only temporarily."

Honey (and apple-cider vinegar, too)

Is honey just a more natural sweetener than table sugar, or does it have healing powers? The results of our survey show that the "effectiveness" of honey as a remedy is about the same as any other sugar pill.

---

*"Three days of an IV in a clinic in Mexico gave miraculous results," writes a retired aerospace engineer from California, "but within six months I had a massive hemorrhage in the abdominal cavity that put me very close to death."

Number of participants who used **honey***   20
Outcome:

"It helped."	7	(35%)
"It did nothing."	6	(30%)
No comment	7	(35%)

*Most of these used honey alone, but six participants combined it with vinegar, and one with willow tea.

"I had an herbalist girlfriend who used to give me willow tea with honey," writes an electronics technician from California. "This does work for a short time, but beware of overdoing it, as too much upsets the tummy." It's quite possible that both the relief and the stomach upset this man experienced had more to do with the willow tea than the honey. Thousands of years before aspirin was created, physicians advised people in pain to chew willow bark for the aspirinlike painkiller it contains.

"We raise our own honey," says a cook/bartender from upstate New York, "and I eat the yellow edge from the comb. It doesn't help."

The popularity of honey with cider vinegar, such as it is, can probably be traced to Dr. D. C. Jarvis's 1960 book titled *Arthritis and Folk Medicine,* in which he aimed to distill some two hundred years of homey Vermont health wisdom into a program of arthritis self-care. That program consisted largely of two teaspoons of apple-cider vinegar and two teaspoons of honey dissolved in a glass of water—or sometimes just the honey, dissolved in a glass of apple juice and sipped like coffee with meals. The advice seems easy to follow, its philosophy is appealingly natural, and Dr. Jarvis himself comes across as an earnest character of great goodwill. Unfortunately, the plan didn't work out for most of our participants who tried it. "I have taken apple-cider vinegar with honey for eight years," writes a retired postal clerk from Georgia, "with no knowledge of any benefit or any harm."

In all, sixteen participants said they had used cider vinegar, either alone or with honey. Most found it unremarkable, such as this retired carpenter from Ohio: "I started drinking Dr. Jarvis's apple-cider vinegar three months ago, and the pains have not gotten worse." An Illinois businessman had a little more luck: "Honey and cider vinegar with water did nothing for the arthritis, but my ulcer got better." The best report comes from a sixty-six-year-old Ohio homemaker who has had arthritis for three years: "I dissolve one-third of a cup of vinegar and one-third of a cup of honey in two quarts of water, and take one glass daily. It seems to work for me. Since I've been drinking this, I've been able to stop taking **Feldene**, which I used successfully for two and one-half years."

Bee venom

Once we dismiss honey, there is still the other end of the bee to consider—the stinging part. It turns out to be sweeter than the honey for several of our participants who found relief in this unusual therapy. "Bee venom cured the crippling arthritis in my toe joint immediately and completely," says a computer consultant from New Jersey. "My husband and I caught a few bees in a mayonnaise jar and shook them gently till they were dizzy and vulnerable. Then we used long tweezers to hold them around the middle and place them within the circle I had drawn in Magic Marker to show the area of pain on my foot. Bingo!"

At least three of the individuals who found relief with bee venom were not seeking therapy at all, but were stung accidentally. "I raise bees," explains a millwright and welder from Maine, "and find that their sting on a hand or arm does seem to help, but I have not tried this on purpose." Another bee-keeper, however, who is a Missouri dairy farmer, writes, "I have received bee stings, of course, but couldn't see that it made any difference in my arthritis."

According to Charles Mraz of Middlebury, Vermont, who has provided free treatments with live bee stings for more than fifty years to the many people with arthritis who visit his home, getting stung accidentally is *not* therapy. Mr. Mraz says that he must sometimes administer as many as two to three *thousand* stings over the course of a year or longer to achieve the desired result.

A few participants got their bee venom from the sting of a hypodermic needle in a doctor's office. One, a retired public school principal from Philadelphia, took shots first in London in the 1930s, and in 1941 from one of the leading American proponents of bee venom for arthritis, the late Dr. Joseph Broadman. "I had to go to New York two to three times a week for several months while Dr. Broadman gave me the injection series," she recalls, "but I never had to return after that. While in his office, I saw people unable to walk across the room, who were walking on their own two weeks later."

Number of participants who tried **bee venom**	23	
Outcome:		
Effective, sometimes dramatically so	11	(48%)
Ineffective	11	(48%)
Made participant feel worse	1	(4%)

Even those participants who seek out bee stings, however, warn of the dangers of allergic reaction and anaphylactic shock. This complication is rare, but it can be fatal, making the treatment entirely too risky for some people. "I had no idea of my allergy to insect venom," writes an air force officer from North Carolina, "until four years ago when I was stung by a yellow jacket and had to be rushed to the hospital emergency room for treatment."

Vitamin therapy

Some people consider vitamins a boon to nutrition and others use them like medicine. In our survey group, more than 70 percent of the participants take some kind of dietary supplement (usually a one-a-day-type multiple vitamin pill) as "insurance," many say, that they're getting all the necessary nutrients. But at least 4 percent take a vitamin, or mineral, or combination product, such as cod liver oil, for its purported benefit in treating their arthritis.

Number of participants using **vitamin therapy**	41	
Outcome:		
Found it helpful	20	(49%)
Found it of no help	14	(34%)
No comment	7	(17%)

Unfortunately, we can't evaluate the individual vitamins here on the basis of these few reports. (See Chapter 15 for a full discussion of the reputed and relative merits of various vitamins for people with arthritis, from ascorbic acid [vitamin C] to zinc.)

Motor oil and more

The brevity of this chapter and the small number of treatments that found even twenty tryers is, again, a testimonial to the caution and good sense exercised by our participants. Based on the research we did before conducting the survey, we had expected to write a much lengthier chapter on quackery, including such exotica as fetal lamb-cell injections and extract of the New Zealand green-lipped mussel—two of the treatments tried by world-famous heart surgeon Dr. Christiaan Barnard and described in his *Program for Living with Arthritis.*

There is nothing laughable or shameful in a person's trying an unproven approach, although there may be danger, or frustration, or both. Sometimes the cost of an unorthodox treatment is so high as to effectively limit the number of people who can try it. For example, Dr. Barnard had to travel to a private clinic in Switzerland for his lamb shots. On the other hand, the cost of conventional medical care may sometimes drive people to seek a cheaper alternative. "My husband died three years ago," writes a housewife from Michigan, "and my insurance was dropped. I had been seeing a rheumatologist and was doing well on **Plaquenil**, but in these past three years I've not been to the doctor or had a prescription filled. I take honey and use **Ben·Gay** and aspirin. I've not had a bad flare-up, but the pain is still there."

For whatever reason, eight of our participants tried to

loosen up their joints with a squirt of a lubricant called WD-40. "In my line of work," says an auto mechanic from Tennessee, "I deal with lots of silicones, and I've used WD-40 for several years. This stuff really works when sprayed on an inflamed joint. Please don't think I'm too silly." The problem is that for each participant who liked the effect of WD-40, another found it useless or worse: "The cold of the spray caused extreme pain," reports the owner of a gift shop in North Dakota, "to say nothing of the smell."

The rest of the survey reports on unproven techniques—including magnets, electricity, turpentine, and uranium rocks—are anecdotes, not supported by enough people's experience to be anything more than interesting stories. Perhaps the most interesting one of all comes from a sixty-five-year-old New York housewife who had to stop gold injections because of a toxic reaction.

"After my gold injections were stopped in 1979, my arthritis got worse, so I answered a newspaper ad which claimed that rheumatoid arthritis could be cured through a 'biotherapeutic neutral-infection absorption' method. This consisted of making a hole in the calf of my leg and inserting a dry chick pea in the hole. Over a period of ten to twelve hours, harmful elements were supposed to drain and be absorbed by the chick pea, and the blood would gradually be cleansed. I was told that in a period of four to six months I would feel improvement and have less pain and stiffness, starting from my shoulders, down my arms, and then my knees and feet last.

"I asked many questions about the risk of infection, blood poisoning, and other unforeseen dangers. I told my rheumatologist about this, and he said it sounded like a fraud and quackery. But he did say there was a new experimental procedure called plasmapheresis, in which a blood protein is removed by machine. To me, the principle sounded similar.

"I started the chick pea treatment in April 1980, while still having regular visits with my rheumatologist. At the end of five days, I felt definite improvement in my shoulders and arms. I found I could carry dinner dishes from the table to the sink with no pain, and wipe the table clean. I continued this treatment for four and a half months, with continuing improvement.

"Then, in August, my gynecologist sent me to the hospital to have a uterine polyp removed. When he discovered the bandage on my leg and learned what it was, he exploded. Didn't I know that this was a medieval practice, and that I was very foolish to use it? He ordered the treatment stopped, had the chick pea removed, and took cultures of the drainage hole. They came back positive for both strep and staph infections. When I left the hospital, I did not wish to risk infection again, so I did not restart the treatment.

"As for the cost—that was limited to the bag of chick peas and a few other supplies, including a bottle or so of hydrogen peroxide. The man who treated me for four and a half months, coming to my home each time, receiving my phone calls, etc., charged me absolutely nothing. Not one penny changed hands. When I would ask him what his fee was, he would say only, 'Don't think about it. Just get well!' "

Summary of Popular Unproven Treatments

Copper jewelry—less than a "placebo effect"
DMSO—of some use to about half those who tried it
Vitamin therapy—helpful to about half its adherents
Honey—no better than a sugar pill
Bee venom—tempting but dangerous

10

THREE WIDELY USED UNCONVENTIONAL TREATMENTS FOR ARTHRITIS:
What Is Their Value?

■ Manipulation ■ Acupuncture ■ Yoga

Somewhere between the mainstream treatments and the fringe therapies lies a large gray area of popular but unconventional approaches to arthritis care. These techniques include manipulation, acupuncture, and Yoga, all of which have a long history and a large following. Indeed, manipulation is the mainstay of chiropractic care, which is the second-largest health-care system in the country. (Allopathic, or medical, is the biggest.) Manipulation is also an important tool in the practice of osteopathy, the third-largest system of health care. Acupuncture and Yoga, both foreign imports, have stood time's test, worldwide, over *hundreds* of centuries. Nevertheless, many people continue to look askance at these unconventional treatments because of their "unscientific" philosophies.

The Arthritis Foundation pretty much pooh-poohs all

three of them. In its brochure *Arthritis Unproven Remedies,* the Foundation relegates acupuncture to a list of harmless but unproven remedies, including copper bracelets and uranium mines. Chiropractic care, which figured on the Foundation's "suspicious" list for years, has been dropped from the latest edition of the brochure.

The Foundation-written book *Understanding Arthritis* (Scribner's, 1984) makes no mention of manipulation, even in a negative way, nor does it mention chiropractic care or osteopathy. Yoga isn't mentioned, either. As for acupuncture, it is dismissed in a single sentence as being temporary, expensive, and of no real benefit.

Several hundred of our 1,051 Arthritis Survey participants ventured down at least one of these alternate avenues, however, and many *found* the help they were looking for. Others were disappointed, and a few were actually injured. In this chapter, you can share their experiences with manipulation maneuvers, with acupuncture needles, and with Yoga positions—and discover their relative risks and benefits. You may be surprised to learn, for example, that acupuncture is *safer* than manipulation, in spite of the needles, and that Yoga is one of the most helpful approaches available.

Manipulation

Hands-on healing that sometimes gets rough

Chiropractors cite 1895 as the year their profession was officially introduced to the world. They created their "natural method of health care" in reaction to what they saw as an overuse of drug treatments by medical doctors of the day, and an overemphasis on *curing diseases,* as opposed to *maintaining health.* The name *chiropractic* comes from the Greek word for hand, and the hand of the practitioner is the primary healing instrument. The hand manipulates and adjusts errant vertebrae in the patient's spine, removing unwanted pressure on the nerves and thus restoring normal "nerve supply" to keep all parts of the body functioning at peak performance.

Osteopathic physicians practice manipulation, too, but

they use the technique more sparingly since they receive the full range of training that medical doctors do and can prescribe medications and perform surgery. In a few cases, our survey participants received manipulation treatments from a physical therapist or a nurse. The manipulation techniques vary widely from one practitioner's hands to another's.

"The chiropractor worked on me while I lay face down on his table," writes a retired printer from Illinois. "The osteopath manipulated my spine while I lay face up, and he put his hands *under* my back. I found I got more lasting results that way." A homemaker from Florida notes, "The chiropractor helped to relieve pain with a new method of using pressure points instead of pushing on my body."

No matter how it was performed, manipulation provided at least temporary relief for more than half of our survey participants who tried it. "I went to a chiropractor when my back was so bad that I could not straighten up," says a housewife from North Carolina with arthritis in her back, knees, wrists, and feet. "He used a sound-wave treatment, applied heat and ice, and manipulated my back—and I walked out of his office standing straight."

Number of participants who tried **manipulation**	190	
Outcome:		
Temporary or lasting relief	116	(61%)
No relief (ineffective)	22	(12%)
Made participant feel worse	22	(12%)
No rating (too soon to tell)	30	(15%)

Despite all the good reports, we endorse this technique with *caution,* since the "Made participant feel worse" rate was higher for manipulation than for most other types of hands-on treatments, *including* surgical procedures. As noted above, the rate was 12 percent for manipulation, compared to 6 percent for acupuncture, 5 percent for physical therapy, 4 percent for massage, and 2 percent for all types of joint reconstruction and replacement combined. Only traction, at 22 percent, caused relatively more misery. The reasons our survey participants give for feeling worse after manipulation include one broken bone and episodes of increased pain that lasted for weeks or months in some cases.

Most of the participants who benefit from manipulation note that they have to go for regular treatments to keep up the improvement. "Spinal manipulation has helped a great deal in allowing me to keep my mobility," says an amateur musician from Michigan. "I see the chiropractor three times a week. If I miss a treatment, I start having difficulty walking." A retired engineer from New York reports, "Manipulation helps me get through the acute attacks of shoulder pain I suffer every one to three months, but it does not prevent the *next* acute attack."

Acupuncture

Ancient medicine, still practiced and still promising

The origins of acupuncture are buried in myth and mystery going back thousands of years, at least to the time of China's Yellow Emperor in the fifth century B.C. One often-told story is that acupuncture was discovered accidentally in battle, when warriors pierced by arrows felt a sudden release from long-standing pain or illness. But no one can verify the story, *or* explain how that chance observation got translated into a complex philosophy of medicine, based on universal harmony, with a whole new view of anatomy. For acupuncture goes beyond the body as Western science knows it. East and West both see the musculoskeletal system, the digestive system, as well as the reproductive, respiratory, and circulatory systems. Acupuncture *also* recognizes a grand independent network of channels called "meridians" that unite all those other systems, and unite mind with body, too. A vital energy courses through these meridians, acupuncturists say, and they can tap into it by stimulating one or more of the 360 distinct acupuncture points charted along the meridian pathways. Inserting needles into these precise points restores energy imbalances, breaks up energy blockages, and charges the body to heal itself.

Even before acupuncture followed President Richard Nixon home from China in the early 1970s, modern medical scientists began trying to explain *how* it works, in their terms, because they simply couldn't live with the concept of "vital energy" moving inside *invisible* anatomic structures.* Electricity makes more sense to them, since the nerves are known to carry electrical impulses, and acupuncture points lie near peripheral nerve endings. Based on their experiments with animals, they suggest that acupuncture electrifies the nerve endings, which then signal the brain and spinal cord to release their own internal pain-blockers and painkillers. Other chemicals that may shower into the bloodstream in reaction to acupuncture are the body's own *anti-inflammatory* agents, and this may further explain why acupuncture sometimes helps people with arthritis.

"I was treated in a hospital by a Korean acupuncturist who was also an M.D.," writes a forty-four-year-old bookkeeper from upstate New York. (She kept up her orthodox treatments, too, which have included **Indocin**, prednisone, gold shots, **Ridaura**, and penicillamine.) "He told me right up front that he could *not* cure my rheumatoid arthritis, but he felt he could help relieve pain. At the time, I was in excruciating pain, and had been for quite a while. So I tried it, and it did indeed help. I went from barely being able to get out of a chair alone—or walk, or use my hands—to feeling enough relief to begin a careful joint-exercise program that helped me become more flexible."

Number of participants who tried **acupuncture**	104	
Outcome:		
Temporary or lasting relief	39	(37%)
No relief (ineffective)	36	(35%)
Made participant feel worse	6	(6%)
No rating (too soon to tell)	23	(22%)

*The ancient Chinese, it is said, did not dissect human bodies, and no modern-day autopsy or surgical procedure has ever revealed any sign of the meridians. The only evidence for their existence comes from French scientists who spent ten years injecting radioactive tracers into the acupuncture points of human volunteers and following the tracers' migrations through the body with detectors called "gamma cameras." Their slides, presented at the World Research Foundation's Congress of Bio-Energetic Medicine in Sherman Oaks, California, in 1986, showed the tracers aligned along the classical acupuncture meridians.

These are not encouraging statistics. In fact, the 37-percent relief rate looks like nothing more than the one-third improvement we might expect from the placebo effect (the good feeling one gets from a treatment one *thinks* is helping). But the ho-hum success rate changes dramatically when we look at what happened to those participants who got acupuncture treatments from bona fide acupuncturists, and not from a chiropractor or an M.D. who was dabbling with the technique.

Number of **acupuncturists** (M.D. or non-M.D.)	37	
Outcome:		
Gave temporary or lasting relief	27	(73%)
Gave no relief (ineffective)	8	(22%)
Made participant feel worse	2	(5%)

If you are going to try acupuncture, then look for a well-versed practitioner. (See Chapter 4 for more information about acupuncturists.)

"When I started seeing the acupuncturist," recalls a sixty-six-year-old retired inventor from Washington, "I couldn't drive, and my wife had to take me to and from his office. After about two months of receiving treatments three times a week, I was doing all the driving on the seventy-mile round trip. I continued taking acupuncture treatments for three years, and it helped a great deal." Aside from the pain relief, he noticed one other benefit: "Soon after I was stricken with rheumatoid arthritis in 1966, I had a terrible flare-up, and couldn't even stand to be touched because I felt like I was being skinned alive. My doctor put me in the hospital and shot me full of cortisone and painkillers for a *month*. The cortisone made my skin as thin as wet tissue paper, with about as much strength, and for years I continued to get sores that took up to twelve months to heal. But after three years of acupuncture, my skin cleared up and my sores healed."

For reasons they cannot explain, some of our participants who enjoy acupuncture find that it helps some joints but not others. "Acupuncture helped my back pain and related leg pain tremendously," reports a fifty-year-old executive secretary from South Carolina, "but I've relied on physical therapy and exercise for my hands, shoulders, and elbows." A thirty-nine-year-old company vice-president from Minnesota tells a similar story: "Physical therapy helps my hands, wrists, shoulders, and knees, but the arthritis in the ball of my foot went away completely with acupuncture." The sixty-two-year-old owner of a yarn shop in Massachusetts says: "Acupuncture was great for my shoulders but didn't do any good for my hands or feet."

The risk of acupuncture is minor. If the needles are sterile,* there is scant possibility of infection, and there are no other known physical side effects. Although six of our participants noted that they felt worse after acupuncture, no one complained of any injury to the joints. For example, a retired machinist from California recalls, "Acupuncture sometimes helped a lot. At other times, I felt worse, but I was never injured."

A few participants did complain about the cost of the treatment, though. "Acupuncture helped for about three or four days after my weekly treatment," writes a forty-six-year-old legal assistant from Oregon, "but I couldn't justify the expense for only a little relief." A fifty-eight-year-old seamstress from Minnesota observes, "Acupuncture helps the most to relieve pain, but I can't afford it often enough." (However, a proportionately larger percentage of participants complained about the cost of prescription drugs.)

Traditional acupuncture is practiced with very fine needles, which may be inserted in places fairly far removed from your painful parts. The acupuncturist may then twirl the needles in place, for added effect, or burn moxa (an herb) in a small cup atop the needle. Some practitioners prefer to attach electrodes to the needles and turn on the juice. Modern acupuncture can even be performed by beaming laser light on the acupuncture points instead of needling them. Another needleless variation, called acupressure, or Shiatsu, substitutes fingertips for the fine needles. The practitioner prods the spot, or spots, or shows you where they are so you can treat yourself. "Acupressure made some difference!" says a heavy-equipment

---

*Check to see that the acupuncturist sterilizes the needles before each use, or uses disposable needles for each patient.

operator from Washington state. "Because it's basically pressure on various nerves, you can do it yourself. I get seven to eight hours of reduced pain this way."

Yoga

A way of exercise, a way of life

Yoga is the living heritage of ancient India. Its philosophy may seem mystical and remote, based as it is on a belief in the unity of all that is. The same energy, or consciousness, exists everywhere and unites everything with everyone. Mind and body, especially, are united. Indeed the word *Yoga* means unity.

But many of the Yoga *postures,* or *positions,* which students of Yoga use to attain relaxation and open themselves to the flow of universal energy, also have a very mundane aspect. They stretch and strengthen the muscles. And they may look *exactly* like the range of motion exercises you received from your doctor or physical therapist. The names have been changed, naturally, from Sanskrit images to modern descriptions. And the movements prescribed for people with arthritis stop far short of the goals in some Yoga texts, which leave you marveling at the way a man can sit with his legs crossed in front of him and his arms crossed in back of him, holding his toes in his fingers! Several of the exercises based on our survey participants' advice (see Chapter 19), such as the Head Roll, for example, have their counterparts in *simple* Yoga movements.

"I do light Hatha Yoga for the lower spinal pain," writes an electrician from Florida. "I feel it really lessens the pain, as long as I am gentle and very, very self-aware. I never do forceful, stressful exercise." Yoga differs substantially from most aerobic exercises in this regard. The emphasis is on slow motions, awareness of your own physical limits, relaxation, and deep and even breathing. There's no bouncing, no panting, no thought of any given number of repetitions of a movement. Still, injuries can and do occur.

"I tried a few Yoga postures that were too advanced," concedes a secretary from California, "and pushed my body too far. I overdid, causing a lot of pain." Usually, novices do better learning Yoga from an instructor instead of a book, so they can have expert guidance on safe positions, but this participant was taking instruction when she was injured. Not all teachers, unfortunately, have the ability to work with people in pain. If you decide to try Yoga, explain your condition to the instructor and find out how much experience he or she has in teaching people with arthritis. An anatomy professor from Missouri recommends, "Find a good Yoga instructor who is easygoing and is not primarily gung ho for Hinduism."

"I stumbled into a course in Hatha Yoga to fulfill a physical-education requirement when I went back to school to finish college," reports a sixty-one-year-old freelance writer from Ohio. "I took it for three years, from 1974 to 1977, then kept it up by following Yoga programs on television, and I enjoyed a total remission of my arthritis that lasted until 1986. The experience with Hatha Yoga carries over into all my everyday activities, which I do at my *own* easy, comfortable pace. I also find I get relief from using good posture, whether I'm standing, sitting, or lying down."

Number of participants who tried **Yoga**	41	
Outcome:		
Temporary or lasting relief	36	(88%)
No relief (ineffective)	2	(5%)
Made participant feel worse	3	(7%)

We are concentrating here on Yoga as a form of *exercise,* but it has other benefits for some participants. "I do believe that Yoga has been *extremely* beneficial for me," writes a childcare worker from South Dakota who began taking Yoga instruction twenty years ago when she lived in a big city. "I have seven sisters, but I am the only Yoga practitioner in my family. At forty-five, I'm third from the oldest, but more limber than all but the 'baby' of thirty. If nothing else, daily Yoga keeps one *thinking* healthy and spry."

Summary of Unconventional Treatments

Manipulation—Is a technique for adjusting the spine so as to remove pressure from the spinal nerves, and thereby maintain health.

Is practiced most often by chiropractors and osteopaths.

Is performed in different styles by different practitioners.

Provides at least temporary relief for about 60 percent of those who try it, according to our survey statistics.

Carries a relatively high risk of injury.

Needs to be repeated frequently to maintain its effect.

Acupuncture—Is a technique for correcting *energy imbalances* or *blockages* in the body by inserting fine needles along the energy pathways.

May bring relief by stimulating the brain and spinal cord to release the body's own internal painkillers.

Provides relief to nearly 40 percent of those who try it, according to our survey findings.

Is more effective when practiced by well-trained acupuncturists, whether or not they are M.D.s.

May bring more relief to one joint than another.

Carries a negligible risk of injury.

Yoga—Is an ancient philosophy of life that includes beneficial exercises.

Differs from aerobic exercises in pace, goal, and physiological effects.

Provides temporary or lasting relief to 88 percent of those who try it, based on our survey participants' experiences.

Carries a risk for those who attempt advanced positions too soon.

11

EXPERIMENTAL TREATMENTS:
Which Ones Hold Real Promise?

■ New uses for existing drugs ■ New anti-in-flammatory agents ■ Animals, plants, and oils that are the natural enemies of arthritis ■ Healing rays ■ Copying the body's own weapons

Not all of the unorthodox, unusual treatments for arthritis are dispensed by charlatans and faddists. Some of them are available only at the most well-established hospitals, from the most highly regarded physicians. These are the therapies at the forefront of medical science—treatments so new that the individuals receiving them are not only patients but human subjects in experimental research. A few of the approaches covered in this chapter have not even reached the stage of development where they can be tried on people, but they have shown their promising effects in treating the painful inflamed paws of laboratory mice.

The world of experimental medicine is a world of hope and daring. Doctors and researchers, frustrated by the relentless course of arthritis, turn to ever-more-potent weapons to conquer it, up to and including anticancer drugs and radiation therapy for rheumatoid arthritis, as you will read in this chapter. Sometimes, the new treatments they explore sound strangely similar to the "quack" remedies they deplore. A tablespoon of cod liver oil as arthritis care, for example, is just another old wives' tale, as far as rheumatologists are concerned, but a handful of fish-oil capsules is serious experimental therapy. Arthritis–fish-oil studies are going on today at hospitals affiliated with prestigious universities, including Harvard Medical School, and are backed by money from the National Institutes of Health.

People like you, who scan the pages of books such as this for some new hope of help, play a tremendous role in medical research. You are the ones doctors turn to, to put their ideas to the test. If you were invited to join a study—to try some new drug cooked up in the laboratory or dredged up from the ocean floor—what would you say? Would you jump at the chance? Or would the fear of unknown consequences make you stick with the standard treatment? There is no right or wrong answer on the horns of this dilemma. But more than 70 of the 1,051 participants in our nationwide Arthritis Survey, faced with the choice, opted to serve in the interest of science, in the hope of improving their own lives. For most of them, as you will see, the risk was well worth taking.

Clinical trials, as these human studies are called, are secretive affairs. Every aspect of them involves one secret or another. When you volunteer to participate, you don't know whether you'll actually get the new therapy being tested or some pretend therapy that looks or feels just like it. That's kept secret from you until the experiment is over. The doctors who actually examine you along the way likewise have no idea which treatment you're getting. It's kept secret from them, too, lest their hopes and expectations color their opinion of your progress.

The secrets come out at the end. Then the code that tells who got what is broken, and the researchers tell the world their results by writing an article for a scientific journal.

If you want to take part in a clinical trial, you practically have to fall into one. Their very existence is a kind of secret, because there's no organized way for you or your doctor to find out who is testing what, where, when, why, on whom, and with how much success. There is no central clearing house for such information—not for arthritis, anyway, although the National Cancer Institute keeps tabs on most trials regarding cancer or

AIDS. What usually happens is that an individual researcher at some institution gets an idea or makes a discovery, then has to get money to study the idea, and then looks around locally for volunteers to participate in a trial. For you, as the would-be participant, it's a matter of being in the right place at the right time. For each topic covered here, we'll give you the name of a clinic or researcher who may be willing to provide more information if your doctor requests it. As a rule, however, researchers working with promising new treatments are beseiged with so many phone calls and letters that they cannot possibly answer them all *and* continue their research.

Once word of an experiment gets out in the pages of the medical literature, however, other doctors are free to use the treatment—if it is available—for selected patients. This is precisely what happened with methotrexate.* A number of our survey participants were taking this technically experimental treatment on their doctors' orders, even though they were not taking part in any formal research project. Not a new substance, methotrexate was originally approved by the Food and Drug Administration as an anticancer drug. Later, it won approval for treating severe disabling psoriasis. But it was still considered experimental for rheumatoid arthritis when we undertook our survey. The Food and Drug Administration has only recently approved the use of methotrexate for rheumatoid arthritis, and Lederle launched a newly packaged, newly named version of the drug, called **Rheumatrex**, in January of 1989.

Methotrexate

From cancer to arthritis with good results

Methotrexate was developed for leukemia therapy in the 1940s, and a report of the first attempt to pit it against rheumatoid arthritis appeared in 1951—more than thirty-five years ago. It has taken all this time for other studies to prove the

*Methotrexate is marketed as **Methotrexate** (pills and solution) and as **Rheumatrex** (pills) by Lederle. Bristol-Meyers markets two injectable solutions, called **Mexate** and **Mexate-AQ**.

claims of that first report. Methotrexate was considered an experimental treatment for rheumatoid arthritis until very recently. Practitioners worried about its severe and potentially lethal side effects (more about these later), which become a tremendous concern for people with arthritis, who, unlike cancer patients, may take the medication for a long, long time.

Within the last ten years, in fact, as more and more rheumatologists have tried methotrexate on patients with the most destructive cases of rheumatoid arthritis, the drug has proved to be safer than they expected. The dread toxic reactions have not shown up as frequently or as severely as had been feared. This is probably because the dosage level used for arthritis is so much lower than the dosages required for cancer chemotherapy—about 1/100 of the amount. What's more, some new studies indicate that methotrexate can be used in even smaller doses if it is combined with another similar drug called azathioprine. The combination approach may not only decrease the dangers of methotrexate, but appears to boost its effectiveness even higher. Still, some experts say that it may take another ten or perhaps twenty years to gather conclusive proof that methotrexate can be used safely over a prolonged period of time.

Methotrexate is by all means a *long-term* treatment. It seems to perform a miracle within the first month or two of use for many people with arthritis, relieving even the most intractable pain and all but eliminating stiffness. A good number of these individuals keep on improving steadily as they continue the treatment over successive months, and they may stay on it for years. Withdraw the drug, however, as doctors have done in studies, and all signs of improvement vanish in a blazing flare-up within a few weeks. At Albany (NY) Medical College, five patients stopped receiving methotrexate in 1987 after three years of steady use. As a group, they suddenly had more than twice as many painful joints as they'd had while taking methotrexate, and their period of morning stiffness *quintupled* in length. Every way the five individuals and attending doctors looked at the situation, their arthritis was definitely as bad as it had been before they began the treatment. The experiment completed, they went back on methotrexate and were feeling much better one month later.

Here's how our survey participants rated methotrexate.

Number who tried **methotrexate**	48	
Outcome:		
Dramatic improvement	24	(50%)*
Moderate improvement over time	3	(6%)
Temporary or minor improvement	1	(2%)†
No improvement (ineffective)	5	(10%)
No rating (too soon to tell, or toxic reaction forced individual off drug before any benefit could be achieved)	15	(31%)

*These percentages have been rounded to the nearest whole number, with the result that ratings for some treatments do not total 100%.
†This participant, a fifty-eight-year-old homemaker from Michigan, actually received methotrexate for her psoriasis, but she also has both rheumatoid and osteoarthritis. "Methotrexate helps my psoriasis a lot," she says, "but gives little help for my pain."

These numbers, drawn from our survey, approximate the results from formal clinical trials. In 1984, for example, in a large study organized at the University of Utah, slightly more than 50 percent of the 189 patients enjoyed a significant reduction of pain and swelling on methotrexate.

Methotrexate works. That's the good news. And it works where all else has failed, because methotrexate is not given to anyone who hasn't already tried a whole series of strategies, typically including aspirin, other nonsteroidal anti-inflammatory drugs, steroids, gold shots, and antimalarial drugs or penicillamine. "Methotrexate is helping me a great deal. It has given me back the strength in my wrists and hands," writes a sixty-two-year-old retired government official from Tennessee who took gold injections for seventeen years until they lost their effectiveness for him. A sixty-seven-year-old medical technician from New York who has had arthritis for twelve years says, "This is the first time that something has worked. I'm on my third year."

How is methotrexate used?

Methotrexate is prescribed in addition to other treatments, not instead of them. Our participants take their anti-inflammatory medication on a daily basis, rest and exercise regularly, undergo physical therapy, apply heat or ice as needed, *and* receive a dose of methotrexate—shots or pills—once a week. Several people who have been relying on large quantities of prednisone find that they can get by with less of it once they are on methotrexate. "I have very little pain and stiffness anymore since I have been on **Methotrexate, Orudis**, and prednisone," a sixty-five-year-old Alabama housewife says. "I lead a very normal life and do almost all of my housework. I even work as an Avon representative. I feel so fortunate, because I remember the times when I couldn't do the simplest chore, and when I had so many sleepless nights due to pain." A forty-six-year-old offset printing pressman and lithographer from California writes: "Since beginning my present regimen of **Orudis**, amitriptyline, and methotrexate, plus physical therapy and exercise, I have gone from being totally bedridden to an up-and-down, mostly painful but self-sufficient person again. I feel the future to be much brighter for me. I am afraid of methotrexate, but it's doing what it's supposed to do, and I have great faith in my doctor."

Just what, exactly, methotrexate does in rheumatoid arthritis remains a mystery; but then, no one can say for sure how most of the common arthritis drugs achieve their benefits. If they *work*, they are used. And while it would be very nice to know *how* they work, scientific understanding has not kept pace with practical experience.

The names applied to methotrexate and the other drugs in its class—they are called, by turns, cytotoxic drugs, immunosuppressives, antimetabolites, and immunomodulatory drugs—all hint at their possible actions in the body. For example, "cytotoxic" means "poisonous to the cells." By interfering with cell reproduction, these drugs can halt the uncontrolled growth that characterizes cancer, or, as in rheumatoid arthritis, the runaway inflammation and destruction of the joints. "Immunosuppressive" means they can damp the immune response. Since rheumatoid arthritis is believed to be an immune-system attack on one's own body, it stands to reason that suppressing the immune system might quiet the disease. Again, the mechanism by which methotrexate brings arthritis relief is simply not known.

What are the side effects of methotrexate?

The most common side effect of methotrexate—in clinical studies and among our participants—is nausea. Eleven survey participants mentioned it, three of whom said the nausea was only occasional or slight. Nausea, unfortunately, is nothing new to people who have run the gamut of nonsteroidal anti-inflammatory drugs, as most methotrexate recipients have done. But that doesn't make it any easier to bear. The nausea from methotrexate, however, often disappears on its own, and if not, it may be controlled by lowering the dose or by spreading it out—that is, by taking the three or four tablets of methotrexate every few hours over the course of the appointed day, instead of swallowing them all at once. Another option is to take the drug as an injection instead of a pill, but that necessitates a weekly trip to the doctor.

A weekly trip to the doctor may be avoidable, but a monthly one is *mandatory* if you are on methotrexate. Every few weeks, you must undergo the tests that show whether the drug is causing any of the more hidden noxious kinds of damage of which it is capable. You need a complete blood count because methotrexate can suppress the production of new blood cells and lead to severe forms of anemia. You also get a blood test to point up possible ill effects in the liver, called a liver-chemistry profile. Liver damage is one of the worst threats of methotrexate, because the damage, once begun, cannot be undone. The blood-chemistry profile, moreover, is not a complete check for liver problems, since the most serious damage does not show up in a blood test. Only an actual biopsy can tell for sure, and if you take methotrexate, you are supposed to undergo a liver biopsy after about two years of treatment. The other worrisome fallout from methotrexate is lung disease. If you take the drug, you are warned to be on the lookout for a dry cough accompanied by fever and shortness of breath. If you notice these symptoms, you need to see your doctor and have a chest X ray *immediately.*

"**Methotrexate** dramatically relieved my arthritis," writes a fifty-six-year-old communications consultant from North Carolina, "but it also brought extreme tiredness, inability to eat, weight loss, lowered resistance to infection, and depressed spirits. I had to discontinue it because the side effects were unacceptable to me." She now manages her arthritis with prednisone and penicillamine.

Some people on methotrexate develop sores on their skin or inside their mouths. These are signs of a toxic reaction to the drug, and mean, "Get off it at once." Others begin to lose their hair. Here's a rundown of the side effects reported by our participants.

Problem	Number Affected	Percentage
Nausea or vomiting	11	23%*
Lowered disease resistance	4	8%
Lost or thinning hair	3	6%
Sores in mouth	3	6%
Liver dysfunction	3	6%
Hives or skin lesions	3	6%
Depression	2	4%
Shingles (herpes zoster)	2	4%
Stomach pain or burning	2	4%
Eye problems	2	4%
Low blood count	1	2%
Anorexia and weight loss	1	2%
Intestinal cramps	1	2%
Bladder ulcers	1	2%
Dry skin	1	2%
Extreme fatigue	1	2%
Dizzyness	1	2%
Swelling of legs and feet	1	2%
Difficulty breathing	1	2%
No side effects	8	17%

*Some participants reported two or more side effects.

Who can take methotrexate?

Arthritis specialists figure that about 10 to 15 percent of the seven million Americans with rheumatoid arthritis—hundreds of thousands of individuals—could be considered candidates for methotrexate because they have "failed to respond" to standard treatment. (Research reports routinely talk about patients who "fail to improve" on this or that therapy, when of course it is really the therapy that fails to help the person in pain.)

Methotrexate is not for everybody. The decision to prescribe it is not made lightly, and the drug is reserved for those with the most severe cases of rheumatoid arthritis. In other words, you have to have a great deal of pain, stiffness, and swelling in several joints, plus fatigue. You also have to have proved yourself a reliable patient, since it takes a fair degree of responsibility on your part to follow the treatment plan, both in taking the drug on schedule and showing up at the doctor's office for frequent checkups to test for danger signs.

You cannot take methotrexate if you are pregnant or planning to have a baby. This warning also applies to men who are planning to become fathers, since the drug may cause birth defects and even sterility. A few other physical conditions would rule out using methotrexate. If you drink a lot of alcohol, for example, the danger of cirrhosis of the liver rises dramatically.

What is the future of methotrexate and other cytotoxic drugs in arthritis?

Now that FDA approval has been granted for use of this drug in treating arthritis, more different types of physicians are likely to prescribe methotrexate for their patients with rheumatoid arthritis.

In the future, methotrexate may be introduced earlier in the course of treating this condition. It is used now for those who have not been helped by existing treatments, including at least one of the slow-acting antirheumatic drugs—gold, penicillamine, and **Plaquenil** (hydroxychloroquine sulfate). Even though these other drugs may not be any safer than methotrexate (see Chapter 5 for a full discussion of their effects and side effects), rheumatologists feel more comfortable prescribing them. "Essentially," explain rheumatologists Richard I. Rynes, M.D., and Joel M. Kremer, M.D., in *The Journal of Musculoskeletal Medicine,* "we would rather deal with the known side effects of slow-acting, antirheumatic drugs than with the unknown and potentially life-threatening side effects of long-term cytotoxic therapy." Some researchers, however, think that methotrexate might do even more good if it were introduced sooner, *before* the disease had a chance to deform the joints or destroy their function.

Another cytotoxic drug, called **Imuran** (azathioprine), is being tested in experimental combinations with methotrexate. In 1987, doctors at the Cleveland Clinic Foundation in Ohio reported that eleven men and ten women who had not been helped by either methotrexate *or* azathioprine were given low-dose combinations of them *both.* Used together, methotrexate and azathioprine worked extremely well, allowing three of the patients to enjoy a complete remission within six months, according to the researchers. Only one man had to drop out of the study because of nausea and sores in his mouth, which signaled a toxic reaction, but the majority of the other patients saw good results by the year's end, including less pain, less stiffness, less swelling, and greater strength. The outcome was so positive, in fact, that this combined approach is being tried on larger numbers of patients at several clinics at once, in the hope of proving its long-term safety. (See Chapter 5 for more information about **Imuran**.)

Other cytotoxic drugs tried experimentally in rheumatoid arthritis also work but appear more toxic than methotrexate, or less effective, or both. These include chlorambucil, cyclophosphamide, and cyclosporine. "I was on **Cytoxan** (cyclophosphamide) for ten years when it was an experimental drug," writes a sixty-year-old homemaker from Arizona who has had rheumatoid arthritis since age eighteen. "But I stayed on it too long. I lost my hair, had an early change of life, and finally lost my bladder with cancer—which may be related to the cytotoxic drug."

Guanethidine

A drug for high blood pressure strikes a blow at arthritis

Like methotrexate, guanethidine is an existing drug with a long history. It has been approved and used for decades to lower high blood pressure. Now it promises to lower the pain of arthritis as well.

In moving from anticancer drugs to blood-pressure pills, it may seem that doctors treating arthritis will try any old treatment that has worked on *anything* else. In one sense, this is true. Gold was originally used to treat tuberculosis; aspirin was intended for short-lived pain and fever; **Plaquenil** was a malaria cure; and penicillamine is the drug of choice for a rare genetic disorder called Wilson's disease. However, the history of medicine—not just arthritis treatment—is full of stories of drugs that were discovered or produced for one purpose and wound up being used for another. Some of the medications that now control the violent behavior of schizophrenia, for example, were a failed attempt to make a good nasal deconges-tant.

Most of the time, there is good reason for turning to an existing drug used to treat another ailment, and guanethidine is a case in point.

It all started a few years ago in San Francisco, where rheumatologist Jon D. Levine and his colleagues at the University of California were experimenting with arthritic rats. They found that the animals' most susceptible joints contained relatively large amounts of something called "substance P." Substance P occurs naturally in animals and humans, and it is known to be a neurotransmitter—one of the chemicals that carries messages from one part of the nervous system to another. What was it doing inside the joints?

The scientists tried injecting the rats with more substance P, in joints that were already inflamed. The shots measurably increased the pain and bone destruction in those joints. This was the first hard evidence that the nervous system played a role in rheumatoid arthritis, which is now widely considered to be a disease of the immune system. "Soft" evidence of the nervous system's role had been available for some time. For one thing, many people with arthritis note that their flare-ups are frequently triggered by stress. Also, doctors had observed that people with arthritis *and* stroke had milder arthritis on the stroke-affected side of the body, as though the injured nerves could no longer aggravate the joints. Now it seemed that substance P was the missing link between the nervous system and the arthritic joint. Block the entry of substance P, therefore, and you should reduce the inflammation and joint deterioration of arthritis.

Levine and his colleagues thought that they might indeed treat arthritis by putting obstacles along substance P's path into the joints. They needed a drug that would block the action of the nervous system near the affected joint. Guanethidine was their choice.

Introduced in 1960, guanethidine is marketed by Ciba-Geigy under the brand name **Ismelin**. It is usually prescribed in tablet form for people with high blood pressure, which it lowers by quieting the part of the nervous system that reacts to stress. The California researchers knew that giving these pills to arthritis patients, however, would probably make them light-headed enough to faint. So when they began a clinical trial with twenty-four men and women, they injected the drug directly into a vein near the subjects' elbows. The one shot relieved the pain in the nearby joints for as long as two weeks in some participants. This is particularly encouraging, since these people all had rheumatoid arthritis for an average of twelve years and were already taking "second-line" drugs such as gold, penicillamine, steroids, and azathioprine. To test the effectiveness of guanethidine, thirteen individuals got the real thing, while the other eleven got a sham shot—and neither the doctors nor the subjects knew who'd received what until the results of the experiment were all in. The guanethidine group fared far better than the others in terms of pain relief, although the drug didn't seem to make too much difference in relieving the amount of stiffness they experienced. Nevertheless, having a pain-free elbow for the first time in years was a most-welcome situation.

After reporting their results in *The Journal of Rheumatology,* the California group next conducted a second trial of guanethidine against knee pain, using a series of four injections, which brought relief to some of the participants for several *months.*

Guanethidine must be injected intravenously near the painful joint or joints, and the only way to do that at this early stage is to ask the patient to report to the hospital for the treatment. In the elbow trial, the drug was kept from moving beyond the target area by wrapping each patient's upper arm with a blood pressure cuff and leaving it on for half an hour after the injection. The researchers know they need a better way to deliver the drug to the problem joints, for convenience sake, but the procedure does seem safe. In no case did the injection lower anyone's blood pressure or cause any other noticeable side effects. (Taken orally for hypertension, **Ismelin** is infamous as a cause of impotence.) What would happen with repeated use, however, remains to be seen. The researchers also need to find out how often guanethidine would have to be injected to keep up its positive effects.

In other work that is still limited to experiments with rats, Dr. Levine and his colleagues have found further proof that blocking some actions of the sympathetic nervous system can offer protection or relief from arthritis. They gave their experimental animals existing drugs known as beta-2 antagonists, which block the action of certain stress-related hormones. As a result, the animals suffered less joint damage than other animals not receiving these drugs. (See Chapter 16 for more information about stress and arthritis.)

New Anti-Inflammatory Drugs

Variations on a theme from laboratories around the world

The drugs commonly used for treating all kinds of arthritis—the nonsteroidal anti-inflammatory drugs, or NSAIDs—have rapidly become some of the biggest-selling medicines ever marketed; and manufacturers keep coming out with more of them. Some physicians yawn at the prospect of new NSAIDs, arguing that there are already enough of these products, while other doctors welcome the newcomers that widen the field of choices. After all, the drugs are so quirky that there's no telling in advance which one is most likely to work for which person. With lots of them on hand, the doctor always has another drug waiting in the wings if the first one or two (or three or four) don't suit any given patient. (See Chapter 5 for a full discussion of these drugs, plus ratings.) About a dozen NSAIDs share the turf in the United States today, with an even greater number already available in Europe, and an unknown number under study or awaiting approval from the Food and Drug Administration. As our survey got under way in 1987, we learned the names of several new drugs in progress, including etodolac from Ayerst, nabumetone* from Beecham, ketorolac from Syntex, isoxicam from Warner-Lambert, oxaprozin from Wyeth, and proquazone from Sandoz. Three more that were on that list, carprofen (**Rimadyl**) from Roche, diclofenac sodium (**Voltaren**) from Ciba-Geigy, and flurbiprofen (**Ansaid**) from Upjohn, have since received FDA approval.

New ways to make NSAIDs easier to take

One NSAID may be easier on your gut than another, but they all have the potential to induce stomach upset and bleeding. Drug makers have yet to design an anti-inflammatory agent that does *not* threaten the stomach lining, so researchers are experimenting with other drugs that can undo the damage NSAIDs cause—or prevent it altogether.

Enter misoprostol (**Cytotec**, Searle), an anti-ulcer compound just recently approved by the FDA in early 1989. The drug was already being used to help heal ulcers in many other countries, including France and Canada. Misoprostol is a fairly close copy of one of the body's own products, called prostaglandin E-1. What's exciting about this drug from our perspective is that it helps the stomach protect itself from

---

*One of our survey participants, a fifty-two-year-old office worker from Wisconsin, is taking nabumetone (**Relafen**) as part of a three-year drug study. She prefers the drug to **Motrin** and **Naprosyn**, she says, because it has helped her more than the others, although she's had no side effects from any of them. Other survey participants report taking diflunisal (**Dolobid**) and tolmetin (**Tolectin**) when these two were experimental—or, in FDA terms, "investigational new drugs."

anti-inflammatory drugs. Aspirin and NSAIDs work by blocking the production of certain substances called prostaglandins,
but misoprostol apparently replaces one prostaglandin the
stomach needs to stay intact. Indeed, misoprostol can now be
prescribed in a preventive fashion, given right along with aspirin or NSAIDs, to keep people with arthritis from ever developing an ulcer. It is the first drug ever approved by the FDA
for this purpose.

On the road to FDA approval, **Cytotec** was the subject of
a large study involving 270 patients at several clinics, including
the Arthritis Center in Phoenix. In the first stage, the volunteers took aspirin alone for four weeks and then underwent
tests to see what shape their stomachs were in. Nearly *90
percent* of them had obvious injuries, including ulcers, and yet
many had *no pain* or other symptoms to warn them or their
doctors that they were heading for serious stomach trouble. At
this point, about half of the volunteers began taking misoprostol along with their aspirin, while the other half received aspirin plus placebo. By the end of eight weeks on the aspirin
combinations, there were startling differences between the
two groups—not in their arthritis but in their stomachs.
Among those on misoprostol, most of the ulcers had healed and
many other stomach lesions had completely vanished. Among
those taking aspirin with placebo, not quite one-third showed
this kind of improvement. Importantly, misoprostol did not
keep the aspirin from getting into the bloodstream and doing
its job, so that all the subjects kept their arthritis under control
in roughly equal fashion.

Endoscopy, the test these research volunteers took *three
times* in the course of the study, is a fairly invasive, uncomfortable procedure that requires you to lie immobile on a table for
about half an hour while a long lighted gastroscope is passed
down your throat and into your stomach to inspect the situation there. It is also expensive (in the hundreds of dollars) if you
have to pay for it yourself. It isn't the sort of test that can be
done casually on someone with no symptoms of stomach trouble. And yet this study suggests that *many* people with arthritis may have "silent," or symptomless, ulcers. The researchers
therefore concluded that it makes sense to give misoprostol as
an ounce of prevention, although it is currently approved only

for people at high risk for ulcers—those over the age of sixty-five and those who have had ulcers before.

The only gut-level complaint from the volunteers taking misoprostol in the study was diarrhea, which troubled a few of them. However, misoprostol apparently poses a special danger for pregnant women, since it may cause miscarriage.

Nature's Gifts

Animals, plants, and oils that are the natural enemies of arthritis

Caribbean sea whip In the blue-green waters of the Caribbean Sea, an elegant-looking soft coral called a sea whip delivers a rude surprise to any fish that try to feed on it. Would-be predators get a taste of noxious chemicals that send them swimming the other way. Such self-defense systems are not unusual in nature, but the sea whip's arsenal contains a unique group of compounds that seem ideally suited to fighting—of all things—arthritis. These compounds may surpass the power of any known analgesic for controlling pain, yet they are not addicting, and they apparently can reduce inflammation more effectively than the one leading arthritis drug they've been tested against: indomethacin.

In 1982, on a special sea voyage aboard the research vessel *Calanus,* scientists from the Scripps Institution of Oceanography took a close look at the sea whip's chemicals to see whether any of them might be medically useful. The discoveries they made were so startling and so exciting that they kept them *secret* for four years while they scrambled to get U.S. and international patents for the sea whip's natural anti-inflammatory compounds. Without a patent, they well knew, there would be no way to protect the use of the promising new drugs, and no financial incentive for any drug manufacturer to take over their development and marketing. The sea whip's promise would remain just so much purple-colored coral on the ocean floor.

Meanwhile, the scientists devised various ways to test the

new compounds, which they named pseudopterosins (pronounced *sue-do-TERR-uh-sins,* with *two* silent *p*'s) after the
sea whip's scientific name—*Pseudopterogorgia elisabethae.*
They found more than a dozen different pseudopterosins in
the sea whip, and every one of them proved capable of controlling pain and inflammation in mice with induced arthritis.
When the University of California at San Diego, Scripps' parent institution, received patent approval in 1986, the researchers finally reported their results in the *Proceedings of the
National Academy of Sciences,* one of the most-respected
scientific journals in the world. The work was directed by Dr.
William Fenical, an organic chemist at Scripps, and Dr. Robert
S. Jacobs, a pharmacologist at the Marine Science Institute of
the University of California, Santa Barbara.

There have been no human trials of any of the pseudopterosins—yet. The Scripps group says that a major drug manufacturer, although they would not divulge the company's
name, has signed an agreement with them to shepherd the
pseudopterosins through the various procedures required to
win FDA approval for testing new pseudopterosin-based
drugs.

Herbal Remedies   In China, an *ancient* herbal remedy with
the imposing name of "thundergod vine" and with a long
history of use in arthritis treatment was tested recently in
clinical trials. The official experiment allows East and West to
meet on the matter, and thundergod vine, or T2, as the active
ingredient is called, may yet find a foothold in the United
States. It takes a few well-conducted clinical trials to move an
herbal remedy out of the realm of folklore and into the world
of orthodox medicine. And thundergod vine, which grows in
southern China and goes by the scientific name *Tripterygium
wilfordii,* has now passed its first test. When the news of thundergod vine's effectiveness against rheumatoid arthritis in two
trials was presented at the 1987 meeting of the American
Rheumatism Association (now called the American College of
Rheumatology), researchers here called the work "interesting
and exciting," and conceded that the herb did seem to have
an effect on arthritis.

In one study, scientists at the Chinese Academy of Medical

Sciences and the Peking Union Hospital, both in Beijing, used T2 from thundergod vine to treat seventy patients with rheumatoid arthritis over a sixteen-week period. For the first twelve weeks, half the participants took T2 tablets every day, and the other half took placebos (look-alike duds). Then, during the last four weeks, the groups switched medications, so that those who had been taking T2 got the placebo and the others had a short trial period on T2. Neither the people in the trial nor the doctors examining them knew who was taking what, or when, until all the results were in. And the results were quite encouraging.

Everyone in the long-treatment group who stayed in the study (twenty-seven of the original thirty-five people) felt at least some improvement, and two of them had a remission. What's more, the good results lasted through the four-week period when they were *not* getting T2 each day, and some of them still felt improved several *months* after the study ended. T2 seemed to affect every arthritis symptom that can be measured: the degree of joint tenderness, the number of swollen joints, the duration of morning stiffness, the strength of the person's grip, and the time he or she takes to walk a certain distance, as well as several laboratory blood tests, including the sedimentation rate and the amount of rheumatoid factor in the blood. The good effects made themselves known after four weeks of treatment. The participants in the short-treatment group, who took T2 for a total of four weeks, also noticed some improvement.

T2, like any herbal remedy or synthetic drug, has its risks and side effects. Indeed, twelve people—eight in the long-treatment group and four in the other group—had to drop out of the study because they couldn't tolerate the side effects of T2. There were lots of skin rashes reported, not all of them serious enough to force the individuals out of the experiment, plus thinning of the skin and nails, and changes in skin color. Several of the women found that the drug stopped their menstrual periods, or, in a few cases, brought on bleeding in women who'd already gone through menopause. And other side effects cropped up, too: diarrhea, loss of appetite, and abdominal pain. No problem seemed life-threatening, and *all* of the problems resolved after T2 treatment stopped, although some of them took a few months to disappear.

Dr. Tao Xue-Lian and her colleagues, who conducted the trials in China, are convinced of T2's benefit. They are now fiddling with the drug to try to make it safer. In current studies, their aim is to isolate the parts of T2 that are *therapeutic* from those that are troublemakers, and thus hone the power of the thundergod vine. As of this moment, however, American herbalists are prohibited by law from prescribing it.

Meanwhile, in England, an herbal remedy used for headache and stomachache since the sixteenth century is showing up in the *Lancet* and *British Medical Journal* as a possible treatment for arthritis and migraine. It is the feverfew plant, or bachelor's button—a pretty flower with a disturbing potential for interfering with women's menstrual periods and inducing abortion in animals. People who use feverfew usually chew a few of its leaves, fresh, every day, but tablets containing dried feverfew are now sold in health-food stores. The few small studies that have been done suggest that feverfew might prevent severe attacks of migraine, but there have been no trials to determine feverfew's safety or effectiveness in treating arthritis.

Fish Oil   The fish story of the century is the tale of the way fish oil went from rags to riches—from a laughable home remedy to a medical marvel used to prevent heart disease, stop blood clots, control blood pressure, improve psoriasis, relieve migraine headaches, slow the spread of cancer (in animals), and reduce the pain and inflammation of rheumatoid arthritis. Although the news sounds too good to be true, there is mounting evidence of real benefit from fish oil for people with rheumatoid arthritis.

The fish oil being tested and touted throughout the country today is not cod liver oil, but omega-3 fatty acids, extracted from the flesh of oily fish. Cod liver oil contains these acids, too, but also packs a dose of cholesterol, which most people try to avoid, plus vitamins A and D, which can be toxic in large amounts.

Smelly, old-fashioned, unpleasant cod liver oil has been

replaced by smooth amber-colored capsules of fish oil that are selling like hotcakes in health-food stores and pharmacies, with names such as **MaxEPA** (R. P. Scherer), **Promega** (Parke-Davis), and **Proto-chol** (Squibb). Most people buy them to ward off heart attacks, on the grounds that the Greenland Eskimos, who consume large quantities of oily fish, have a strikingly low incidence of heart disease. (Although it isn't talked about as much, the Eskimos also have a low incidence of arthritis.) Even as the fish-oil capsules have created a multimillion-dollar industry, however, medical debates rage over several issues: How much fish oil, if any, should the average person take per day? What are the long-term effects of daily fish-oil supplements? Is it safer to eat fish three times a week than take fish oil in pill form? Some experts argue that the Eskimos' healthy lifestyle (they don't smoke and they get a *lot* of exercise) is at least as important as their diet in preventing heart disease.

For arthritis, for once, the situation is more clear-cut. The studies already completed have defined the dosage level of fish oil that may bring relief—about fifteen to twenty capsules a day, taken in small batches with meals. While few doctors or researchers are openly recommending such a regimen as yet, many of them are genuinely excited about the results they've seen so far.

Perhaps the most compelling of the recent studies on fish oil for arthritis took place at Albany (NY) Medical College, where doctors gave fish-oil capsules to forty men and women.* As usual, the participants were divided into two groups, but instead of giving fish oil to one group and placebo pills to the other, *everyone* got equal time on each. Half the participants took fish oil for the first fourteen weeks, while the other half took an identical-looking pill, made by the same manufacturer but containing no fish oil. Then, for a period of four weeks, everyone took placebos, although the participants were not told when they were being switched from one type of pill to the other. In the next stage, the group that had taken fish oil for fourteen weeks started fourteen weeks of placebo capsules,

---

*One of the benefits of participating in a clinical trial is getting your medication free. In this study, for example, the doctors not only "gave" the fish oil, in the sense that they prescribed it, but actually gave it away to their research subjects, thanks to the interest of R. P. Scherer Corporation, makers of **MaxEPA**.

and those who had taken placebos all along received fourteen weeks of fish-oil capsules. The experiment ended with another four-week period when everyone took the placebo version.

If you're wondering what it would be like to swallow fifteen pills a day *in addition* to your other medication(s), as these individuals had to do, you may be interested to learn that five of the original forty participants dropped out of the study because of the inconvenience of it all—downing handfuls of capsules and making regular visits to the clinic for tests. Two more were kicked out by the experimenters because blood tests showed they were not really taking the pills. Research is hard work for everyone involved—subjects and scientists alike.

At the end of the thirty-six weeks, after averaging the experiences of the thirty-three volunteers who completed the study, the researchers found that fish oil had helped the participants a lot. On the whole, they felt less pain while taking it; they had fewer tender joints; and they didn't get tired until later in the day. What's more, these benefits stuck with them for weeks after they stopped taking the fish oil. Reporting their work in *The Annals of Internal Medicine,* the researchers allowed that higher doses of fish oil, given over a longer period of time, might have done even more good. (A later study, conducted in Australia and reported in the October 1988 *Journal of Rheumatology,* supported this idea.)

What does this mean for you? Should you start popping fish-oil capsules? Dr. Joel M. Kremer, who headed this research project as well as an earlier study that *also* showed rheumatoid arthritis could be improved with fish-oil supplements, does not recommend it; not yet, anyway. More research needs to be done, and he surely will be doing it. What Dr. Kremer *did* recommend, when interviewed for newspapers and magazines after he announced his findings in 1987, was more fish on the dinner plate. "The doses of fish oil given," *Prevention* magazine quoted him, "were roughly equal to a salmon dinner or a can of sardines." In *Medical Tribune,* a weekly newspaper for health professionals, Dr. Kremer said, "It is very, very interesting. Just the fact that diet can change anything, I think, is fascinating."

Dr. Richard I. Sperling, who headed a related study at Harvard Medical School, also has said that eating more fish "couldn't hurt." (See Chapter 14 for a full diet plan that is based, in part, on this body of research.)

Thirty of our survey participants take fish-oil capsules, mostly for general (heart and blood) health. Nine participants, however, make it clear that they use fish oil, or tried using it, as arthritis therapy. We can't formally rate a treatment on the basis of nine reports, but we *can* say that five of these people find it from moderately to magnificently beneficial. By far the most enthusiastic report comes from a fifty-one-year-old Missouri waitress, who writes: "Fish oil is a wonder drug—or should I say a wonder food? The medicines the rheumatologist gave me all helped my rheumatoid arthritis, but the side effects nearly killed me. I took aspirin, **Motrin**, and **Disalcid**, and I lost twelve pounds and wound up in the hospital for five weeks with an ulcer, liver problems, heavy periods, and ringing in my ears to the point of deafness. He was about to put me on gold when I found out about fish oil *on my own*. I started taking fifteen capsules a day two years ago, and I can live again. I can move. I work five days a week as a waitress, with no stiffness, even. I get around like a sixteen-year-old."

Among the other four participants using fish oil, two judge it useless, one gives it a cautious "maybe," and one says he has just started on "megadoses of fish oils" with no results yet. (As is true with many of the orthodox arthritis treatments, fish oil may take several weeks to produce any noticeable effect.)

Fish oil has side effects, too, of course. Some of them are good side effects, such as a presumed lowered risk of heart attack. But those same Greenland Eskimos—the ones with the legendary lack of heart disease—have a comparatively long bleeding time after injury, due to the blood-thinning effects of omega-3 fatty acids. This could be a real problem for anyone taking aspirin, as so many of our participants do, or other drugs that also thin the blood. Fish oil may pose special dangers for people with diabetes, who have been known to lose control of their blood-sugar levels after taking relatively small daily doses of fish oil for just one or two months. It is also known that the Greenland Eskimos have a higher rate of stroke than Americans have, which may or may not be related to their fish-heavy diet. (A Greenland Eskimo typically eats more than three hundred pounds of fish a year, while the average American eats only about ten to fifteen pounds per year, according to *Medical Tribune.*)

Diarrhea or other bowel changes sometimes bother people taking fish-oil capsules. Indeed, diarrhea forced one person to drop out of a recent Harvard study, in which all fourteen volunteers took twenty fish-oil capsules a day.

The only side effects our survey participants mention are "fishy burps" and heartburn. "I took fifteen capsules of **Max-EPA** daily for about two months," says a fifty-six-year-old California housewife with osteoarthritis. "They seemed to help the stiffness in my body and legs, and allowed me to do more walking temporarily. This would only last several hours and then I was back to being really stiff again. But I began burping up a fish-oil taste, which I didn't care for, so I stopped." Eating citrus fruits may help this problem—provided you can tolerate them. Chlorophyll-rich greens such as parsley, watercress, and romaine lettuce, some nutritionists say, should help to chase away the fishy aftertaste.

Given the promising results of the early trials and the low incidence of side effects seen in these studies, fish oil seems to be *the* treatment to watch.

Healing Rays

Shooting at arthritis with radiation, magnetic pulses, and lasers

Radiation Therapy   Borrowing an idea that has worked on Hodgkin's disease (cancer of the lymph system), a few researchers have tried treating rheumatoid arthritis with radiation therapy. So far, fewer than one hundred men and women worldwide have had total lymphoid irradiation, or TLI, as the technique is called, for treatment of arthritis.

Like methotrexate and other cytotoxic drugs, TLI takes for its target the immune system—the self-defense network that protects the body from outside assault. Rheumatoid arthritis is thought to be one of several so-called "autoimmune diseases," in which the body becomes its own enemy. The goal of

TLI is to knock out the self-destructive activity of the immune system by blasting large doses of radiation at the hotbeds of immune-system activity: the thymus gland, the lymph nodes in the neck, chest, and abdomen, and the spleen.

TLI was first developed at Stanford University School of Medicine in California, nearly thirty years ago. And it was there, in the 1970s, that Dr. Samuel Strober and his colleagues decided to try the technique on eleven of their patients with severe cases of rheumatoid arthritis who had not been helped by other approaches. At exactly the same time, on the other side of the country, a team of investigators at Harvard Medical School, led by Dr. David E. Trentham, also used TLI experimentally to treat ten people with chronic intractable rheumatoid arthritis. Since these first attempts were reported in the *New England Journal of Medicine* in 1981, another ten or twelve people have undergone the treatment each year as the experiments continue.

Wherever TLI has been given for rheumatoid arthritis—at Stanford and Harvard, as well as in Ireland and Germany—the results have been good but the costs have run high. In the various trials, from one-third to three-quarters of those treated enjoyed great relief, while others had at least some measure of relief, and the good effects tended to last for a year or longer after the treatment ended. Four people died of infections they could not fight off, however, presumably because of the radiation therapy. The more common side effects, well known from twenty-plus years' experience with treating Hodgkin's disease, include fatigue, nausea, vomiting, loss of appetite, dry mouth, skin irritations, and hair loss, which come on during or shortly after the treatment period but tend to go away on their own. TLI, however, also carries a risk of cancer. Its advantage, as compared to methotrexate, is that each course of treatment seems to bring about very long-lasting improvement.

In the trials already done, TLI therapy lasted anywhere from several weeks to several months, with four or five treatments per week during that time, on top of any regular medications the participants were taking. Most of the people in these studies received a total of two thousand rads in each of two or three body areas, depending on the experiment.

Instead of giving a sham radiation treatment to half the

participants in each group, the placebo in these trials was a course of low-dose radiation, totaling either 200 or 750 rads. In a few cases, the people in the low-dose groups *also* felt much improved—and also suffered some of the bad side effects, such as herpes zoster (shingles).

TLI will undoubtedly remain experimental therapy over the next several years as researchers try to answer a host of questions through more clinical trials. For example: What is the least amount of radiation that can be of help in treating rheumatoid arthritis? Who are the people most likely to benefit from the treatment? How can the side effects be minimized? Which other treatments given simultaneously might make TLI more effective—or more hazardous?

Magnetic Pulses　In Poland, according to a report in the journal *Reumatologia,* hundreds of people with osteoarthritis and rheumatoid arthritis have apparently been helped by a much less dangerous burst of energy—high-frequency magnetic-field pulses from a Polish-made machine called a Terapuls GS-200.

Once they had tailored the right dose to fit each individual in the experiment, scientists at Sniadecki Hospital in Wloszczowa say that treatment was a relatively simple matter of placing an electrode right on an affected joint, then turning on the juice for twenty to twenty-five minutes.* Each person had one or two joints treated this way at a time, every day for about two weeks. They sometimes felt a "delicate warming," they said, while receiving the treatment. Pain began to disappear by the third session for some people, and inflammation died down soon afterward. Minus their pain and swelling, the participants became more active and found that the good effects lasted for several *months* after the treatment ended. The placebo therapy in this trial was a course of short-wave diathermy—a form of heat treatment used widely in the United States by physical therapists, chiropractors, and others.

The results were less pain and greater mobility and flexi-

---

*They figured out the right duration, intensity, and frequency (in hertz) for each person's every joint by factoring in the size of the joint (hip versus toe, for example), the amount of fat covering it, and the degree to which it had been damaged by arthritis.

bility for the group as a whole (159 people with osteoarthritis and 189 with rheumatoid), although those with rheumatoid arthritis seemed to enjoy a slightly higher rate of improvement.

Magnetic-pulse therapy seems extremely safe. No one in the trial had any unpleasant sensations or side effects to report. In fact, the Sniadecki researchers maintain that the treatment is even safe for people with all kinds of additional medical problems, such as heart disease, poor circulation, high blood pressure, and varicose veins. While many of the other treatments we've discussed in this chapter are reserved for those people who are the most disabled by arthritis, high-frequency magnetic-pulse therapy probably could be used on anyone at any stage of the disease. If accepted here, it would most likely become part of the realm of physical therapy.

Laser Beams   The superfocused beams of laser light have been used medically to do everything from circumcise an infant with hemophilia to clear a blocked coronary artery in a forty-year-old man. In arthritis, laser light directed at a painful joint can bring relief. This was first demonstrated about ten years ago, when Dr. John Goldman of Medical Corridors in Atlanta, Georgia, studied the effect of laser light on thirty people with rheumatoid arthritis. Since 1980, several more studies in the United States and abroad have also shown lasers capable of reducing the pain and stiffness of arthritis, but their use is still considered experimental. Beyond pain relief, lasers may work some mysterious change on the immune system itself. Some rheumatologists admit they have a prejudice against lasers because there's no conclusive proof of what, if anything, the light beams *do* inside the joints to bring relief. But, as we've seen repeatedly, the lack of a good explanation has never prevented the use of a therapy that works.

Most proponents claim that laser therapy has no side effects, but the intense light of some lasers can threaten a person's eyesight unless proper precautions (protective goggles) are used. The "soft lasers" get around this risk and seem to be just as effective in reducing pain, some researchers say. In a few instances, people receiving laser treatments complain of a burning sensation in the joints that may last a few hours. The good effects, on the other hand, may carry over for a full month after one treatment.

Three of our survey participants received laser therapy— two of them from American chiropractors and one from an M.D. at a Canadian pain clinic—and all three deemed them helpful. "I find my joint pain and stiffness are greatly reduced with monthly acupuncture and soft laser-beam treatments," writes a seventy-one-year-old retired banker from British Columbia who has had rheumatoid arthritis for twenty years. "Most of the other treatments I've taken, including forty-one gold injections, have all led to unacceptably low white-blood-cell counts."

If you want more information about laser treatments for arthritis, or the names of doctors who use them, you can write to the American Society for Laser Medicine and Surgery, 425 Pine Ridge Blvd., Suite 203, Wausa, WI 54401.

The Body's Own Weapons

Human hormones and immune boosters

Hormones   Perhaps it struck you that some of the experimental treatments covered here are guilty of sex discrimination. Women may have to avoid them, at least part of their lives, because they interfere with menstruation, conception, or pregnancy. However, numerous women with rheumatoid arthritis, including several of our survey participants, notice that they feel greatly improved during pregnancy, which may hint at a therapeutic role for the high levels of certain hormones circulating in their blood. Also, some women trace the onset of their arthritis, or flare-ups of it, to the time *immediately following* the birth of a child, when the hormone balance shifts dramatically. It is also possible that the improvement during pregnancy is due to the subtle damping of the immune system that keeps the mother's body from attacking the half-foreign tissue of the baby inside her.

Sex-hormone treatments for arthritis have long been considered quackery, but there is some medical-research interest now in the possible antiarthritis action of birth control pills, which are mixtures of female sex hormones. As Dr. Jan P. Vandenbroucke of Erasmus University in the Netherlands reported in *JAMA* (The Journal of the American Medical Association), women who use oral contraceptives may actually be protected from developing rheumatoid arthritis. In these studies, the researchers reached their conclusions by interviewing more than one thousand women attending several arthritis clinics, to see whether there was any connection between taking "the pill" at some point in their lives and the type and severity of their arthritis. The researchers did not prescribe birth-control pills for any of these women. They just wanted to establish the fact that such a link exists. Meanwhile, other studies are exploring the effects of sex hormones on arthritis in animals.

Interferon   When it was first isolated, this potent product of the human immune cell was seen as the possible cure for the common cold and perhaps even the ultimate answer to treating many forms of cancer. Doctors in Germany and Mexico have tested it against rheumatoid arthritis—and with some success. We also have some information about an American interferon trial from one of our survey participants, a thirty-four-year-old nurse from Pennsylvania who has been giving herself daily injections of interferon for the past year.

When she first joined the trial, at her rheumatologist's invitation, she had had rheumatoid arthritis for nine years and had tried a variety of treatments, including high doses of aspirin (with an ulcer to prove it), several NSAIDs, gold injections, two total joint replacements (her left hip at age twenty-nine and right wrist at thirty-one), and periodic cortisone shots. She felt she'd been extremely well cared for by her rheumatologist ("If I'd seen him from the beginning, I don't think I would have lost my hip.") and was eager for the chance to try the new treatment. As it happened, she spent twelve weeks taking what later turned out to be placebo injections.

Once the initial phase of the trial was over, however, the interferon manufacturer offered to provide the drug, free of charge, to anyone in the study who wanted to take it, for as long as they found it helpful. "During the actual experiment, I had to travel to the doctor's office—about an hour's drive for me—five days a week to get a shot," she explained. "But those of us who chose to keep on the interferon were taught how to mix it with sterile water and inject ourselves. We use a special type of syringe that isn't hard to work, even if your hands hurt. I give myself a shot five days out of seven, and I see the rheumatologist once a month to get blood tests and the next month's supply of medication. I also have to have a complete physical every three months. But I feel really good. I have less pain by far, and my stiffness lasts only about half an hour in the mornings, whereas it used to last clear through lunchtime. Also, I'm not so tired now. I can remember feeling so exhausted most of the time that I could have slept all day. But the interferon has enabled me to go back to work."

She has not been troubled by any side effects, she says, although one of the other nineteen volunteers in the research project dropped out because of nausea. Flulike symptoms, with fever, aches, and chills, also occur. "We're supposed to take **Tylenol** half an hour before each injection to ward off these side effects. It seems strange that the interferon, which is helping my arthritis, would produce these symptoms, which are just like the fevers and chills the arthritis sometimes gives me. Also, I needed a cortisone shot in my ankle recently. I don't know if this means the interferon may be losing its effectiveness for me, or if my being back at work and on my feet so much is the problem."

In the Mexican study, led by Dr. Mohan V. Peddinani at the University of Guadalajara, forty people took daily injections of interferon or a placebo. Half the group got interferon for the first nine weeks, and then nine weeks of placebo, while the other half started out on the placebo and later switched to the interferon—never knowing, of course, which came when. The researchers periodically checked both groups for pain, swelling, stiffness, and range of motion. They also evaluated how well the participants could manage daily activities, from bathing and dressing to walking, writing, and climbing stairs. What they saw was a rapid and constant improvement while the people were receiving interferon. As a whole, the group that started on interferon fared better and better until they were switched to the placebo, when they steadily lost all the ground they'd gained. The group that started on placebo stayed about the same for the first part of the study, then quickly improved when they began taking interferon.

The Mexican researchers believe that the powerful effect of interferon seen in this trial suggests something even more exciting than a new treatment for arthritis. They see the possibility of a vaccine that could be used to *prevent* the disease.

At the Weizmann Institute of Science in Rehovot, Israel, Dr. Irun R. Cohen and other biologists are already trying a vaccination approach on a type of arthritis they can give to rats. They take cells from the animals' own immune systems, alter them under pressure, and then return them in the form of live vaccines. The animal work is promising, but the ultimate question driving these scientists is: Can we use a similar technique to vaccinate people? And will it work?

Summary of Experimental Treatments for Arthritis

Treatments that have just been, or are about to be, approved as standard therapy for arthritis
—Methotrexate (**Methotrexate, Rheumatrex**)
—New NSAIDs
—Misoprostol (**Cytotec**)
Treatments that involve existing products or technologies, and which seem extremely safe, extremely promising, or both
—Fish oil
—Laser therapy
—Interferon
Treatments that will likely require further investigation
—Guanethidine (**Ismelin**)
—Total lymphoid irradiation
Treatments that have not been tested in clinical trials in this country
—T2 from thundergod vine
—Feverfew
—Magnetic-pulse therapy
—Hormones

Techniques that are still limited to laboratory or animal experiments
   —Pseudopterosins from Caribbean sea whip
   —Beta-2 antagonists
   —Autoimmune vaccination

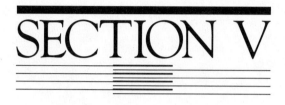

SECTION V

NUTRITION
AND ARTHRITIS

What rheumatologist has not been asked about the role of diet in the treatment of rheumatoid arthritis? Who among us has not responded that there is no evidence that diet treatment works?

> —Nathan J. Zvaifler, M.D., from an editorial in *Arthritis and Rheumatism,* April 1983

Surprisingly, despite the fervor of advocates and skepticism of rheumatologists, little objective information exists about nutritional therapy for rheumatic diseases, and virtually all conclusions have been based on inadequate data or improper study design.

> —Richard S. Panush, M.D., from an editorial in *Annals of Internal Medicine,* April 1987

The doctor said what I eat doesn't affect arthritis, but I know better.

> —Survey Participant #664, a carpenter from Texas

12

A REVOLUTION IN MEDICAL THINKING ABOUT NUTRITION AND ARTHRITIS

■ Diets for arthritis ■ Supplements that control symptoms ■ Fasting for periodic relief ■ Food allergies that aggravate arthritis

This is an unprecedented moment in the history of arthritis care. For the first time, many mainstream practitioners are exploring the role of nutrition in arthritis prevention and treatment, *and* calling for stepped-up research efforts in this area.

Arthritis is perhaps the last bastion of medical prejudice against nutritional approaches to disease management. Cardiologists and oncologists once scoffed at the notion of diet as treatment for heart disease or cancer, but they take it quite seriously now. And they take pains to take their message to the public. In its most recent effort, the American Heart Association has begun putting a special seal of approval on various items in the supermarket to help consumers identify the foods that are lowest in fat and cholesterol. And the American Cancer Society, in one of its popular magazine advertisements, pairs a doctor in a lab coat and stethoscope with a greengrocer holding an armload of fresh fruits and vegetables. The captions explain that "the best defense against cancer" is to see the doctor once a year and the greengrocer once a week. Indeed, the cancer-preventive powers of vitamins A and C and the importance of a low-fat diet are now getting as much press as was once devoted to the evils of smoking.

But, as you well know, there is no comparable message being broadcast by the Arthritis Foundation about what *you* should or should not eat.

For years, the Foundation's firm position had been a blanket rejection of any dietary approach to the prevention or control of arthritis, except for the one form of arthritis where the dietary connection was well established—gout. Today, at last, a revolution in medical thinking about diet and arthritis is under way. The Arthritis Foundation has already revised its brochure about diet, mentioning some of the exciting new research and recommending dietary guidelines such as: "Avoid too much fat and cholesterol. Avoid too much sodium." The Foundation is also funding some of the research efforts that are upending its longstanding antidiet stance.

It's about time. In 1983, when the revolution was just getting started, distinguished rheumatologist Dr. Morris Ziff of the University of Texas Health Science Center wrote knowledgeably about the "growing literature" offering "cogent evidence that diet may affect inflammation," and he noted how "disconcerting" this evidence might prove to rheumatologists who were "informing their patients that diet has no role in their disease."

Full-length articles, case reports, and doctors' letters about nutrition and arthritis appear routinely now in the medical literature, including *Annals of Internal Medicine, Annals of the Rheumatic Diseases, British Journal of Rheumatology, Lancet,* and *Arthritis and Rheumatism,* which is the official journal of the American College of Rheumatology. In this chapter, we will page through some of these journal articles with you, examining the ideas and experiments that are pushing the boundaries of respectable research into the arena of food and food supplements—where people with arthritis have always wanted them to go.

"Every rheumatologist," Dr. Ziff wrote in *Arthritis and*

Rheumatism, "knows how intent the rheumatoid patient is in asking about the possible role of diet in the disease, and with what doubt accepts the answer that diet is not a factor."

That widespread, well-documented patients' doubt has finally entered the medical community. As Dr. Ziff sums up, "All things considered, there appears to be a case for the investigation of diet in the treatment of rheumatoid arthritis." The breadth of current research ranges from specific diets that may help relieve arthritis pain, to specific food supplements that may work with a diet or by themselves, to the role of food allergy in causing or aggravating arthritis symptoms.

Is There an Arthritis Diet?

There are *hundreds* of arthritis diets, and up until very recently, rheumatologists have been content to brand them all "quack therapy" and pay no attention to their individual differences. But in 1981, Dr. Richard S. Panush and his colleagues at the University of Florida College of Medicine decided to put one popular arthritis diet to the test. They chose the diet laid out in two books by Dr. Collin H. Dong and Jane Banks—*The Arthritic's Cookbook* and *New Hope for the Arthritic,* published by Thomas Y. Crowell in 1973 and 1975, respectively. It was a strict diet that ruled out all dairy products, all fruits, all meats, all alcoholic beverages, and all preservatives, among other things. They selected it, they said, because it had won tremendous media attention, and not for any particular promise they could see in it. In fact, they judged the diet deficient in certain vitamins and minerals, and they beefed it up with a daily vitamin-plus-iron supplement.

Having chosen a diet plan, the researchers had to devise a way to study its effectiveness. They decided to test it against a mock diet of their own creation that ruled out certain foods arbitrarily—sour cream, turkey, bananas, cornflakes, and others—while allowing red meat and white wine. They would ask half the people in their study to follow one diet, half to follow the other, and they would watch and see what happened. But first they had to round up a group of volunteers who all had arthritis and who would all promise to follow a strict diet *to the letter*—for ten full weeks—in the interest of science.

Luckily for the doctors, the average person with arthritis is so open to the idea of diet therapy that they were able to attract thirty-three highly motivated men and women who had rheumatoid arthritis and were willing to give nutrition a whirl. Importantly, none of these people had read the Dong-Banks books or heard about the diet. Experimental science, like justice, is *blind.* Volunteer subjects must have *no idea* whether the pill or the diet they ingest is the real object of study or some sham or placebo pill that is tested for the sake of comparison. All these volunteers knew was that they were following a diet different from their usual one and that it *might* help. And the doctors who periodically examined them every two weeks over the course of the experiment were likewise *blind* as to which diet which patient was on.

Only the dietitian knew who was eating what. The dietitian, after all, was the one who gave each participant detailed personalized instructions, including menu plans and recipes, who telephoned all the participants several times a week to encourage them in their efforts, and who dropped in at their homes, unannounced, *eighty-seven times* at lunch or dinner hour, just to make sure they weren't cheating. But the dietitian was *blind* as to which individuals showed signs of improvement in terms of their blood-sedimentation rate, for example, or the strength of their grip. (They had all been in pretty much the same shape, on these and other measures, when the study began, and every subject's medical treatment continued unchanged throughout.)

Partway through the study, seven of the original thirty-three volunteers dropped out. It was too dull or too difficult to follow the diet, or too hard to keep track of what they ate in their food diaries, as the experiment demanded. The other twenty-six stuck it out the whole ten weeks. And here's how it ended up.

Five of the eleven patients on the experimental diet got better during the study. But so did *six* of the fifteen patients on the placebo diet. What was going on here? Was there some feature common to both diets that could have been responsible? The researchers say they couldn't identify one. More likely, the participants were having a remission for some other reason. Maybe their hopes were buoying them, making them feel better and appear better on examination. If the diet were *really* therapeutic, scientific thinking holds, then it would have had obvious benefit compared to the placebo diet; and it did not.

But one man and one woman on the experimental diet completed this study feeling so greatly improved that they chose to stay on the diet indefinitely. Nine months later, when the researchers completed their report for the April 1983 issue of *Arthritis and Rheumatism,* these two individuals were *still* following the diet. Every time they went off it—she for an ice cream or a candy bar, he for a spicy meat dish or a beer—their arthritis symptoms flared. "Without further study," the researchers said of them, "it is uncertain whether their course was indeed modified by diet or merely reflected the natural history of disease."

It is hard to imagine how a months-long trend of well-being, interrupted only by an occasional binge on a forbidden food item, could reflect "the natural history of disease." Why won't the researchers admit that the diet scored two cures? Because the standards of scientific proof are *rigorous,* and two out of eleven is a scientific bust. If five or six of the people on the experimental diet had gotten better, and one or none on the placebo, then the scientists might have had something approaching preliminary proof. As it is, we are left with two isolated cases, interesting to be sure, that "support, but do not prove, the suggestion that individualized dietary manipulations may be beneficial for selected patients."

Diet Instead of Drugs

More "observation" and "support" were soon to follow, when doctors in Surrey, England, tested a diet as *sole therapy* for rheumatoid arthritis. They took the fifty-three patients in their study *off* their regular medications for two weeks before even starting them on the diet. During this prediet period, the volunteers got placebo pills, although they didn't know what they were, of course, along with two tablets of a nonaspirin painkiller (acetaminophen, which you may know as **Tylenol**) four times a day.

In the next step, half the group began to follow the special diet, which consisted of excluding various foods that might aggravate arthritis. Then, after one week, the foods were gradually reintroduced, a few at a time, beginning with those least likely to offend. Any food that fomented the symptoms of arthritis was quickly eliminated again. Thus, each volunteer's treatment became unique over the six weeks of diet therapy.

Meanwhile, the other half of the volunteers continued, without any change in their normal diet, on placebos and nonprescription painkillers for six more weeks—a total of *two months* away from their standard treatment. (This proved too difficult for some, and in all, eight people dropped out of the study before its completion.) Only then did they begin their six weeks of diet therapy—identical to what the first half of the subjects had tried. The researchers designed the study this way so they could compare people on diet therapy to people on placebo therapy for six weeks, *and* compare some people to *themselves* in two different situations, to see whether and how they changed when they made the switch from placebo pills to diet.

No matter how the researchers looked at it, the diet wrought improvements that were swift and dramatic. Within the first week of diet therapy, the first group of participants had less pain, shorter periods of morning stiffness, fewer painful joints, and a stronger grip. Over the next five weeks, they enjoyed continued relief. The second group, too, despite their longer wait before starting the therapy, responded to the diet with markedly reduced pain and stiffness. On all comparisons, diet therapy proved superior to placebo therapy, from group to group and within the same individuals over time. What's more, nearly everybody in the study lost weight and felt the better for it.

Reporting their results in the *Lancet* of February 1, 1986, Dr. L. G. Darlington and his co-authors wrote, "It is one thing to describe improvement with dietary therapy in patients with rheumatoid arthritis and quite another to explain how it may work." They had a few ideas, though.

- The people may have had genuine *food intolerances,* so that not eating certain food(s) brought relief.

- The *weight loss* alone might have changed the course of the disease.

- Taking the people off their *prescription medications* may have solved some drug-related intestinal problems and made them better able to keep irritants from entering the bloodstream through the gut.

- Eating more of some foods containing certain *fatty acids* (more about these later) may have reduced joint inflammation.

- The *power of suggestion* from being involved in a dietary experiment could have produced the very real improvement seen.

- Perhaps a combination of two or more of these factors was at work.

"For some physicians the use of diet in rheumatoid disease has a disturbing flavor of fringe medicine," they concede, and they suggest that "perhaps the greatest need now is for more careful and well-designed research so that preconceptions may be put aside and any role of diet . . . may be determined."

In other words, caution is crucial, for the scientist who uses anything short of the most exacting standards in diet studies will undermine the revolution and wind up being dismissed as just another quack.

Do Certain Foods Aggravate Arthritis? And If So, Which Ones?

That's what Dr. Deepa Beri and fellow researchers at the All India Institute of Medical Sciences in New Delhi sought to learn in 1987. On the road to discovery, they asked their research subjects to stop taking their nonsteroidal anti-inflammatory drugs (NSAIDs) and try to get by on acetaminophen. Under the circumstances, nearly half the group—thirteen people out of twenty-seven—were *unable* to make it through even the first phase of the study, which put them on a two-week diet of nothing but fruit, vegetables, sugar, and refined oil. (Later on, a fourteenth person dropped out. Despite the fact that he had moved on to a slightly less stringent diet *and* was doing well, he simply stopped going to the clinic, and the doctors couldn't find him.)

The study stretched out over *ten months* and required the patients to persevere through six variations of the diet. Their first two weeks on fruits and vegetables excluded all the foods that the researchers suspected might be arthritis-aggravating, such as milk, wheat, and meat. By the end of this period, ten of the fourteen subjects (71 percent) showed significant signs of improvement. Now they were ready to add on one of the staples of the Indian diet—pulses, which are the edible seeds of certain plants, such as peas, beans, and lentils. Almost immediately, one patient suffered a rapid flare of arthritis symptoms, and two others also grew worse.

On to the third phase and the introduction of wheat and wheat products. Again, there were instant reactions to the foods from some of the volunteers. This pattern repeated itself through each successive stage, in which each added food item decked one or more of the participants. Some could tolerate no rice, others no milk. Unfortunately, some of them proved to be so sensitive to so many foods that the researchers had no choice but to start them on drug therapy, since it seemed impossible to restrict their diets as severely as their symptoms suggested.

"The results showed that a high proportion of patients improved on dietary manipulations," the doctors concluded in 1988 in *Annals of the Rheumatic Diseases,* "and that there was marked individual variation in response to the elimination of different dietary items." Yes, certain foods clearly do aggravate arthritis. But the "certain foods" change from one person to the next. (See Chapter 13 for a list of foods that our survey participants found most likely to be arthritis-aggravating.)

What About Not Eating at All?

Diet studies that include a period of fasting show that arthritis almost always improves in the absence of food. This may sound like a sick joke, since starvation is hardly the way to health, but the finding is a strong argument for the existence of some aggravating factor in food.

"About five years ago," writes a retired industrial designer from Florida who participated in our survey of 1,051 people with arthritis, "I tried a one-month fast from solid foods. I had only vegetable and fruit juices, with vitamins, and enemas to clean out my system. I lost forty pounds in ten days. After being very weak for the first seven days, I began to feel better. After another ten days, I felt cured and even the rheumatoid nodules were disappearing. As the weight returned, so did the arthritis. But I was afraid of damage to my heart if I continued fasting, and I didn't have a doctor who would agree to supervise me, so I stopped."

Unlike our survey participant, the twenty Swedish men and women who fasted for science in 1982 *were* under a doctor's supervision *and* inside a hospital during their two-week fast. Then they stayed for another three weeks, following a strict vegetarian (vegan) diet with no eggs or dairy products. The researchers observing them modeled this experimental fast and diet after popular programs at Swedish health resorts, which were promoted as being particularly helpful for people with arthritis and other diseases.*

Of the ten people in this study who had arthritis, eight said they felt much better while fasting. For eleven days, they had nothing but vegetarian broths, juices made from vegetables or berries, and herbal teas every two or three hours, and their symptoms seemed to wash away.

Fasting studies are not blind, obviously, since there is no way to keep people from knowing that they're not eating; but not everyone had the same reaction to the fast. Two members

---

*These "health farm" treatments, involving fasting and vegetarian diets, spurred doctors in Sweden to conduct, by our count, at least a half-dozen separate scientific investigations between 1979 and 1986—several of them aimed at answering patients' questions about nutrition and arthritis.

of the group grew *worse,* even though they continued taking their regular medications all through the experiment.

After the Fast Is Over

No sooner did the subjects start to eat solid food again than their symptoms began to creep back. Even so, they finished the study feeling slightly better than they had at the outset, and one person felt *considerably* better.

The doctors observed that "fasting seems to have a fairly potent anti-inflammatory effect," (*Acta Dermato-Venereologica,* 1983), although they could not explain why. A few years later, however, other Swedish scientists watched fourteen women with arthritis improve during a one-week total fast, and they began to piece together the reasons.

The *fact* that the women in the study felt better while fasting was obvious from the degree of pain relief they enjoyed—despite having dropped their drug treatments (NSAIDs) two weeks before entering the study. But the *explanation* for their well-being came from intensive analysis of their blood before, during, and after their week of consuming nothing but water.

As Dr. Ingiäld Hafström and others pointed out in May 1988 in *Arthritis and Rheumatism,* fasting changes the blood chemistry of people with arthritis. It slows the action of certain enzymes and blocks key steps in the chain of events leading to painful inflammation. Although aspirin and other anti-inflammatory drugs also block these events, they don't create quite the same changes as fasting does.

No one in the study suffered any kind of side effects from fasting, except for a little passing weakness, weight loss, and light-headedness. This is *light stuff* compared to the side effects of the majority of arthritis treatments, even over-the-counter ones, which often cause nausea, vomiting, indigestion, ulcers, and diarrhea or constipation.

"Thus," the researchers concluded, "fasting is one possible way to induce rapid improvement in rheumatoid arthritis." And although fasting could never be used, of course, for any appreciable length of time, volunteers who fast so that others may learn are revealing the healing processes involved.

A Fish Tale

One promising possibility for gaining some of the advantages of fasting without forgoing food is by supplementing the diet with fish oil—or rather, the omega-3 fatty acids that fish-oil supplements contain, especially eicosapentaenoic acid, or EPA. Dr. Joel M. Kremer and other scientists at Albany Medical College have looked long and hard at this possibility, as have Drs. Richard Sperling, Michael Weinblatt, and K. Frank Austen at Harvard Medical School.

Inspired by a long line of animal and human experiments, Dr. Kremer's group set out to discover whether changing the source of fat in the diet could change the course of inflammation in arthritis.

Their subjects were thirty-eight willing and able patients, who followed dietitian's orders and took special supplements for twelve weeks. And as you know, *they* did *not* know who among them followed the experimental diet and took fish-oil supplements or who followed the sham diet and took placebo pills.

The experimental diet in this case was specially tailored to deliver a high ratio of polyunsaturated fat (the kind found in many types of fish) to saturated fat (the kind you find in butter). Volunteers on the experimental diet were told to eat fish wherever and whenever possible. They could eat red meat twice a week *at most,* and only if they stuck to lean cuts with *all* visible fat removed. Chicken was okay, too, provided they took the skin off. Under no circumstances could they indulge in sausage, bacon, hot dogs, or other lunch meats. Other no-nos included whole milk, butter, and cheese. If they cheated, they had to say so in the food diaries they kept, where they entered everything they ate all day. On top of all that, they had to take ten **MaxEPA** capsules daily.

The volunteers in the control group had dietary restrictions, too, which turned their mealtimes, likewise, into assignments of sorts. For example, they were told to avoid foods high in polyunsaturates, such as corn oil and safflower oil, and they also took ten capsules a day (all duds, however, made of nondigestible paraffin wax). *Both* groups had to *balance* their diets and try not to gain or lose any weight, and both groups continued their regular drug regimens, which ranged from NSAIDs and steroids to the more potent "second-line" treatments such as gold, penicillamine, and hydroxychloroquine.

The kinds of changes the researchers could hope to see in their subjects would take at least six weeks to emerge on the changed diet, and the experiment lasted twice that long. By the twelve-week point, there were indeed differences between the two groups in terms of morning stiffness and the number of painful joints they had. The people in the experimental group were better off. But when the follow-up exams came around a month or two after the study ended, the people in the experimental group had lost all the ground they'd gained, while those in the control group felt *improved.*

The researchers saw these aftereffects as further proof of their theory. In other words, the experimental group grew worse when they went off the diet and stopped taking fish oil because they were no longer getting the combination's anti-inflammatory effect. As for the control group, the rebound relief they enjoyed in the weeks after the experiment was probably the result of dropping the diet high in saturated fat and returning to a more healthful way of eating. Just going back to a polyunsaturated cooking oil, which they had been told to avoid during the study, could have made an appreciable difference, the researchers said (*Lancet,* January 26, 1985), as too much saturated fat may affect the immune system and aggravate arthritis symptoms.

Are Supplements Sufficient?

One of the questions that came out of the Albany diet study was this: What would happen if people with arthritis took the fish-oil supplement and didn't change their diet at all? Would they still notice an improvement? The doctors lost no time in setting up a *new* experiment with another group of volunteers to see whether supplements could make *all* the difference. (This study is described in detail in Chapter 11.)

To make a thirty-six-week-long story very short, the experimenters and those who were experimented upon succeeded in showing that fish oil alone *could* and *did* bring about important improvements.

The next wave of studies will try to set "dosages" of fish oil, and attempt to explain precisely how it works against arthritis.

Fish or Flower?

The evening primrose, whose yellow flowers open at nightfall, yields an oil from its seeds that is the plant world's answer to fish oil. Evening primrose oil, like fish oil, contains an essential fatty acid that can fight against inflammation. It is called gamma-linolenic acid, or GLA. Indeed, some researchers suspect that the *combination* of fish oil and evening primrose oil could be potent enough to *replace* NSAIDs in treating people with arthritis. Doctors at the Royal Infirmary in Glasgow recently tried to do just that. They enrolled forty-nine patients with mild rheumatoid arthritis in a study that lasted more than a year, and they watched many of their subjects decrease or altogether drop their drugs, while controlling their arthritis symptoms with evening primrose oil alone, or a combination of evening primrose oil and fish oil.

For the first three months of the experiment, the participants stayed on whatever NSAID they had been taking, and began swallowing an extra twelve capsules a day. Unbeknownst to them, only sixteen of the volunteers were receiving evening primrose oil in these capsules. Fifteen got identical-looking pills that contained a mixture of evening primrose oil and fish oil, while eighteen took yet another look-alike that was a placebo.*

After the first three months, the patients all tried to cut down on their drugs. (Actually, four of them had stopped taking their NSAIDs by themselves, even before the study began, because they were suffering more drug-induced stomach upset than they could bear.) The doctors' orders were to take less of the drugs, or none at all—but *only* if they could do so

---

*The capsules for the experiment came compliments of Efamol Ltd., one of the leading marketers of evening primrose oil. A dozen evening primrose oil capsules delivered a total of 540 milligrams of GLA, while the total daily dose in the combination capsules was 450 milligrams of GLA with 240 milligrams of EPA. The placebos were made of liquid paraffin. All the pills, placebos included, also contained vitamin E to keep the oils from being oxidized.

without making their symptoms worse. Here's what happened.

- Twenty-eight people in the study were able to reduce or stop their NSAIDs.

- Eleven of these people were taking evening primrose oil at the time.

- Twelve were taking the evening primrose/fish oil combination.

- Five were taking the placebo, although these five didn't reduce their drug dose as markedly as the others.

During this phase of the study, which lasted nine months, thirteen patients dropped out because their arthritis grew worse. And *ten* of them turned out to be on the placebo pills. Of the other three, one was taking evening primrose oil, one was taking the combination, and one wasn't taking anything! Routine blood tests given as part of the experiment proved that he was cheating by not using the capsules he'd been given, and he was dropped from the study.

At year's end, all the remaining patients spent three *more* months trying to maintain themselves on their new low dose (or no dose) of NSAIDs. Meanwhile, their daily dozen capsules were *all changed* to placebos (containing no vitamin E), although the subjects didn't know that this had happened. Gradually, everybody who had been doing fine on evening primrose oil began to feel worse, as did most of those who had been taking the combination capsules. By comparison, the group that had been on placebos all along continued about the same.

"In conclusion, therefore," the doctors wrote in 1988 in *Annals of the Rheumatic Diseases*, "we have shown that it is possible to decrease or stop NSAIDs in some patients with rheumatoid arthritis by introducing evening primrose oil or evening primrose/fish oil treatment." They added that the best use of the oils might be for patients who couldn't take

NSAIDs because of ulcers or kidney problems that would only be aggravated by the drugs.

They didn't make the next leap, though, and suggest that the oils replace the drugs generally. After all, the patients in the study didn't do *better* on the oils than on the drugs. They simply did *as well.*

The study didn't try to determine which oil was more effective as a treatment. Perhaps another experiment will do that soon.

Was It Something I Ate?

A thirty-eight-year-old mother of three made medical history when her severe chronic rheumatoid arthritis—which could not be controlled with aspirin, with NSAIDs, with gold, with penicillamine, with prednisone, or even with the immunosuppressive drug azathioprine—responded to a simple change in diet. Eleven years of suffering ended abruptly when she stopped eating milk, cheese, and butter.

The strange thing about this pale sickly looking woman, according to doctors at the Royal Postgraduate Medical School in London who treated her and reported her case history in the *British Medical Journal,* was that she had none of the usual symptoms of food allergy. No foods upset her stomach, gave her diarrhea, made her skin break out, or brought on a headache. She had no reason to believe that her passion for cheese—she often ate as much as a pound of it in a day—was fanning the flame in her joints. However, she had been through so many medical treatments with so many toxic reactions that she willingly agreed to try the doctors' suggestion to stop eating dairy products.

After three weeks on her new diet, she began to feel better, with less pain and swelling and a shorter period of stiffness in the mornings. As the months passed, most of her symptoms completely disappeared.

The doctors were delighted, but they couldn't let it go at that. They had to show that her case was truly an example of food-induced arthritis. And so they invited her to check into the clinic, where they fed her three pounds of Hammersmith

Hospital cheddar cheese in as many days, along with seven pints of milk. The effect was awful. Within twenty-four hours her old stiffness was back, she could barely make a fist, and her fingers swelled until some of them were two whole ring sizes larger.

There was no question that she met two of the most important criteria for food allergy: Her symptoms went away when she stopped eating certain foods and came back with a vengeance when she ate them again. The results of the allergy tests the doctors gave her weren't so clear-cut, however. In fact, such tests may be inadequate to discover food sensitivities in people with arthritis. There seem to be no good shortcuts—yet—around the difficult but definite route of excluding this or that from the diet for weeks at a time and watching for signs of improvement.

This woman's case is not the only documented case of food-aggravated arthritis on record, but it is one of very few. Swiss rheumatologists recently tried to raise the number of cases by mailing a food-allergy questionnaire to three hundred of their patients with arthritis. Only 158 people filled out and returned the form, however, and only 52 of them believed that certain foods increased their symptoms. When the doctors examined six of these people in person, testing them and challenging their symptoms to flare by feeding them the foods they avoided, *nothing happened.*

"It seems, therefore," the researchers concluded in a 1987 report in *Clinical Rheumatology,* "that true allergic reactions in joints of rheumatoid arthritis patients are rare." Maybe so. Or maybe, as the London doctors suggested, allergies that cause arthritis symptoms work in ways that are not yet fully understood.

Mystery Capsules

Dr. Panush of the University of Florida, who tested a popular diet on a group of his patients (see pages 213–215), looked into the question of food allergy in an ingenious way. He solicited people who noticed that their symptoms got worse after eating certain foods, and then, instead of openly offering them the foods they feared, he disguised various foodstuffs in capsules, with no telltale aromas or appearances. Some of the capsules contained the aggravating items, but some of them contained foods that had never caused these people a lick of trouble. Would the people react to the foods if they were "blind" as to what they were eating?

Dr. Panush and his colleagues began their investigations with a middle-aged woman who couldn't eat milk, milk products, red meat, or dry beans. Her rheumatoid arthritis flared from these foods, she had found, and so she limited herself to fish, chicken, vegetables, and fruits. Her arthritis and her certainty that food affected it made her just the person Dr. Panush and his colleagues were looking for.

After examining her twice and getting her enthusiastic consent to go along with a rather taxing sort of study, they took her out to lunch at a nearby restaurant, where they ordered her the house specialty, containing milk *and* beef *and* beans. Before the afternoon was over, the poor woman literally lost her grip. Her grip strength weakened by 40 percent from the morning's measurement, and she felt much worse. Several of her joints became tender, while other joints swelled. And her walking slowed way down. The luncheon had been a success, and three months later the woman checked into the clinic to go through the rest of the study as an inpatient.

About a week into her hospital stay, the doctors asked her to fast for three days. Within twenty-four hours of starting the fast, she felt worlds better. Her morning stiffness, for example, which usually lasted about half an hour, disappeared altogether while fasting. Then, for the next *month,* she lived on **Vivonex**, a liquid diet, only marginally more appetizing and satisfying than being fed intravenously. But **Vivonex** was not the least bit arthritis-aggravating, and she continued to feel and function almost as well as she had while fasting. She was a great good sport about all of this, too, the doctors reported in *Arthritis and Rheumatism* (February 1986), describing her as "extremely cooperative and motivated." She was also a model subject because she proved to the scientists' satisfaction that her arthritis was most definitely aggravated by food. She even passed the mystery challenge test.

At most of her "mealtimes," she drank her **Vivonex** with

a capsule that contained some disguised food item. Some of the capsules contained milk, others had chicken, beef, rice, lettuce, carrot, or nothing (placebo). She didn't know what was in them, of course, but her body reacted unerringly to the milk every time—with tender joints, with swollen joints, with morning stiffness, and with weakening grip.

Buoyed by this experience, the researchers went on to work with several other people in a similar fashion. Out of fifteen subjects who were tested this way, three felt their symptoms flare every time the capsule delivered one of the offending food items, which included milk, shrimp, and nitrates. Another two people reacted some of the time, and ten didn't react at all. Dr. Panush suspects that only about 5 to 10 percent of people with arthritis have true food sensitivities. However, he wrote in a commentary in *Annals of Internal Medicine* (April 1987), "The notion that food or food-related environmental antigens induce or perpetuate symptoms, at least for some patients, is novel, logical, and potentially enlightening."

More Questions Than Answers

Some of these studies raise more questions than they answer, but they have broken new ground, at last, making nutrition a reasonable and respectable field of inquiry for rheumatologists and other scientists interested in arthritis.

You have no doubt noticed that all the reports covered here deal with rheumatoid arthritis, and none with osteoarthritis. Unfair as it may seem, the revolution hasn't yet spread to osteoarthritis, except for a few studies of certain nutrients that may control pain, such as vitamin E. (See Chapter 15.) Dr. Panush actually intended to include people with osteoarthritis in his study of the Dong-Banks diet—he even had eleven patients picked out—but he dropped the idea when he saw that the diet wasn't working out all that well for the volunteers with rheumatoid arthritis.

As for now, we salute the scientists who stuck their necks out to initiate studies in this area, putting their reputations on the line. We also salute the people who helped them carry out their investigations—the subjects in their research.

Over and over in the reports of these studies, we've seen people willingly give up their freedom of choice in matters of food, staying on highly restricted diets for weeks, even months at a time. Sustained by the encouragement of researchers and by the hope that their efforts will help themselves and others, they are the army of the revolution. And it is an all-volunteer army.

Early nutrition studies, by comparison, such as the ones at the beginning of this century that started to define minimal daily requirements for certain nutrients, didn't have to rely on volunteers. In those days, before research subjects were protected by the doctrine of informed consent, doctors were free to experiment on captive populations in hospitals, asylums, reformatories, and prisons.

Today, doctors know they can *expect* a certain number of people to drop out of a diet study, and this makes their job harder. To take Dr. Kremer's earlier trial, for example, in which the participants had to change their diet *and* take ten capsules a day, three people dropped out because they couldn't stick to the diet, two quit because they couldn't swallow the capsules, another two left when their arthritis got worse, and one suddenly required chemotherapy for cancer. On top of these problems, Dr. Kremer found that six more people, who weren't voicing any particular complaints, were simply *not taking* the capsules as they were supposed to. He was forced to drop them.

In one report we reviewed of a study on food allergy and arthritis, the researchers got openly disgusted with the people who had promised to be their subjects. "The most noteworthy point of this trial," they said, "has been the frequency with which patients have abandoned their declared interest in dietary management once faced with a controlled and demanding protocol of this kind. . . . The self discipline demanded by the trial comes as a harsh antidote to the facile optimism of so many glib theories about food allergy and arthritis."

Nutrition studies make demands of people that most scientific studies do not. If you're asked to take a new drug in the interest of science, then you take it, or you take the placebo, and you let the doctors chart your symptoms for a time. But if you agree to take a diet as treatment, you either consent to being hospitalized so the researchers can control exactly what you eat, or you're stuck keeping a written record of every mouthful. From our own personal experience as volunteer research subjects, we can say that it is sometimes *easier,* in these situations, to go a little hungry than to start taking tests or making notes every time you want a snack.

Summary of Recent Research on Nutrition and Arthritis

Date	Published Findings
1981	London doctors successfully treat a woman with severe rheumatoid arthritis, who had not been helped by any standard treatments or even accepted experimental ones, by putting her on a diet free of dairy products.
1983	Researchers at the University of Florida test a popular diet on their patients. They fail to prove its value, but two people in the study group improve so much that they continue the experiment on their own.
	Doctors in Sweden give patients a version of a spa program, asking them to fast for two weeks and then follow a vegetarian diet for three weeks. People with arthritis improve while fasting, but their symptoms return when they start the vegetarian diet.
1985	Scientists at Albany Medical College find that a diet high in polyunsaturated fats, coupled with supplements of fish oil, can reduce the period of morning stiffness for their participants, as well as the number of tender joints.

1986   English rheumatologists substitute diet for drug treatment with fifty-three patients and observe that they fare better on the diet than on placebo treatment.

            Rheumatologists at the University of Florida use capsules to disguise foods their patients name as arthritis-aggravating. A few people react to the mystery capsules with obviously worsening symptoms.

1987   Swiss rheumatologists send out patient questionnaires to find people whose arthritis is aggravated by certain foods, but they fail to discover a true food allergy in any of them.

            Building on their earlier work, researchers at Albany Medical College observe that giving large daily doses of fish oil to subjects with arthritis, without changing their diet, improves their condition.

            Doctors at Harvard Medical School study blood samples from subjects taking fish-oil supplements, and they describe the chemical changes by which fish oil may work an anti-inflammatory effect.

1988   Scientists in India seek to identify foods that aggravate arthritis. Their study reveals that certain foods do make the symptoms worse, but different foods affect different people. They embark on a follow-up study.

            Swedish rheumatologists determine that fasting reduces the disease activity in rheumatoid arthritis, and they suggest that brief periods of fasting may be used to bring rapid improvement during flare-ups.

Researchers in Scotland find that supplementing patients' diets with evening primrose oil, or a combination of evening primrose oil and fish oil, enables them to take lower doses of anti-inflammatory drugs or to stop using the drugs altogether.

13

EXPERT, EXPERIENCED ADVICE ABOUT NUTRITION AND ARTHRITIS

■ What doctors won't tell you ■ What weight loss can accomplish ■ What foods are most likely to aggravate arthritis pain

Every day, the following scene is acted out in countless doctors' offices. Maybe you've played a role in it yourself.

Patient: Tell me, Doctor, is there any special diet I should follow, or any particular foods that would make my arthritis better or worse?

Doctor: No, there is no known connection between nutrition and arthritis.

The trouble with the doctor's part in the drama is that it is unconvincing. Most people with arthritis find it simply incredible that nutrition could have nothing to do with the disease—especially when they are bombarded with messages about nutrition's importance in other common illnesses, such as diabetes, heart disease, hypertension, cancer, and osteoporosis. It is even more unbelievable if their own experiences show them that diet *does* make a difference in the amount of pain they feel.

"Most of the rheumatologists I have seen," writes a twenty-nine-year-old teacher from Texas who's had rheumatoid arthritis for ten years, "dismiss nutrition, other than to say it is important to eat balanced meals and not to become overweight. But personally, I find that whenever I eat a lot of sugar products I will feel pain in one or more joints. So I try not to indulge my sweet tooth too often. And although I believe it is important to follow a doctor's advice, ultimately I am the judge of what is best for my body, because I know my body better than anyone else does." Her doctor is helping her dramatically, she tells us, through a very effective treatment combining the anti-cancer drug **Methotrexate** with prednisone and **Naprosyn**. Excluding certain foods from her diet is something helpful that she can do for herself.

Nearly half of the 1,051 participants in our Arthritis Survey—495 individuals, or 47 percent of the group—say they have changed the way they eat because of arthritis. A few others made a change because of some other health problem. "After my heart attack," reports a retired executive from Michigan with a twenty-year history of osteoarthritis, "I lowered my cholesterol and fat intake. I eat less red meat, more fish and chicken. This seems to have helped the arthritis, too."

Does nutrition play a role in arthritis care? The short answer is: *Yes, it does.* But the full answer—the one that addresses your surprise or pleasure or disgust at the very idea of a nutritional approach to arthritis; the one that explores the issue with awareness of the hundreds of "arthritis diets" laying false claim to a cure; and the one that serves up the fruits of our participants' experience as specific information for your use—that answer will take the rest of this chapter to explain.

Nutrition's Role in Arthritis

The word *nutrition* is a shorthand way of saying many different things. When we state that nutrition plays a role in arthritis care, we have three definitions in mind: (1) your *general ap-*

proach to diet, whether you are extremely health-conscious or an avowed "junk food junkie"; (2) the *amount* you eat, whether that makes you overweight or undernourished; and (3) the *specific food items* you may try to avoid or consume in quantity, because they either aggravate or ameliorate your arthritis pain. As you will see, some survey participants have succeeded in making themselves feel better by adopting a more healthful, well-balanced diet, by losing weight, by identifying certain foods as friend or foe, and by combining two or three of these approaches. Overall, the changes in their eating habits add up to a more healthful, sensible diet that their families can enjoy with them.

The participants who have eased their arthritis pain by changing their food habits include people with osteoarthritis and rheumatoid arthritis, many of whom had been seriously afflicted for years and had already undergone a wide variety of advanced treatments, from "second-line" drugs such as penicillamine and gold injections to joint-replacement surgery.

It is more than likely that you, too, can benefit from a change in diet.

Conflicting, Confusing Claims

If doctors have been taciturn on the subject of nutrition (and they have), self-styled experts have more than made up for medicine's silence by generating dozens of diets and dietary theories about arthritis. The result, our survey participants report, is mass confusion. Even those participants who are *receptive* to the help nutrition may bring are frustrated by the welter of conflicting opinions. "I have tried to put the suggestions on diet and nutrition which abound in the books and magazines into practice," writes a housewife from New York. "But because much of this information is so contradictory, it is hard to know what is valid and what is not. For just about every group of foods, there is a practitioner who will approve its use, and on the other side of the issue, one who will suggest that it be avoided or eliminated completely.

"Some nutritionists," she continues, "stress the importance of the acid-alkaline or the calcium-phosphorus balance, or balancing the complete body chemistry. Others stress proper food-combining or a raw foods diet. And most nutritionists advise gradually eliminating medications once nutrition therapy is started. I once wanted to try a combination of zinc and manganese supplements I had read about that was supposed to have the same effect as the penicillamine I was taking. But when I described the plan to my doctor, he called the idea quackery and said he could not be responsible for my condition if I went ahead with it, and I did not. As for the diets, I have kept notebooks and charts for myself so I could follow the effects of various ones without losing my mind."

Her perseverance paid off: "Over the years I have worked out a diet plan for myself through trial and error that seems to keep my severe rheumatoid arthritis from getting worse."

What the Doctor Ordered

Although about half of our participants heard *nothing* from their doctors about nutrition, several hundred did get *some* advice, even if it was just a casual suggestion to lose weight, or to try to eat more fiber or less salt. Here's a summary of what our participants were told.

Advice	Number of Participants Given This Advice
Nothing (no advice) / "There is no connection."	583*
"Avoid fats." / "Eat more greens." / Other specific dos and don'ts	146
"Eat a well balanced diet." / "Get proper nourishment."	112
"Lose weight." / "Don't gain weight."	95

*These are numbers of participants, not the numbers of doctors who advised them. Many participants heard the same advice (or lack of it) from several doctors. Thus, the 583 participants who report that their doctors told them nothing about nutrition may be referring to several thousand physicians.

It's not hard to understand why the most common advice is no advice. Most medical doctors have little or no training in nutrition and are hard put to offer such counsel. They could, of course, *refer* their patients to experts on nutrition, and some of them do, but most M.D.s don't see any reason to refer—because they don't see any connection between nutrition and arthritis. Some of them are prejudiced against nutritional approaches as a result of watching their patients try faddish and even exploitative diets, to no avail. And, since medical research has ignored the role of nutrition in arthritis until very recently (see Chapter 12), doctors have felt justified in ignoring it, too. Doctors' no-comment stance on nutrition evoked lots of comments from our participants, however. Here's a sample.

A retired graphic artist from Florida: "Doctors avoid talking about nutrition, and very often, when questioned, will just snicker."

A Naval officer from California: "Doctors don't give such information. One has to beg or force this data."

A retired college professor from Minnesota: "I have learned that rarely does an M.D. know much about nutrition."

An archaeologist from Tennessee: "Most know less about this than I do."

A former research chemist from Pennsylvania: "I don't think there is enough known about the relationship between nutrition and arthritis. Most doctors seem to know very little about nutrition. I would like to know what foods are hurting me and what foods would help my condition."

The bulk of the specific dietary advice from doctors, such as it was, did not relate to arthritis per se, but to improving our participants' general health or to applying a nutritional solution to some other health problem they had, whether it was high cholesterol ("Eat fewer eggs.") or high blood pressure ("Stay away from salt.").

The Importance of a Well-Balanced Diet

Many of our participants and the doctors who advised them stressed the importance of a well-balanced diet. But *well-balanced diet*, like *proper nutrition*, is a vague term that leaves too much unsaid. After all, the diet that was long synonymous with good living in the United States—full of meats, whole milk, and lavish desserts—was well balanced. But now it turns up unhealthy on several counts, and gets blamed for a variety of unwanted conditions that are all too prevalent in this country, such as obesity and clogged arteries.

While it seems obvious that anyone stands to benefit from a well-balanced diet, people with arthritis need to take *extra care* to eat well, because the illness creates its own special obstacles to good nutrition. For example, you may find, as nearly two hundred of our participants report, that pain often interferes with your food shopping or cooking. Nausea and other gut reactions to medications may kill your appetite, while *requiring* you to eat something each time you take a pill. And there is evidence that arthritis, especially rheumatoid arthritis, interferes with the way your body absorbs nutrients from foods. Indeed, doctors at the University of Alabama's Spain Rehabilitation Center found that twenty-seven of thirty-eight hospitalized patients with rheumatoid arthritis were malnourished, and that the malnutrition *alone* made these individuals fare worse in the long run than their peers who also had rheumatoid arthritis. What's more, several arthritis medications can rob your body of one or more vitamins and minerals. (See Chapter 15 for specific drug–nutrient interactions.)

The details of a healthful well-balanced diet are spelled out in our Arthritis Survey Diet and Thirty-Day Meal Plan (see Chapter 14). A registered dietitian worked with us to create this diet. It combines our participants' successful strategies with the best available medical wisdom on general nutrition, and it translates the information into tasteful menus that you can prepare easily—with the least amount of peeling or dicing and the shortest possible time at the stove.

"I can't prove that nutrition directly helps or relieves arthritis," concedes a homesteader from Wisconsin. "I simply believe a healthy dietary program has given me a basis for good health—even with some arthritis."

There are several other benefits of healthful eating that our participants enjoy. "I get a better sense of well-being from eating fresh, well-balanced meals," says the coordinator of an antipoverty agency in Maryland, "and this helps to counteract the depression and anger that often accompany arthritis." A former manager and lecturer for Weight Watchers in Delaware writes, "A light diet of fruits, vegetables, and seafood, chicken, turkey, or veal makes me feel more alert and in control." And a librarian from West Virginia finds, "When I eat well-balanced meals low in salt and full of vegetables, fruit, and fiber, I feel much more active and happy."

The (Relative) Value of Weight Loss

Excess body weight undoubtedly puts an extra burden on joints already stressed by arthritis. Most participants who adopted a weight-loss diet to take the load off their joints were extremely pleased with the outcome. "My doctor told me to lose thirty-five pounds or there was no sense in my seeing him for treatment," says a thirty-seven-year-old insurance agent from New York. "He encouraged me along the difficult road, and I have managed to keep my weight down because I know I am being helped. Diet and weight maintenance go hand in hand with my arthritis. When I was heavier, I felt more uncomfortable. I did not realize then how the extra weight was pulling on my spine."

A few participants bemoan the fact that they have been *un*able to shed excess weight, and even wonder what's the use of trying. "My doctor insists I lose weight," writes a lab technician from New Jersey. "This is easier said than done, because if I could, I would. Nobody likes to be fat. It makes sense to take the pressure off my knees by losing weight, but there is no such pressure on my finger joints—and look how they ache."

True, there is a limit to what weight loss can do for arthritis pain.* It seems most helpful for the weight-bearing joints— the spine, legs, and feet. But weight loss has also improved conditions in the *non*-weight-bearing joints of some of our participants. This may have come about because the dietary changes they made to cut calories removed some offending foods from their dinner plates and replaced them with others that may have had positive effects. A case in point is the substitution of fish for red meat.

Before the fact, avoiding excess weight may help people avoid osteoarthritis of the knees, according to doctors at the Boston University Arthritis Center who studied the connection between obesity and arthritis.

Foods to Avoid

Food allergies are sometimes at the root of arthritis. The fire
in the joints turns out to be an allergic reaction to some food—
milk, for example—and cutting the food out of the diet
amounts to curing the disease. The arthritis goes away, but the
allergy remains, and drinking milk again will bring the arthritis back. Although true food allergies can masquerade as arthritis, such cases are thought to be quite rare. A more common
phenomenon, observed by roughly 10 percent of our survey
group, is food *intolerance* or *sensitivity.* If you are sensitive to
certain foods, they may trigger pain when you eat them, even
though your body does not mount an allergic reaction to them.
It would be great to avoid pain by avoiding those foods, but
how do you learn which ones are the culprits?

One way is to seek them out systematically—by keeping
a food diary, in which you write down everything that goes
down, and a pain diary, where you track the course of your
arthritis pain. By comparing the two records, you may be able
to discover telling patterns. Suppose, for instance, that you are
sensitive to tomatoes. Then each mention of tomatoes in the
food diary should match up with a note about extra discomfort
in the pain diary. But, as you might imagine, this kind of record
keeping is *a lot* of work. And even if you are meticulous with
your notes, you may be stymied by other factors that blur the
relationships between food and pain. Was it the tomato salad
on Tuesday that gave you grief on Wednesday? Or was it the
fact that you exercised too vigorously? And wasn't that the
night you didn't get enough rest?

Another way is to take advantage of our participants' findings. Since many of them agree on the identity of certain food
troublemakers, we can post a "most *un*wanted" list of items.
You could start by avoiding or cutting down on your consumption of one or more of these and see how you feel as a result.
It will likely take several weeks for you to notice any difference
in the way you feel. In scientific studies of dietary changes for
people with arthritis, results have followed within one to six
weeks, depending on the kind of changes made.

Beef and other red meat

More people in our survey avoid red meat than any other single staple. It's not that all 155 of these individuals are vegetarians, since most of them do eat fish and fowl. Some avoid red meat simply because cutting out the beef enables them to cut down on calories and consume less fat and cholesterol. Others have found that eating meat aggravates their pain. "Red meat seems to increase pain and stiffness," writes a homemaker from Michigan, "so I have virtually eliminated it from my diet. I eat more fruits and vegetables, and have increased my intake of calcium-rich foods, such as low-fat milk. I wish more research were being done into the relationship between diet (especially the chemicals used in growing and processing foods, the hormones given to animals, etc.) and the level of pain and crippling. I don't think these things cause arthritis, but they may exacerbate the symptoms."

Some participants discovered the aggravating effect of meat by accident. "My daughters are vegetarians," says an accounting clerk from New York. "This past year I've followed a mainly vegetarian diet, and I find I feel better and seem to have less arthritis pain."

"I decreased my red meat intake at the suggestion of a nurse," reports a program secretary from Florida. "I have less swelling of my knees and toes since that time."

A photojournalist from Massachusetts says her medicines made her give up meat: "Since I started taking anti-inflammatories, I have been unable to eat meat. My idea of bliss used to be a totally fatless, medium-rare roast beef sandwich on super caraway rye. When I threw up seven times after eating one, I began to catch on that something had changed in my system."

Switching to a strict vegetarian, or vegan, diet proved helpful to a group of Swedish men and women with rheumatoid arthritis who took part in a diet study. They learned how to cook vegetarian cuisine from Dr. Lars Sköldstam and his staff at Sweden's Sundsvalls Hospital, and they stayed on the diet for four months. After that many weeks without meat, twelve of the twenty patients said they felt better, although by

Dr. Skoldstam's more rigid criteria, only eleven (55 percent) had really improved. "Many patients with mild or moderate rheumatoid arthritis benefit from eating the vegan diet," Dr. Skoldstam concluded in the *Scandinavian Journal of Rheumatology* (1986), "in that they will feel subjectively better. However, the diet does not seem to significantly suppress the rheumatoid disease. . . ." This is high praise for vegetarianism, since most prescription drugs for arthritis *also* make people feel better *without* squelching the disease.

Sugar . . . and sweets in general

A sweet tooth is an added handicap for a person with arthritis, claim 148 of our survey participants. "When my arthritis was at its worst," recalls a twenty-eight-year-old registered nurse from Texas, "the main thing that aggravated it was sugar." Many others echoed the same theme, including this magazine editor from New Jersey: "I avoid processed sugar in high concentration because it seems to make me flare." And a retired teacher from California says, "I changed my eating habits many years ago because of high cholesterol. Now I find that if I go off my diet and eat sweets, my fingers become swollen and inflamed."

Fat and fried foods

Public enemy number three in our participants' estimation is fat, forsworn by 135 of them. "After seeing a rheumatologist and an internist, I went to a nutritionist who changed my diet and eased the pain," writes an aluminum welder from upstate New York. "I eat nothing fried. I cook vegetables in a wok with a small amount of oil. My fish is baked or broiled."

Please be sure not to throw out the good fats with the bad. Tuna and salmon, for example, are fatty fish, but theirs is the good kind, or highly unsaturated fat, which has been shown in scientific studies to help control joint inflammation for some people with arthritis. Bad fat is the saturated kind found in butter, palm oil, and untrimmed meat—the fat condemned by the 1988 Surgeon General's Report on Nutrition and Health.

To find out about the amount of fat in many of the foods you eat, just read the labels. It takes a little time to get familiar with the format, but the food labeling required by the Food and Drug Administration is the most accessible and reliable source of information about what's in what you eat. The label tells you, among other things, the number of calories per serving and the amount of protein, carbohydrate, and fat in the food. These amounts are given in "grams per serving," and the fewer grams of fat, the better. (A gram is the metric system's equivalent of $\frac{1}{28}$ of an ounce.)*

Salt

Salt aggravates pain or swelling for ninety-eight survey participants. "Salt is one of the worst things for arthritis," maintains a corporate vice-president from Iowa. To cut it down or out of your diet, you not only have to stop using the saltshaker at the table but leave this ingredient out of your cooking, and avoid it when you shop, the way this masonry contractor from Pennsylvania does. "I eat low-sodium-chloride foods, low- or no-fat foods, low sugar. I buy low-sodium, low-fat cheese. When my knee is most inflamed, eating foods that are high in salt or refined sugar will intensify the arthritis and prolong the pain."

A Pennsylvania researcher finds that salt exacerbates the side effects of her medication. "I avoid salt because prednisone encourages water retention and swelling, and the low-sodium diet reduces the swelling." Since it is the sodium in salt that causes most salt-related problems, look for the sodium content in foods when you read labels.

---

*Food labels let you calculate the number of calories from fat in any food, if you remember that fat gives you 9 calories per gram. The label on a quart of skim milk, a very low-fat food, shows that it contains 1 gram of fat per serving. That's 9 calories worth of fat in each glass of skim milk. Whole milk, by comparison, contains 8 grams of fat per serving, or 72 calories' worth of fat. And the fat is what gives a glass of whole milk almost twice as many calories as there are in a glass of skim milk.

Caffeine

Of the fifty-six participants who avoid caffeine, twelve mention coffee in particular, and eight single out tea. Other sources of caffeine are cola-type sodas and chocolate. If you are really sensitive to caffeine, watch your drugstore purchases, too, since several over-the-counter medicines, including **Anacin**, **Excedrin**, and **Vanquish**, contain caffeine. A retired aerospace engineer from New York, who once drank seven to ten cups of coffee a day, made several helpful changes in his diet: "I quit drinking so much coffee and began avoiding the nightshades [see pages 245–246] as much as possible. After I started on this diet, the pain diminished and has mostly disappeared. But two or three cups of coffee will bring the pain back to my hips within twelve hours.

"My younger brother has arthritis in his hips, knees, and hands," the engineer continues. "He was in the same environment and business as I was. He usually spends a month with us each summer on board our boat, eating our diet, and feels and acts much better. But I can't convince him to change his diet."

Scientists at Washington State University found that caffeine makes people lose calcium in their urine faster than they usually do. Since the health of your bones may already be threatened by arthritis itself or some of the drugs used to treat it, *losing* calcium is a bad idea. This study suggests a rationale for switching to decaffeinated brews.

Dairy products

Adding the number of participants who avoid dairy products altogether (nineteen), or milk alone (sixteen), or cheese alone (fifteen), gives a total of fifty individuals. One, a student and math tutor from Washington, was forced off milk by her inability to digest milk sugar—a condition known as lactose intolerance. But several participants blame dairy products for arthritis pain. A California waitress finds, "If I eat any dairy product or calcium-rich food, I become immobile! My fingers and ankles swell and I cannot walk. I worry about osteoporosis, but the arthritis pain is too great if I eat these foods. I never noticed any milk sensitivity before four years ago. And as long as I don't drink it, I remain fairly pain free and mobile." The same is true for a few people whose stories have been told in the medical literature because their severe chronic arthritis all but vanished when they banished milk from their diet. (See Chapter 12.)

Cheese avoidance often has as much to do with the fat and salt in cheese as the milk it contains. Likewise, the four additional participants who avoid ice cream may be offended by the fat, the sugar, the cream/milk, or all three.

Nightshade vegetables

Although hundreds of survey participants advocate eating more vegetables, forty-eight steer clear of one or all vegetables in the family known as the nightshades—tomatoes, white potatoes, eggplant, and bell peppers of all colors. The black pepper used for seasoning is *not* part of this problematic family, but paprika *is*.

"I do not eat any of the nightshade vegetables," writes a retired dressmaker from New York. "If I do, I get red hot and swollen knuckles on both hands. It takes a week or two for this to clear up." Some participants sacrificed these foods willingly, while others mention how much they miss eating the produce from their summer gardens. "I eliminated the nightshade vegetables, which helped relieve the discomfort," reports a sales associate from New Jersey, "but it is very difficult cooking for my Italian family without tomatoes, peppers, and eggplant."

The 48 people in our survey who avoid nightshades account for about 5 percent of the entire group of 1,051 participants. This statistic is in line with the estimate made by Dr. Norman Childers, who first observed the irritating effect of nightshades on his own arthritis and later concluded that only 5 to 10 percent of all people with arthritis could be helped by dropping these foods from their diet. If you are one, you must be especially careful to read labels on prepared foods, from soup to chips, because flakes of tomatoes, starch from potatoes, and pieces of peppers can crop up *anywhere.* It may take six weeks for you to notice an improvement on a no-nightshades diet. And remember that tobacco is *also* a nightshade, or solanaceous plant, so you can't smoke it or chew it.

Pork and smoked or processed meats

Whether they mention pork by name or make a blanket rejection of smoked or processed meats such as bacon and bologna, thirty-seven survey participants stay away from them. Pork is a pain-inducer for some, while others find it too fatty. Smoking and processing add carcinogens to these insults. Nitrates, which often show up on lunch-meat labels as preservatives, were found to aggravate some people's arthritis in a food-allergy study at the University of Florida.

Alcohol

Several of the thirty-four participants who curtailed or cut out alcohol consumption say they understand the temptation to drown out pain by having a few drinks. The irony, they say, is that the alcohol can actually make things worse. "Alcohol makes my joints swell," writes a visiting nurse from New Hampshire. "I avoid alcohol and foods that will upset my stomach, since the medicines do enough damage."

Another reason to avoid alcohol is that heavy drinking (more than two drinks per day) can weaken your bones. Indeed, the Arthritis Foundation now warns that alcohol may contribute to osteoporosis.

Junk food

With deference to those who believe a balanced meal is a fast-food special in each hand, thirty-two participants gave up junk food for more healthful diets featuring lots of fresh fruits and vegetables.

Starches

Highly processed starches such as white bread, white flour, and white rice fell by the way for thirty-one participants, who replaced them with whole-wheat bread and flour and brown rice. Most of them were after the fiber that whole-grain products preserve. Some find that the fiber works better than taking a laxative for the constipating effects of various arthritis medications.

An additional sixteen participants avoid any and all wheat products, including cereals and pasta, because they find these foods aggravate pain and inflammation.

Additives and preservatives

Do you ever feel you need to study chemistry to understand the ingredients in foods? Twenty-nine of our participants studiously avoid the chemicals put in foods to give them longer shelf lives. Colorings are also suspect for some. "U.S. yellow #4 makes my joints swell," says a receptionist from Washington. "I avoid all medicines colored with this. I eat a high-protein, high-fiber diet, avoiding grease and saturated fats, and find this gives me increased general health and enhanced response to pain medications and anti-inflammatories."

Acid foods

Twenty-three survey participants avoid foods with a high acid content, such as tomatoes and vinegar. "I find acid-heavy foods produce a reaction and increase my pain level," writes the manager of an automobile dealership in Massachusetts, "so I try to monitor my acid intake."

Another seventeen participants specify citrus fruits, high in citric acid, as items to avoid. "By trial and error, by eliminating certain foods over a period of more than two years," reports a retired bookkeeper from Florida, "I have found that I must avoid members of the nightshade family, as well as wheat and citrus."

Chocolate

Chocolate stands in a class by itself. In addition to the 148 participants who avoid sweets in general, 21 must make it a point to turn down chocolate. Chocolate is not only sweet but high in fat, and also contains caffeine, so it's hard to say which element is the offending one. "I try to avoid an overload of chocolate," says a homemaker from Michigan, "which I've found tends to make my hands and fingers feel stiff and achy."

Purines

If you've ever been told that diet plays no role in arthritis, you've probably also heard the tag line, "except for gout." Gout is the one form of arthritis that everyone knows can be controlled by diet. The pain of gout is caused by crystals that accumulate inside the joints. The crystals come from uric acid, and much uric acid comes from eating certain foods, such as liver and kidney, and drinking certain drinks, such as beer and wine. If you have gout, you can help keep the crystals from lodging in your joints—and protect yourself from painful attacks—by avoiding foods that contain *purines,* which break down to form uric acid in your body. Thirteen of our survey participants have gout in addition to rheumatoid or osteoarthritis, and sixteen say they avoid foods with a high purine content. It is ironic that anchovies, herring, and sardines, which may be so beneficial for people with other forms of arthritis, can actually aggravate gout because of their high purine content. Other types of fish, however, have no more purines than equivalent portions of chicken, turkey, or nonorgan meats.

A List of Foods Avoided by
Our Participants

Item	Number of Participants Who Avoid It
Red meat	155
Sugar	148
Fats	135
Salt	98
Caffeine	56
Nightshades	48
Alcohol	34
Junk food	32
Starches:	
Refined (white) flour and rice	31
All wheat products from cereal to pasta	16
Additives and preservatives	29
Acid foods	23
Citrus	17
Pork	20
Smoked or processed meats	17
Dairy products:	
All	19
Milk	16
Cheese	15
Ice cream	4
Soda (colas/carbonated beverages)	16
Purines (liver, etc.)	16
Mixes, prepared or processed foods	20
Canned vegetables	11
Spices	14
Eggs	13
Yeast or fermented foods	6

Having listed the foods most likely to offend, let us reiterate that these sensitivities are a personal matter. "I do believe in my case that there is a correlation between food allergy and a flare-up of pain with my rheumatoid arthritis," writes a thirty-two-year-old registered nurse from South Dakota who sees an allergy specialist because she also has asthma. "But even if arthritis is food-related for everyone, not everyone is allergic to the same food substances. Milk, eggs, and chocolate cause my problem. Someone else could be allergic to peanuts!"

Foods to Favor

Just as they have learned to avoid certain substances, many of our participants seek out other foods for their good features, from high-fiber and low-calorie content to extra bounties of vitamins, minerals, and essential fatty acids. They choose some items as more healthful substitutes for others they must avoid, such as eating chicken or turkey *instead of* red meat. Perhaps even more interesting are the foods they pile in because they see them as a form of treatment, whether it's calcium disguised as a glass of skim milk or an anti-inflammatory that looks like fillet of sole. Here are the items our participants eat more of, and the reasons why.

Vegetables

Green, leafy, raw, and *fresh* are the words most commonly used by the 204 survey participants who have added more vegetables to their diet. "My doctor told me that nutrition *can* help with arthritis," reports a retired accountant from California whose rheumatologist is treating her with a combination of experimental and standard treatments. "I eat more leafy green vegetables, more fruit, and fewer dairy products. After paying more attention to my eating habits, I find a marked difference in the inflammation of my joints."

Fruit

Fresh fruits follow right behind the vegetables in our survey, with 174 participants eating more of them, or drinking more fruit juice, or both. "I notice a lot of what I eat depends on how I feel on certain days," says an Idaho homemaker who has cut out fats, curtailed sugar, and now eats more raw vegetables and fresh fruit. "The fresh fruits are so refreshing when you don't feel so perky."

Fruits, like vegetables, are also a good source of dietary fiber. An additional forty-two participants say they eat more high-fiber foods now, including fruits, vegetables, and whole grains.

Fish

Fish never figured as a really popular food for many Americans, until recently, when its heart-helping and anti-inflammatory effects captured headlines. "I try to eat more fish," writes a personnel specialist from Illinois, one of eighty-nine survey participants who has made this change. Why? "I read an article that suggested the oils from cold-water fish have a beneficial effect on some forms of arthritis." There is indeed a great deal of research interest now in fish-heavy diets and in dietary supplements of fish oil. (See Chapter 12 for research on diets, and Chapter 11 for studies regarding fish-oil supplements for arthritis.)

"My husband and I are vegetarians," says an executive secretary from California, "but we have recently added fish to our diet because of current information."

Although fish has always been a healthful, if unpopular, alternative to meat protein, the big news in fish now is the high content of omega-3 fatty acids in certain cold-water varieties, such as Norway sardines, Atlantic mackerel, herring, salmon, and Greenland halibut. One of our participants, a retired airplane pilot from Alaska, reports that he has been following this hot new trend for more than thirty-five years: "I got off sugar and salt in 1953," he writes. "As a bush pilot I often had trouble getting green or fresh vegetables, but I ate a high percentage of fish, heavy on omega-3—lots of king salmon—and the red meat of wild game like moose and caribou." Omega-3 fatty acids, which are thought to protect the heart and relieve inflamed joints, can also be found in the wild-growing green vegetable called purslane, and in several kinds of beans, as well as walnuts and chestnuts. Two of our participants say they have begun to eat more tofu, or soybean curd, which is yet another omega-3 source.

Chicken and turkey

Fowl is a fine low-fat alternative to beef and other meats, particularly if you remove its skin before cooking. Sixty-one survey participants say they eat more chicken and turkey now.

Milk

Milk, especially low-fat milk, is the favorite way of getting more calcium for thirty-seven participants. It's also the best drink to take with many medications, including aspirin, because it can protect your stomach from some drug side effects. Another five participants eat more yogurt, and seven prefer to get their calcium from cheese.

Calcium-rich foods

Not counting the more-milk drinkers, another twenty-two participants tell us that they seek out calcium-rich foods to ward off osteoporosis. Participants who have taken prednisone and other steroids are particularly worried about thinning bones as a side effect of the drugs. And arthritis alone can do a fair degree of bone damage at selected sites.

We tend to think of dairy products as the prime providers of calcium, and most of them are, but sardines or salmon (eaten with the bones), and oysters are also rich sources. So are selected vegetables, such as spinach, collard greens, and broccoli.

Water

Whether it comes from the tap or an imported bottle, twenty-two participants advocate drinking more water because it performs so many vital functions, from aiding digestion to helping the kidneys eliminate the end products of various arthritis drugs.

A List of Foods Our Participants Favor

Item	Number of Participants Who Eat More of It
Vegetables	204
Fruit	174
Fish	89
Fowl	61
Fiber	42
Milk	37
Whole grains	34
Calcium-rich foods	22
Water	22
Protein, including *lean* meats	14
Garlic	7

Summary of Nutrition Advice from Survey Participants

Although opinions vary widely on the subject of nutrition and arthritis, our survey participants' experience supports these ten recommendations.

1.   At the very least, you may improve your overall health by reevaluating your eating habits and trying to improve your diet to make it more nutritious.

2.   Take care to avoid faddish or extreme diets that may leave you open to vitamin deficiencies or other nutrition problems.

3.   Question any diet or any advisor who urges you to stop taking your prescribed medications.

4.   Don't expect a lot of nutrition advice from your doctors, but do inform them of any significant change in diet that you plan to make.

5.   If you are overweight and are troubled by arthritis in your weight-bearing joints, you can likely gain mobility and comfort by losing the extra pounds.

6.   If you decide to lose weight, do it slowly, by adopting a more healthful style of eating, rather than following a "crash" diet for a quick loss.

7.   Try to discover your own food sensitivities by eliminating some of the food items voted by our participants as the most likely to be irritating. The top five offenders are red meat, sugar, fat, salt, and caffeine.

8.   Try eating more of the foods our participants find the most beneficial. The five top favorites are vegetables, fruits, fish, fowl, and high-fiber foods such as whole-grain breads and brown rice.

9.   Choose fresh foods over prepared items that are smoked, canned, or highly processed.

10.   Read all you can, think it over carefully, experiment cautiously, and observe yourself to prove the value of any dietary measures you take.

14

THE ARTHRITIS SURVEY™ DIET AND THIRTY-DAY MEAL PLAN

■ *A sensible new diet based on participants' experience and current research* ■ *General dietary guidelines* ■ *Specific thirty-day menu plan with recipes*

The healthful diet laid out in this chapter is a blending of our survey participants' successful experiments with nutrition and the exciting new research that indicates an important role for dietary changes in the treatment of arthritis. If you follow the plan, you can be sure that you're heeding your doctor's advice to "Eat well balanced meals." You'll also have the kind of low-fat, high-carbohydrate diet that is endorsed by researchers and physicians for the prevention or control of heart disease, diabetes, and certain forms of cancer. You'll be getting a rich supply of the fish oils that have been shown to control arthritis symptoms. And, although the diet is not a calorie-counting, weight-loss program, you'll find that you can indeed lose excess weight by following it.

Nutritionist Kathleen Pratt, M.S., R.D., of Olympia, Washington, worked with us to translate the survey findings on nutrition into the meal plans you see here. The recipes she created are all designed for ease of preparation, too, so that you don't have to stand and fuss for long, or do a lot of peeling, chopping, or other activities that might strain your hands.

We present the Arthritis Survey Diet in two forms—guidelines and specifics. The guidelines sketch the basic principles and give suggestions for putting them into practice. The specifics are just that—thirty days' worth of detailed menus and recipes that you can follow to the letter or modify to meet your own particular needs.

General Guidelines

Eat less fat. Foods that are low in fat generally have fewer calories and are more healthful and nutritious. Fruits, for example, contain almost no fat. Choose naturally low-fat items over fatty foods and snacks. If you drink milk, make it skim milk. Always look for low-fat alternatives to things you normally eat, such as light margarine (Imperial and Fleischmann's are two brand names you can look for), light sour cream (Land O Lakes makes one), low-calorie mayonnaise (such as Hellmann's or Kraft), and tuna fish packed in water instead of oil. Try to reduce the amount of fat (oil, shortening, butter, or margarine) that you use in cooking.

Cook smart. Broiling, baking, poaching, and grilling are all low-fat cooking techniques. Even stir-frying uses less fat than pan-frying. And a microwave oven, if you have one, can cook many items in a fat-free way. If you must fry, try using a nonstick pan or a cooking spray instead of butter or oil. To keep as many vitamins in your vegetables as possible, steam or microwave them instead of boiling in water. You can also sauté vegetables in a small amount of water and oil, or in a low-salt broth.

Eat more vegetables. Eat fresh ones especially, and raw vegetables in salads. Try to eat at least one meatless, vegetable/pasta dinner per week. If you wash carrots carefully, you can save yourself the aggravation of peeling them.

Eat less red meat. Substitute poultry and fish for meat as often as possible. When you do prepare red meat, select the leanest cuts and remove the visible fat before you cook it. Avoid pork altogether, if possible.

Eat more fish. Aim for a minimum of three fish dinners per week and at least two fish lunches. If you can't get fresh fish, look for frozen fish without breading. Pick the varieties that have the highest content of omega-3 fatty acids, such as Norway sardines, Atlantic mackerel, lake trout, Atlantic herring, albacore tuna, anchovies, Atlantic salmon, bluefish, pink salmon, and Greenland halibut. When you buy canned tuna, choose water-packed, as the oil used in canning is vegetable oil, which contains no omega-3 fatty acids.

Eat more poultry. When you prepare chicken for cooking, remove the skin from the individual pieces, since the skin contains much of the fat. Then prevent the meat from drying out by cooking in a covered dish or using a sauce for basting. If you roast chicken, remove the skin as you carve.

Cut down on sodium in general, and salt in particular. You can drastically reduce your sodium intake by cutting down on lunch meats, salty snacks, and prepared processed soups and sauces. In your own cooking, try substituting various herbs and spices for salt, such as rosemary on chicken, sage on cooked carrots, nutmeg on spinach, basil on peas or green beans, and fresh-squeezed lemon juice on broccoli. When you shop, look for low-salt alternatives to foods you usually buy, including low-sodium or low-salt cheeses, snack crackers, soy sauce, tomato sauce, and tomato paste.

Use sugar in moderation. You can reduce the amount of sugar in most dessert recipes without hurting the taste at all. Sugar substitutes are easily obtained, if you crave them, but you may find that you *enjoy* the taste of low-sugar or no-sugar-added jams and jellies, and canned fruit packed in its own juice instead of heavy syrup.

Eat lots of fiber. The complex carbohydrates that have a high-fiber content, as well as important vitamins and minerals, are whole-grain breads and cereals, fruits, vegetables, and dried beans and peas.

Don't skip breakfast. Your first meal of the day, ideally, should supply about one-quarter of your daily requirement for calories and nutrients. If you take medication with meals, a good breakfast may help you minimize some of the drug's side effects.

Learn your own food sensitivities. Many people with arthritis find that certain foods aggravate their symptoms. Chocolate is the culprit for some, while others avoid citrus fruits or the nightshade vegetables—tomatoes, white potatoes, green peppers, and eggplant. Try to determine whether you have a food sensitivity (Chapter 13 tells you how), and then avoid that food at all costs. The recipes in this section offer alternatives for most ingredients that our participants singled out as problem foods.

Read labels. Let the rich trove of information on food-package labels lead you to the most nutritious items. Since ingredients are always listed in order of their concentration, with the most abundant ones first, you'd do well to pass up foods that list sugar or salt among the top three. You can also rely on the labels to alert you to hidden enemies in prepared or processed foods. Potato starch, for example, shows up in more items than you would imagine. Also check the protein, carbohydrate, and fat contents, which are listed as grams per serving, and select items that have the least fat. Low-fat foods are lower in calories, too, because fat contains more than twice as many calories per gram as protein or carbohydrate.

Make it easy on yourself. Look through the frozen foods at your grocery for nutritious convenience items that you can store for a day when you are unable to cook. Frozen vegetables are almost as good as fresh, and come to you already washed, peeled, and diced. If you can't comfortably crush a clove of garlic, by all means buy a jar of peeled, chopped garlic or use one-eighth of a teaspoon of garlic powder for each clove mentioned in a recipe.

Drink lots of water, milk, and juice. Everyone needs about eight glasses of water a day, and medications may require you to drink even more than that. Milk (skim) is generally considered the best chaser for many arthritis drugs because of its stomach-coating action. Try to have at least two glasses a day for the calcium milk provides—provided, of course, that dairy products sit well with you. If citrus is your enemy, you can still drink other fruit juices such as apple, grape, apricot, and pear. If you find caffeine irritating, stick to decaffeinated coffee and herbal tea. Postum (made from bran, wheat, and molasses) is another caffeine-free alternative in the hot-beverage department. As for alcohol, several participants report they must avoid it altogether. Alcohol's effect on the stomach is reason enough to skip it if you take aspirin or related anti-inflammatory drugs, not to mention the many other problems associated with drinking. A couple of our recipes call for small amounts of sherry or wine in sauces, but these are added before heating, so that the alcohol cooks away.

Enjoy your meals. This is neither a starvation diet nor a fad diet. For example, although we say whole-wheat bread is the best choice for toast or sandwiches, our breakfast suggestions include English muffins, bagels, and biscuits. You need to eat nutritious foods, but you also need to have some variety and enjoy your meals within sensible guidelines. A very strict limited diet is impossible to stick with for long, and our goal is to give you a lifetime plan.

The Arthritis Survey Diet: Thirty-Day Meal Plan

Recipes for each day's specials (marked with an asterisk) are included right below the meal suggestions. If you read through the whole plan, you'll see we've tried to anticipate and use up leftovers where possible. Snack and dessert items are listed at the end of the chapter. Unless otherwise stated, the recipes serve four—so your family or friends can enjoy sharing these meals with you.

Day 1

Breakfast *Oatmeal with raisins; whole-wheat toast with no-sugar-added jam; skim milk; fruit juice*

Lunch *Wild rice and chicken salad*; whole-wheat roll; melon slices; skim milk (juice)*

Dinner *Poached fish with snow peas*; Steamed broccoli, carrots, and onions; baked (sweet) potato with light margarine, plain yogurt, or light sour cream*

Wild rice and chicken salad

⅔ cup light mayonnaise
⅓ cup skim milk
2 T lemon juice
 (optional)
¼ t dried tarragon
3 cups cooked cubed
 chicken
⅓ cup finely sliced
 scallions

3 cups cooked wild rice
1 (8 oz.) can sliced water
 chestnuts, drained
½ t pepper
1 cup seedless green
 grapes, halved
1 cup unsalted
 cashews

Blend mayonnaise, milk, lemon juice, and tarragon, and set aside.
In large bowl, combine chicken, scallions, wild rice, water chestnuts, and pepper.
Stir in mayonnaise mixture until blended.
Cover and refrigerate for two to three hours.
Just before serving, fold in grapes and cashews.

Poached fish with snow peas

2 T dry sherry
2 T light (low-salt) soy
 sauce
½ t grated fresh ginger
1½ lb. fish fillets

2 scallions, split and cut
 into 2-inch sections
16 snow peas
1½ T toasted sesame
 seeds†

Prepare sauce by combining sherry, soy sauce, and ginger in small bowl.
Place fish in 10-inch fry pan, cover with scallions, snow peas, and sauce.

---

†To toast sesame seeds, spread them in a pan and bake at 350°F. for 10 to 12 minutes, shaking the pan often to prevent burning.

Cover and cook over medium heat for 10 minutes, or until fish flakes.

Garnish with sesame seeds.

Day 2

Breakfast *English muffin with jam; berries (fresh, or frozen ones defrosted and warmed slightly) served over vanilla yogurt; skim milk (juice)*

Lunch *Tuna with pineapple salad*, served on lettuce leaf as salad, or in pocket (pita) bread as sandwich; celery and carrot sticks; skim milk (juice)*

Dinner *Spaghetti with lean ground beef and tomato sauce or white clam sauce; tossed green salad with creamy vinaigrette dressing*; (whole-wheat) Italian bread*

Tuna with pineapple salad

1 can (20 oz.) crushed, unsweetened pineapple, well drained†
1 can (12 ½ oz.) water-pack tuna, drained‡
½ cup sliced scallions

1 medium red pepper, chopped (optional)
¼ cup light mayonnaise
¼ cup light sour cream
1 ¼ t lemon juice (optional)

In large bowl, combine pineapple, tuna, scallions, and red pepper.

In small bowl, combine remaining ingredients, stirring until smooth.

Add dressing to tuna mixture and toss until well mixed.

Cover and refrigerate at least one hour before serving.

†If you cannot eat citrus fruits, substitute seedless green grapes.
‡Rinsing tuna in a sieve under cold water, then pressing it dry, removes much of the salt added in packing.

Creamy vinaigrette dressing

1 T olive oil
1 T red wine vinegar
1 T fresh lemon juice
(optional)
1 T plain yogurt

1 T water
1 clove garlic, crushed (or
1 t prepared garlic, or
⅛ t garlic salt)
¼ t pepper

Combine all ingredients in a jar with a tight-fitting lid. Shake well, and refrigerate until ready to serve. (The oil may harden when chilled, so shake the jar or stir the dressing before you serve it.)

Day 3

Breakfast   *Frozen waffle with light syrup or pureed fruit; skim milk; fruit juice*

Lunch   *Vegetable and lentil soup*; unsalted wheat crackers; apple or other fresh fruit; skim milk (juice)*

Dinner   *Sliced turkey breast; rice pilaf; steamed carrots; fresh fruit salad*

Vegetable and lentil soup

2 cups lentils
2 t Bac-Os (optional)
1 cup chopped onion†
1 cup chopped celery†
1 cup chopped carrots†
3 T parsley

1 clove garlic, minced
½ t pepper
½ t dried oregano
1 can (1 lb.) or 2 cups
tomato puree‡
2 T vinegar

†If chopping is difficult, use frozen diced vegetables.
‡If you avoid nightshades, substitute chicken broth.

Rinse lentils, drain, and place in soup kettle with 8 cups of water.

Add remaining ingredients except tomato and vinegar. Simmer, covered, for 1½ hours.

Add tomato puree and vinegar, and cook 30 minutes longer.

Day 4

Breakfast *Shredded-wheat cereal with blueberries; bagel with cream cheese; skim milk (juice)*

Lunch *Tuna salad on whole-wheat bread; celery and carrot sticks; canned peaches (in juice); skim milk (juice)*

Dinner *Shrimp with lemon and garlic*; baked (sweet) potato wedges; steamed broccoli, cauliflower, and carrots*

Shrimp with lemon and garlic

2 lbs. raw, peeled,
    deveined shrimp
½ cup light margarine
2 cloves garlic, chopped
¼ cup fresh lemon juice
    (optional)

¼ t pepper
1 T chopped fresh
    parsley (or flakes)

Bring 6 cups water to boiling, add shrimp, bring to boil again, then lower heat and simmer about 1 to 3 minutes until shrimp turn pink. Drain.

Melt the margarine in a skillet, add garlic, and sauté a minute or two.

Add the shrimp, lemon juice, and pepper; sauté about 5 minutes.

Sprinkle with parsley just before serving.

If you have a *microwave oven,* try preparing the dish this way:

In small bowl, cook garlic in margarine on HIGH for 30 seconds.
Stir in lemon juice and pepper.
Arrange shrimp in a single layer in a flat baking dish.
Pour sauce over shrimp and cover with wax paper.
Microwave on HIGH for 6 minutes, stopping once to stir and baste shrimp.
Let stand for 2 minutes. Sprinkle with parsley.

Day 5

Breakfast *Bran muffin with honey; soft-boiled egg; canned pears packed in fruit juice; skim milk*

Lunch *Minestrone soup; crackers with unsalted tops; bagel with light cream cheese; orange or other fresh fruit; skim milk*

Dinner *Baked fish fillets*; stir-fried rice*; steamed green peas; Waldorf salad prepared with low-calorie salad dressing*

Baked fish fillets

2 T light margarine
½ cup slivered almonds
1½ T lemon juice (optional)
½ t onion powder (or powdered mustard)

Dash of pepper
1 t paprika (optional)
1 lb. fish fillets

Melt the margarine in a baking dish, stir in the almonds, and toast them in the margarine in a 350°F. oven until almonds are golden brown.
Add the lemon juice, onion powder, pepper, and paprika.
Arrange fish fillets in the mixture, turning to coat each side.

Bake in 350°F. oven for about 25 minutes, or until fish flakes.

Stir-fried rice

1 onion, chopped
1 green pepper, chopped†
2 cloves garlic, pressed
⅓ cup bouillon or broth
1 egg, slightly beaten
2 cups cooked brown rice (can be made the day before and refrigerated)

1 cup frozen peas and carrots
2 T light (low-salt) soy sauce

In a wok or large fry pan, stir-fry the fresh vegetables in the bouillon until tender.
Push the fresh vegetables aside, add the egg, stirring as it cooks.
Add remaining ingredients.
Heat until peas and carrots are hot.

Day 6

Breakfast   *Cream of Wheat, or Wheatena, with raisins; whole-wheat toast with jam; fruit juice; skim milk*

Lunch   *Turkey with lettuce on whole-wheat bread; skim milk (juice); banana or other fresh fruit*

Dinner   *Vegetable linguine*; fruit salad; French bread*

---

†Nightshade-avoiders can use celery instead of green pepper.

Vegetable linguine

8 oz. linguine or other
pasta, uncooked
4 cups vegetables in
bite-size pieces (peas,
broccoli, snow peas,
zucchini, mushrooms)
1 ½ t light margarine
¼ t minced garlic

1 cup low-fat ricotta
cheese
2 T grated Parmesan
cheese
2 T skim milk
1 egg yolk
½ t oregano, crushed
⅛ t pepper

Cook pasta according to package directions, drain, and place in large serving bowl.

Blanch vegetables in boiling water until crisp-tender (2 to 3 minutes).

Drain vegetables, add to pasta, toss gently, and cover to keep warm.

In small sauce pan, melt margarine.

Add garlic and sauté until golden. Remove from heat.

Stir in ricotta, Parmesan, milk, egg yolk, oregano, and pepper.

Cook, stirring, over low heat until hot (about 3 minutes). Do not boil.

Blend until smooth and creamy, pour over pasta mixture, and toss gently.

Day 7

Breakfast *Biscuits with no-sugar-added jam; canned peaches in their juice; low-fat cottage cheese; skim milk*

Lunch *Chicken and vegetable soup; whole-wheat toast; grapes or other fresh fruit; skim milk (juice)*

Dinner *Fish fillets with stir-fried broccoli*; brown rice pilaf; shredded apple, carrot, and raisin salad (store-bought, if the preparation taxes your hands too much)*

Fish fillets with stir-fried broccoli

1 T vegetable oil
1 (16 oz.) package frozen
    broccoli
1 small onion, sliced
½ cup celery
1 clove garlic, minced (or
    ⅛ t garlic powder)

½ t oregano
1 lb. fish fillets
dash of pepper
2 t lemon juice (optional)
Lemon slices, for garnish
    (optional)

Put oil in 10-inch fry pan, add vegetables, garlic (powder), and oregano.
Cook, stirring frequently, over medium-high heat until vegetables are crisp-tender (about 5 minutes).
Remove from heat.
Add fish to fry pan with ¼ cup water, pepper, and lemon juice.
Bring to a boil over high heat.
Reduce heat to low, cover, and simmer 5 to 10 minutes until fish flakes.
Garnish with lemon.

Day 8

Breakfast Oatmeal with nectarines; English muffin with jam; fruit juice; skim milk

Lunch Toasted Muenster cheese on whole-wheat bread; cucumber spears; fresh or frozen melon balls; skim milk (juice)

Dinner Fish and apple kabobs*; whole-wheat noodles; steamed peas and carrots

Fish and apple kabobs

1 green pepper, cut in   *6 cherry tomatoes†*
1½-inch squares†   *2 t lemon juice (optional)*
1 Golden Delicious   *1 T light margarine,*
  apple, thickly sliced   *melted*
½ lb. fish steak, cut in   *dash of pepper*
  1½-inch cubes   *dash of thyme*

On 6 skewers, alternate green pepper, apple, fish, and tomato.

Combine remaining ingredients and brush over all surfaces of kabobs.

Broil 3 to 4 inches from heat, 2 minutes per side (8 minutes total), or until fish flakes easily with fork.

Day 9

Breakfast *Whole-wheat pancakes with strawberries; fruit juice; skim milk*

Lunch *Sardines on whole-wheat bread; tossed green salad; fresh fruit cup*

Dinner *Poached chicken breast with fresh vegetables*; baked (sweet) potato; fresh fruit salad with yogurt dressing*; skim milk*

Poached chicken breast with fresh vegetables

4 chicken breasts   *1 medium onion,*
2 cloves of garlic, minced   *chopped*
Dash of pepper   *1 large green pepper,*
Dash of onion powder   *chopped‡*
2 medium tomatoes,   *2 cups mushrooms,*
  chopped‡   *quartered*

†If nightshades are a problem for you, substitute onions, pineapple chunks, and sweet-potato wedges for the green pepper and tomatoes.
‡To avoid nightshades, substitute zucchini and yellow squash for tomatoes and green peppers.

In 10-inch fry pan, bring 1 cup of water to a boil.
Add chicken and spices.
Cover and reduce heat; simmer for 15 to 20 minutes, until chicken is partially cooked, adding more water if needed.
Add vegetables; simmer 10 to 15 minutes, until vegetables are cooked.

Fruit salad with yogurt dressing

Apples
Bananas
Seedless grapes
Oranges (optional)
Raisins
Kiwi fruit

Blueberries
Strawberries
Vanilla yogurt
Shredded coconut
(unsweetened)

Use any combination of fruits you like.
Wash and prepare fruit by cubing, slicing, or separating into sections. Leave grapes, raisins, and small berries whole. Combine them in large serving bowl, cover, and refrigerate until ready to serve.
Spoon yogurt over fruit at last moment. Sprinkle with coconut.

Day 10

Breakfast *Puffed-rice cereal with banana; English muffin with jam; fruit juice; skim milk*

Lunch *Pasta vegetable salad; whole-wheat roll; melon slices; skim milk (juice)*

Dinner *Baked salmon; steamed asparagus; baked (sweet) potato wedges; marinated cucumbers; cinnamon apple ring*

Day 11

Breakfast   *Oat'n'fruit muffin*; scrambled egg; canta-loupe; skim milk*

Lunch   *Tuna salad in pocket (pita) bread; vegetable soup; unsalted crackers; skim milk (juice)*

Dinner   *Beef (or chicken) and vegetable kabob; rice pilaf; fruit salad with yogurt dressing*

Oat'n'fruit muffin

1 cup whole-wheat flour	*2 eggs, beaten*
1 cup rolled oats	*2 T honey*
½ cup bran flakes	*2 T molasses*
2 t baking powder	*1 cup chopped apples,*
1 t cinnamon	*pears, or nectarines, or*
½ t nutmeg	*use prepared chopped*
½ t salt (optional)	*dates, or raisins.*
1 cup skim milk	
¼ cup light margarine,	
melted	

In large bowl, combine dry ingredients. Preheat oven to 375°F.

Combine milk, margarine, eggs, honey, and molasses; stir into dry ingredients, along with fruit, until flour is moistened.

Fill baking cups in muffin pan ⅔ full.

Bake at 375°F. for 25 minutes, or until muffins test done. Remove to wire rack to cool. (Leftover muffins freeze well.)

Day 12

Breakfast *Cooked wheat cereal; bagel with jam; skim milk; fruit juice; applesauce*

Lunch *Herring salad plate; whole-wheat roll; melon slices*

Dinner *Fast turkey pie*; tossed green salad; fruit cup; skim milk (juice)*

Fast turkey pie

2 cups cooked turkey or
    chicken pieces
1 (4½ oz.) can sliced
    mushrooms, drained
½ cup sliced scallions

1 cup shredded Swiss
    cheese
1½ cups skim milk
¾ cup Bisquick
3 eggs

Layer turkey, mushrooms, scallions, and cheese in pie plate.

Beat remaining ingredients until smooth (about 15 seconds in blender at high speed) and pour into pie plate over turkey combination.

Bake at 400°F. for 30 to 35 minutes, until golden brown and knife inserted into pie comes out clean.

Let stand 5 minutes before cutting.

Day 13

Breakfast *Low-fat cottage cheese; canned peaches (in fruit juice); raisin toast; fruit juice; skim milk*

Lunch *Turkey in pita; celery and carrot sticks; kiwi or other fresh fruit; skim milk (juice)*

Dinner *Poached fish fillets*; whole-wheat pasta; steamed asparagus; fruit salad*

Poached fish fillets

4 cups water *1 ½ lbs. fresh fish fillets,*
1 ½ t salt *or frozen ones, thawed*

In a 10-inch fry pan, bring water to a boil.
Add salt and place fish in a single layer in the hot water.
Cover, reduce heat, and simmer for 8 to 10 minutes, or until fish flakes easily with fork.
Drain fish before serving.

Day 14

Breakfast *Apple oatmeal*; whole-wheat toast with jam; fruit juice; skim milk*

Lunch *Vegetable and lentil soup; rice and spinach salad*; pear or other fresh fruit; skim milk (juice)*

Dinner *Broiled salmon with mustard dill sauce*; steamed cauliflower; whole-wheat roll; fresh fruit salad*

Apple oatmeal

½ cup diced Golden *Dash of cinnamon*
Delicious apple *Dash of nutmeg*
⅓ cup apple juice *⅓ cup quick oats,*
⅓ cup water *uncooked*

Combine apples, juice, water, and seasonings, and bring to a boil.
Stir in oatmeal and cook for one minute.
Cover and let stand several minutes before serving.

Rice and spinach salad

*1 cup brown rice,
   uncooked
½ cup low-calorie Italian
   dressing
1 T light (low-salt) soy
   sauce*

*2 cups fresh spinach
½ cup sliced celery
½ cup sliced scallions
A few Bac-Os (optional)*

Cook rice according to package directions.
Transfer cooked rice to bowl and cool slightly.
Combine dressing and soy sauce, and stir into warm rice.
Cover and chill. Fold in remaining ingredients just before
serving.

Broiled salmon with mustard dill sauce

*1½ lb. salmon steaks
   (1-inch thick)
1 cup plain low-fat
   yogurt*

*2 T Dijon mustard
½ t dried dill weed*

Spray broiler rack with nonstick spray. Preheat broiler.
Remove skin from salmon steaks.
Mix together yogurt, mustard, and dill weed.
Place steaks on broiler rack and brush each with sauce.
Broil 6 inches from heat for 8 to 10 minutes, brushing with
more sauce as needed.
Turn steaks, brush other side with sauce, and broil 8 min-
utes, or until fish flakes easily with fork.

Day 15

Breakfast   *Fruit and nut muffin*; poached egg; fruit juice; skim milk*

Lunch   *Sardine salad plate; crackers or rice cakes; kiwi or other fresh fruit*

Dinner   *Fast vegetable pie*; tossed green salad with dressing; fresh or frozen melon balls; skim milk*

Fruit and nut muffin

2 cups flour
1/2 cup sugar
2 t baking soda
1/2 t salt (optional)
1 t cinnamon
1 t nutmeg
1 cup grated carrots

1 cup grated apple
1/2 cup raisins
1/2 cup chopped pecans
3 eggs, slightly beaten
1/2 cup vegetable oil
2 t vanilla

Combine flour, sugar, soda, salt, cinnamon, and nutmeg. Stir in carrots, apple, raisins, and pecans.
Combine eggs, oil, and vanilla until blended; add to flour-fruit mixture, and stir until blended.
Spoon into baking cups in muffin pan.
Bake in preheated 350°F. oven for 20 to 25 minutes, or until muffins test done with a wooden toothpick.
Let muffins cool in pan on wire rack for 5 minutes. (Freeze the extras.)

Fast vegetable pie

3 cups vegetables (A cau-
liflower-broccoli-carrot
mixture works well.)
1 (4½ oz.) can sliced
mushrooms, drained
½ cup sliced scallions

1 cup shredded Swiss
cheese
1½ cups skim milk
¾ cup Bisquick
3 eggs

Steam the vegetables briefly.

Layer vegetables, mushrooms, scallions, and cheese in pie plate.

Beat remaining ingredients until smooth (about 15 seconds in blender at high speed) and pour into pie plate over vegetable combination.

Bake at 400°F. for 30 to 35 minutes, until golden brown and knife inserted into pie comes out clean. Let stand 5 minutes before cutting.

Day 16

Breakfast   *Whole-wheat toast with apple butter; canned peaches (in fruit juice) with low-fat, low-salt cottage cheese; fruit juice; skim milk*

Lunch   *Clam chowder; cheese melt on bagel; celery and carrot sticks; juice*

Dinner   *Turkey broccoli bake*; cooked noodles; tossed salad; whole-wheat roll; skim milk*

Turkey broccoli bake

1 (16 oz.) package frozen
   broccoli
1½ lbs. cubed cooked
   turkey
4 T light margarine
1 medium onion, diced
4 T flour

2 cups skim milk
1½ T lemon juice (op-
   tional)
½ t curry powder
¼ cup cheddar cheese,
   shredded

Steam broccoli, drain, and place in baking dish. Arrange turkey on top.

Melt margarine in small saucepan over medium heat.

Add onion and cook until tender, stirring occasionally.

Reduce heat; blend in flour.

Add milk all at once. Add lemon juice and curry powder. Cook quickly, stirring constantly, until mixture thickens and bubbles.

Pour sauce over turkey and broccoli. Sprinkle with cheese.

Bake in preheated 375°F. oven for 30 to 40 minutes.

Day 17

Breakfast   *Cream of Wheat, or Wheatena, with raisins; bagel with jam; fruit juice; skim milk*

Lunch   *Tuna and apple salad*; whole-wheat toast with light margarine; raw vegetables (broccoli, carrots, zucchini); skim milk (juice)*

Dinner   *Beef (or chicken) Stroganoff prepared with lean meat and yogurt; noodles or rice; steamed green beans; sliced tomatoes or cucumbers*

Tuna and apple salad

1 red or Golden Delicious
  apple, cored
1 can (6½ oz.) water-
  pack tuna, rinsed and
  drained
¼ cup sliced water chest-
  nuts

¼ cup chopped scallions
Lettuce leaves
4 t lemon juice (or water)
1½ t vegetable oil
2 t light (low-salt) soy
  sauce

Chop half the apple; slice the other half.
Combine chopped apple with tuna, water chestnuts, and
scallions.
Arrange apple slices on leaves; top with tuna mixture.
To make dressing, combine remaining ingredients and
mix well.

Day 18

Breakfast *Frozen waffle with peaches; fruit juice; skim milk*

Lunch *Peanut butter and banana on whole-wheat bread; apple or other fresh fruit; skim milk (juice)*

Dinner *Stovetop fish steaks*; tossed green salad; corn on the cob; whole-wheat roll; cinnamon apple ring*

Stovetop fish steaks

¼ cup light (low-salt)
  soy sauce
¼ cup rice-wine vinegar
1 clove garlic, crushed
2 T sesame oil
1 t grated fresh ginger
  (¼ t powdered)

1½ lb. fish steaks (fresh
  tuna, halibut, or other
  thick fish)
1 T margarine

Combine soy sauce, vinegar, garlic, sesame oil, and ginger.
Marinate fish in above mixture for 30 minutes at room
temperature.
Melt margarine in skillet.
Add fish, with marinade, and cook about 8 minutes on
each side, or until fish flakes easily.

Day 19

Breakfast *Puffed-rice cereal with banana; blueberry muffin; skim milk; fruit juice*

Lunch *Potato soup (or corn chowder); turkey sandwich; pear or other fresh fruit; skim milk (juice)*

Dinner *Broiled fish with tangy dressing*; brown rice; steamed broccoli and carrots; fruit salad with yogurt dressing; whole-wheat roll*

Broiled fish with tangy dressing

¼ cup light mayonnaise
2 T Dijon mustard
2 T white wine
2 T lemon juice (optional)

1 clove garlic, crushed
¼ t pepper
1 to 2 lbs. bluefish or other fresh fish
2 T chopped scallions

Combine mayonnaise, mustard, wine, lemon juice, garlic,
and pepper.
Spray broiler rack with nonstick coating and place fish,
skin side down.
Spread dressing thickly over top of fish.
Broil 8 to 10 minutes, or until fish flakes easily with fork.
Top with scallions.

Day 20

Breakfast *Low-fat, low-salt cottage cheese; canned pears (in fruit juice); raisin toast; fruit juice; skim milk*

Lunch *Salmon salad plate; rice cakes; carrot/pineapple/ raisin salad; banana or other fresh fruit; skim milk (juice)*

Dinner *Broiled chicken; rice; steamed asparagus or zucchini; orange wedges or grapes; applesauce*

Day 21

Breakfast *Pancakes with light syrup or pureed berries; cantaloupe; fruit juice; skim milk*

Lunch *Crab and shrimp salad; soft bread sticks; apple wedges; skim milk (juice)*

Dinner *Broiled fish fillets with sauce*; tossed green salad; baked acorn squash; steamed green beans*

Broiled fish fillets with sauce

4 mackerel fillets
Sauce #1
⅓ cup lemon juice
½ t garlic, minced
1 T olive oil
½ t dried basil, crumbled
or

Sauce #2
⅓ cup light (low-salt) soy sauce
1 T rice vinegar
½ t garlic, minced
2 t fresh ginger, minced (½ t powdered)

Rinse mackerel, pat dry with paper towels, and place in baking dish.
Prepare either one of the sauces and drizzle it over the fish.

Refrigerate, covered, for 1 hour.
Arrange fillets, skin down, on broiler pan coated with non-stick spray.
Sprinkle with pepper, if you like.
Broil 6 inches from heat until fish flakes easily with fork (about 5 to 7 minutes), basting once with marinade.

Day 22

Breakfast *Bagel with light cream cheese; cantaloupe; fruit juice; skim milk*

Lunch *Turkey sandwich; raw vegetables (celery, etc.); nectarine or other fresh fruit; skim milk (juice)*

Dinner *Spinach quiche*; whole-wheat roll; steamed broccoli, carrots, onions; fruit salad with yogurt dressing*

Spinach quiche

2 T shallots, onions, or
   scallions, minced
2 T light margarine
1 (10 oz.) package frozen
   chopped spinach,
   cooked and well
   drained
1/8 t pepper

1/8 t nutmeg
1 cup low-fat cottage
   cheese
3 eggs
1/4 cup shredded Swiss
   cheese
1 9-inch pie shell (un-
   baked)

Sauté shallots in margarine.
Add spinach and stir over moderate heat until water is evaporated.
Remove from heat. Add spices.
Blend cottage cheese and eggs in electric blender.
Stir in spinach mixture and Swiss cheese. Pour into pie shell.

Bake at 425°F. for 12 minutes; reduce heat to 375°F. and bake another 25 to 30 minutes until set.

Day 23

Breakfast *Oatmeal with raisins; bran muffin; honeydew melon; skim milk (juice)*

Lunch *Chicken salad sandwich; cucumber spears (and tomato slices); grapes or other fresh fruit; skim milk (juice)*

Dinner *Seafood fettucine*; steamed broccoli, cauliflower, carrots, and zucchini; fruit salad with yogurt dressing; whole-wheat roll*

Seafood fettucine

2 cups fresh or frozen scallops, shrimp, and crab meat
1 clove garlic, minced
¼ t white pepper
½ t nutmeg
1 T parsley, chopped (or flakes)
8 oz. fettucine or other pasta (uncooked)

1 ½ t light margarine
1 cup low-fat ricotta cheese
1 egg yolk
2 T skim milk
2 T grated Parmesan cheese

Combine seafood and garlic in a bowl, sprinkle with pepper, nutmeg, and parsley; toss gently, cover, and refrigerate for 10 to 15 minutes.

Cook pasta according to package directions, drain, place in large serving bowl, and cover to keep warm.

In large sauce pan, melt margarine, then sauté seafood over medium heat for 3 to 4 minutes, stirring constantly. Remove from heat.

Blend ricotta cheese, egg yolk, and milk in electric blender until smooth and creamy.

Add cheese mixture to seafood and cook until thoroughly heated.

Add to fettucine and toss gently. Sprinkle with Parmesan cheese.

Day 24

Breakfast   *Poached egg on whole-wheat toast; canned peaches (packed in fruit juice); skim milk (juice)*

Lunch   *Mushroom barley soup; toasted cheese sandwich; apple or other fresh fruit; skim milk (juice)*

Dinner   *Crispy baked fish fillets*; steamed green beans; baked (sweet) potato wedges; coleslaw*

Crispy baked fish fillets

1 lb. fish fillets   *2 T vegetable oil*
Black pepper   *⅓ cup cornflake crumbs*

Wash and dry fillets.
Season, brush with oil, and coat with crumbs.
Arrange in a single layer in a lightly oiled shallow baking dish.
Bake at 500°F. for 10 minutes.

Day 25

Breakfast *Shredded-wheat cereal with banana; blue-berry muffin; fruit juice; skim milk*

Lunch *English muffin pizza; lettuce wedge with dressing; fresh fruit cup; skim milk (juice)*

Dinner *Whole fish with vegetable stuffing*; three-bean salad; brown rice; melon slices*

Whole fish with vegetable stuffing

1 T light margarine
1 small onion, minced
½ stalk celery, minced
2 medium zucchini, diced
1 T lemon juice (optional)

¼ t pepper
4 red snappers (1 lb. ea.), Coho salmon, or trout
1 small lemon, in 4 wedges (optional)

Melt margarine over medium heat in 2-quart saucepan.
Add onion and celery and cook for 5 minutes, stirring occasionally.
Add zucchini, ¼ cup water, lemon juice, and pepper; heat to boiling.
Reduce heat to low; cover and simmer for 10 minutes until tender.
With slotted spoon, fill cavity of each fish with vegetable mixture, saving the vegetable liquid. Close each cavity and fasten with toothpicks.
Arrange stuffed fish in roasting pan; spoon remaining vegetable mixture around fish and pour vegetable liquid over fish.
Bake in preheated 350°F. oven for 30 to 40 minutes, basting occasionally with pan juices until fish flakes easily with fork.
Remove toothpicks and garnish with lemon wedges.

Day 26

Breakfast *Raisin toast; fresh or frozen blueberries with yogurt; skim milk*

Lunch *Sardine sandwich; spinach salad; orange or other fresh fruit*

Dinner *Vegetable pasta; Waldorf salad; whole-wheat roll; skim milk (juice)*

Day 27

Breakfast *Puffed-rice cereal with blueberries; English muffin with jam; fruit juice; skim milk*

Lunch *Salmon sandwich*; tossed green salad; grapes or other fresh fruit; juice*

Dinner *Grilled chicken; rice pilaf; steamed peas and carrots; applesauce; skim milk*

Salmon sandwich

*1 can (7½ oz.) salmon,
  rinsed and drained
2 T chopped dill pickle
2 T reduced-calorie salad
  dressing*

*1 t lemon juice (optional)
thin slices of cucumber
  or zucchini
whole-wheat bread*

Combine salmon, pickle, salad dressing, and lemon juice; mix well.

Spread salmon mixture on whole-wheat bread, top with cucumber or zucchini.

Serve as open-face sandwich, or top with another slice of bread.

Day 28

Breakfast   *Oatmeal; biscuit with jam; fruit juice; skim milk*

Lunch   *Chicken salad with nuts*; whole-wheat toast; cantaloupe or other fruit; skim milk (juice)*

Dinner   *Broccoli and fish bake*; brown rice; steamed peas and carrots; grapes or other fresh fruit*

Chicken salad with nuts

*2 cups cubed cooked
   chicken breast*
*¾ cup seedless green
   grapes, halved*
¾ cup sliced celery
½ cup chopped pecans

Dressing
*½ cup low-calorie salad
   dressing*
¼ cup light sour cream
*½ t grated fresh ginger
   (or ⅛ t powdered)*
⅛ t pepper

Combine chicken, grapes, celery, and pecans in bowl and set aside.
In another bowl, combine ingredients to make dressing. Mix well.
Stir dressing into chicken mixture; cover and refrigerate 1 to 2 hours before serving.

Broccoli and fish bake

*1 (10 oz.) package frozen
   broccoli*
1 lb. fish fillets
*1 T lemon juice (op-
   tional)*
2 T light margarine

2 T flour
¾ t dried dill weed
⅛ t pepper
1 cup skim milk
*1 T grated Parmesan
   cheese*

Cook broccoli according to package directions; drain.
Place fish fillets in baking dish; top with lemon juice and
broccoli.
Melt margarine in saucepan over low heat; add flour, dill
weed, and pepper, stirring constantly over low heat until
smooth.
Whisk in milk and bring to a boil, stirring constantly.
Boil and stir one minute, pour sauce over broccoli.
Sprinkle with cheese. Bake at 350°F. for 25 minutes, or
until fish flakes.

Day 29

Breakfast   *Cream of Wheat with raisins; bagel with jam;
fruit juice; skim milk*

Lunch   *Meat loaf or tuna sandwich; tossed green salad;
grapefruit or other fresh fruit; skim milk (juice)*

Dinner   *Shrimp and vegetable stir fry*; rice; Waldorf
salad; melon or papaya slices*

Shrimp and vegetable stir fry

*1 lb. fresh or frozen
   shrimp, washed and
   deveined*
1/2 t cornstarch
*1/2 t light (low-salt) soy
   sauce*
1/8 t sesame oil
dash of white pepper
*4 oz fresh or frozen snow
   pea pods*
1 T cornstarch
1 T cold water
1 T vegetable oil
*1 clove garlic, finely
   chopped*

*1 t ginger root, minced
   (1/4 t ground)*
2 T vegetable oil
*8 oz. bok choy (4 or 5
   stalks), sliced diago-
   nally*
*1 cup fresh mushrooms,
   quartered*
*2 T light (low-salt) soy
   sauce*
1/4 cup chicken broth
*3 scallions, cut in 2-inch
   pieces*

Combine first five ingredients; cover and refrigerate for 30 minutes.

For fresh pea pods, remove strings, then cook, covered, in boiling water for 1 minute; drain. Rinse immediately under cold water, drain, and set aside.

Mix 1 T cornstarch and 1 T cold water, and set aside.

Heat wok or large fry pan. Add 1 T vegetable oil, then garlic and ginger, and stir fry until garlic is light brown. Add shrimp and stir fry until shrimp is pink. Remove shrimp.

Add 2 T vegetable oil to wok; add bok choy and mushrooms and stir fry for one minute.

Stir in 2 T soy sauce and the chicken broth, and heat to boiling.

Stir in cornstarch/water mixture; cook and stir about 10 seconds until thickened.

Add shrimp and pea pods; cook and stir for another 30 seconds.

Garnish with scallions.

Day 30

Breakfast   *Banana-bran muffin*; soft-boiled egg; orange or other fresh fruit; skim milk*

Lunch   *Turkey soup; spinach-avocado salad; apple or other fresh fruit; skim milk (juice)*

Dinner   *Chicken chow mein; rice; fresh fruit salad*

Banana-bran muffins

1 1/4 cup whole-wheat
   flour
1/4 cup sugar
3 t baking powder
1 1/2 cup whole-bran ce-
   real or bran

3/4 cup skim milk
1 cup mashed ripe ba-
   nana
1 egg
1/4 cup vegetable oil

Sift together flour, sugar, and baking powder. Set aside.
Combine bran cereal, milk, and banana in bowl and set
aside to soften.
Add flour mixture, egg, and oil to cereal mixture; mix until
all ingredients are moist.
Spoon into baking cups in muffin pan.
Bake in preheated 400°F. oven for 25 minutes or until
muffins test done with a toothpick.
Cool on wire rack for 5 minutes before removing muffins
from pan.

Snack Items

*Fresh fruit; dried fruit; low-salt crackers (with low-salt,
low-fat cheese); fruit drink*; raw vegetables—plain, with
creamy cottage dip,* or yogurt and dill dip* (celery, carrots, broccoli, cauliflower, cucumber, zucchini, snow peas,
etc.); unsalted nuts; air-popped popcorn; mineral water or
seltzer*

Fruit drink

*1 cup unsweetened straw-
   berries or raspberries
1 cup orange (or apple)
   juice*

1 banana

Blend fruits and juice until smooth in electric blender.
If your blender can crush ice, add a few ice cubes for a
frothier drink.

Fruit shake

1 banana
1/2 cup low-fat yogurt
1/2 cup skim milk
1 cup fresh fruit
(peaches, berries,
crushed pineapple)

Ice cubes (if blender can
crush ice)

Blend all ingredients until smooth in electric blender.

Creamy cottage dip

1 (12 oz.) container low-
fat, low-salt cottage
cheese
6 T skim milk

1 1/2 T minced onion
1 T chopped pimento
1 T chopped parsley

Combine cottage cheese, milk, and onion in a bowl; blend
with electric mixer.
Stir in pimento and parsley.
Cover and refrigerate.

Yogurt and dill dip

1 cup plain low-fat yo-
gurt
1 t dried dill weed
1 clove garlic, pressed (1/4
t powder)

2 T chopped fresh chives
(or 1 t dried)
Dash of pepper

Combine all ingredients and blend thoroughly.
Cover and refrigerate.

Dessert Suggestions

Ginger snaps (2); vanilla wafers (up to 5); angel food cake (thin slice) with fruit; arrowroot cookies (up to 3); fresh fruit (apple, orange, grapes, banana, kiwi, melon, berries, peach, etc.); fresh fruit with yogurt dip*; graham crackers (1 whole, or 4 small sections)

Yogurt dip for fruit

*1 cup peach- or rasp-
    berry-flavored yogurt*
⅛ t almond extract

*coconut topping (un-
    sweetened)*

Combine all ingredients.
Cover and refrigerate.

15

HOW AND WHEN TO SUPPLEMENT YOUR DIET WITH VITAMINS AND MINERALS

■ *Countering the effects of arthritis itself* ■ *Countering the effects of the drugs used to treat arthritis*

What could be more appealing than a cheap bottle of pills—made from the same natural ingredients found in good food—that promises pain relief or overall better health, with hardly any risk of side effects? That is the inimitable appeal of dietary supplements, from vitamins and minerals to yeast, amino acids, and herbal essences such as ginseng or black cohosh root, all of which have been tried by our participants.

In all, 771 of the 1,051 participants in our Arthritis Survey, or 73 percent of the group, take supplements of some kind. Most rely on the shotgun approach of a multivitamin and mineral tablet manufactured by a reputable company. But many seek out a single nutrient for its particular virtues, or combine a few carefully chosen correctives in a regimen tailored to meet their own special needs.

In this chapter, we'll examine all these strategies, giving you our participants' winning combinations, with support, where possible, from medical research on the value of nutritional supplements for people with arthritis. We'll translate these ideas into specific recommendations that you can discuss with your doctor. And don't worry about being laughed at for broaching the subject. Indeed, some arthritis specialists seen by our participants are already incorporating dietary supplements into their treatment plans.

"My rheumatologist sent me to a nearby medical school for a vitamin assay," reports a writer from New Jersey who has osteoarthritis in her hands, ankles, and knees. "Despite my lust for grapefruit, I turned out to be low in vitamin C, as well as several of the B vitamins. Adding supplements has been most helpful. The rheumatologist increased my C to a minimum of 1,000 milligrams daily, and double or triple that for flare-ups."

Others have received no professional counsel, and they try this or that supplement because of its rumored benefits, with varying degrees of success.

"Cod liver oil—YUK!" exclaims a registered nurse from South Dakota. "I don't think this dietary punishment helped my arthritis, but it did make me feel so nauseated that it took my mind off all other aches and pains."

What Survey Participants Say About Supplements

Although close to three-quarters of our participants use one or more supplements regularly, only about 160 of them chose to *comment* on the advantages of doing so. Here's a summary of what they said.

Comment	Number of Participants Saying So
I feel supplements help/seem to help my arthritis.	77
I take them for help with a specific problem, not necessarily arthritis-related, such as C for colds.	32
They give me more energy.	26
I feel my general health is better as a result of taking them.	26

Several of the 280 participants who take *no* supplements say that they rely on a good nutritious diet for the vitamins and minerals they need. This may be the safest, surest course for people enjoying perfect health, but the fact that you have arthritis makes it *likely* that you might need some kind of supplement—especially if any of the following statements could have come from your lips.

- I use aspirin or other NSAIDs daily to control pain and inflammation.

- I find that arthritis drugs upset my stomach.

- I have taken lots of prednisone or other steroid drugs.

- I take penicillamine or immunosuppressive drugs for rheumatoid arthritis.

- I am about to have (or have just had) surgery.

- I am over sixty-five.

- I bruise easily.

- I frequently skip meals because of pain, and just get by on snacks.

- I am on a restricted diet.

All of these statements apply to at least some of our participants, and here are the supplements they rely on, beginning with the most popular ones.

Supplement	Number of Participants Taking It
Daily multivitamin with minerals	429
Vitamin C (including rose hips, bioflavonoids, and rutin)	279
Calcium	270
Vitamin E	191
Vitamin B complex	113
Vitamin A	62
Zinc	61
Vitamin D	55
Cod Liver Oil	55
Vitamin B_6 (pyridoxine)	51
Iron	43
Vitamin B_{12} (cobalamin)	40
Magnesium	39
Potassium	38
Fish Oil (such as **MaxEPA**)	33
Lecithin	31
Alfalfa	30
Garlic Capsules	28
Herbal Teas (including nettle, comfrey, and willow)	20
Selenium	19
Bee Pollen	17
Beta Carotene	14
Brewer's Yeast or Yeast Tablets	14
Vitamin B_3 (niacin, nicotinamide, or nicotinic acid)	12
Multiminerals	12
Kelp	10
Lysine	10
Yucca	8
Vitamin B_1 (thiamin)	7
Pantothenic Acid	7
Ginseng	6
Vitamin B_2 (riboflavin)	5
DLPA (DL-phenylalanine)	5
Folacin (folic acid)	5
Tryptophan	5
Wheat Germ Oil Capsules	5

Supplement	Number of Participants Taking It
Chromium	4
Evening Primrose Oil	4
Aloe Capsules	3
Manganese	3
PABA (Para-aminobenzoic acid)	3
Protein Powder	3
S.O.D. (Superoxide Dismutase)	3
Anti-Oxidants	2
Barley Green	2
Black Cohosh	2
Chapparal	2
Copper	2
Co-Enzyme Q10	2
Horsetail Grass	2
Iodine	2
Liver	2
Royal Jelly	2
Safflower Oil	2
Wood Betony	2
Ammonium Molybdate	1
Arginine	1
Biotin	1
Choline	1
Vitamin K	1
Ornithine	1
Phosphorus	1
Tyrosine	1

A Little of Each

Taking a multivitamin and mineral supplement, our survey participants' favorite way to augment their diets, is surely the simplest solution to deficiency worries for most people. The brands mentioned most often in our survey are **One-a-Day, Centrum, Theragran,** and **Stresstabs,** in that order, but we have no evidence to suggest that one is better than any of the others.

To get an idea of the range of opinions on multivitamins, consider the comments from our participants about **Theragran** and **Theragran-M**, both made by Squibb.

A housewife from Utah: "I take **Theragran** and I seem to have more energy."

A foster grandparent from Oklahoma: "I take **Theragran** and I think it helps."

A high school English teacher from South Dakota: "I have taken **Theragran-M** for twenty-five years, and I'm experiencing arthritis at a much older age, and less severely than my grandmother, mother, and younger sister."

A retired production vice-president from Pennsylvania: "I take **Theragran** on the advice of my neurosurgeon, but I don't notice any difference if I stop taking it."

Based on our participants' experience and our reading of the medical literature, we highly recommend that you take a multivitamin and mineral supplement that provides 100 percent of the U.S. Recommended Daily Allowances (U.S. RDA). Although it is no substitute for a healthy diet, the supplement can fill in some of the gaps for you. It is a well-documented fact that many people with arthritis are at least marginally malnourished, with deficiencies in one or more nutrients, according to studies in the United States and Europe. For some, the disease itself is to blame. You yourself may have experienced pain and swelling in your hands that make cooking difficult, or jaw pain that turns eating into a chore. Arthritis also seems to interfere with the way your body utilizes some of the nutrients from foods, so that you may need supplements as a safety net, even though you eat well. Other people find that the drugs they take for arthritis treatment can rob the body of one or more essential nutrients (more about this later), or affect the gut in such a way that it can't properly absorb the nutrients from food.

Although you can buy a multivitamin over the counter (or through the mail), it's a good idea to talk to your doctor before starting any new supplement regimen. Unpleasant side effects from taking multivitamins according to package directions are extremely rare, but a California social worker in our survey, for example, has been advised *not* to take vitamins since her stomach hemorrhage. A retired mechanical engineer from Florida notes that vitamins cause his mouth and lips to break out in blisters.

Taking extremely large quantities, or *megadoses,* of vitamins and minerals, on the other hand, is risky business. This is especially true of the fat-soluble vitamins A and D, which can build up in your body and lead to assorted horrors. Megadoses of vitamin A have been known to *cause* joint pain in some people, and too much vitamin D, ironically, can *weaken* your bones.

A Vitamin to (Almost) Every Purpose

The last of the thirteen known vitamins was identified more than forty years ago, yet various ones come to the forefront of attention from time to time, like changing fashions, as more of their actions are understood—vitamin C for colds in the 1970s, vitamin A for cancer prevention in the 1980s. Although no vitamin has yet been scientifically proven to alter the course of arthritis, some of our participants say they have found pain relief from taking vitamin C, vitamin E, or one or more of the B vitamins.

Vitamin C

Of the 270 participants who use vitamin C (ascorbic acid), 24 explain why: 13 find that it helps relieve pain or swelling; another 7 cite prevention of colds and infections as their rationale; 2 take it for general well-being; and 1 says it keeps him from bruising. Two British physicians recently documented this antibruising effect while trying to treat the spontaneous skin bruises that often accompany rheumatoid arthritis. They gave 500 milligrams of vitamin C a day to three of their patients who had been troubled with this problem, and all three stopped getting bruises. Writing in the *British Journal of Rheumatology,* the authors explain that the three elderly women in the trial were poorly nourished and actually deficient in vitamin C, and, further, that inflammation reduces the body's store of this vitamin.

Indeed, the fact that people with rheumatoid arthritis have lower-than-normal levels of vitamin C in their joints and in their blood has been known since the 1930s. However, the (few) studies conducted in the past fifty years have failed to set an *amount* of vitamin C that might produce improvement.

Dr. Richard S. Panush, working with colleagues at the University of Florida College of Medicine, has shown that vitamin C can enhance the immune response for people with rheumatoid arthritis, although he isn't convinced it really helps their arthritis.

Vitamin C may also boost the effectiveness of aspirin in your body. This action has not been shown in human subjects, but there is some test-tube evidence from researchers at Simon Fraser University in British Columbia. Another aspect of the aspirin–C interaction is that aspirin may literally dump C out of your system, causing you to excrete it much faster than people who don't take the drug regularly.

The recommended dose of vitamin C varies from 60 milligrams a day, as the U.S. government advises for average adults,* to three hundred times that much, or 18 grams, which is what Dr. Linus Pauling recommends for life extension and general disease prevention. We suspect that 500 milligrams—the most popular amount mentioned in our survey—is adequate for most people with arthritis. More may be required for those undergoing the physical stress of surgery, since vitamin C helps the body heal. Some people can't tolerate a C supplement at all, however, because it upsets their stomachs. Vitamin manufacturers have tried to meet this challenge with buffered C tablets, but there is always the natural vitamin C in citrus fruit, if you can eat it, in papaya and other melons, and in dark-green vegetables. Several members of the nightshade family—tomatoes, peppers, and potatoes—are good C sources for those who can enjoy them.

---

*A 60-milligram dose of vitamin C is the Recommended Dietary Allowance (RDA) for healthy adults. RDAs are determined by the Food and Nutrition Board of the National Academy of Sciences–National Research Council. The RDAs specify the necessary amounts of certain nutrients for groups of people at different age levels (from under six months to over fifty-one years) and life stages (adolescent boys, for example, or pregnant women). In turn, the Food and Drug Administration uses this information to construct the more general U.S. Recommended Daily Allowances (U.S. RDA) that appear on food labels.

Vitamin E

Vitamin E is swallowed regularly by 191 of our participants, for several different reasons, two of which have to do with side effects from arthritis drugs. "I have cornea damage in both eyes as a result of taking **Butazolidin** thirteen years ago," writes a housewife from New Jersey. "Vitamin E seems to improve my vision."

"My skin condition has gone downhill since I started gold treatments about a year ago," reports a draftsperson from Pennsylvania. "Vitamin E seems to help it." A plumber from Wisconsin also takes vitamin E for his skin, although not for any specified drug reaction.

Two participants increase their E intake because of concern for their heart and circulation. Two more find it heightens their energy and sense of well-being. One believes it boosts her body's natural cortisone, and eight say it helps, or seems to help, their arthritis. How might it accomplish this feat? No one knows for sure, but in animals, vitamin E shows promise of keeping the immune system operating at peak performance. One theory about the way vitamin E may boost immunity is by interfering with the action of the prostaglandin called E_2, or PGE_2, which can curtail immune function. But PGE_2 is also a known inflammatory agent. So it is just *possible* that the vitamin exerts an anti-inflammatory effect by blocking PGE_2.

Scientists in Israel, who tested vitamin E on a group of twenty-nine people with osteoarthritis, concluded their report in the *Journal of the American Geriatrics Society* by suggesting a possible anti-inflammatory role for E. Without that possibility, they were at a loss to explain the good results of their experiment. Fifteen people—more than half the group—had significant pain relief while taking vitamin E.

Most adults are thought to need 30 international units of vitamin E every day. Most of our survey participants who specify the amount they use take 400 international units, although a few take 800 or more—amounts that threaten to bring on headaches, blurred vision, and extreme fatigue.

No arthritis drugs are known to deplete the body of vitamin E, but diet can increase your need for it. If you follow a diet that is high in polyunsaturated fats—such as the Arthritis Survey Diet and Thirty-Day Meal Plan (see Chapter 14) and other experimental diets that have been shown to help reduce some symptoms of arthritis—your vitamin E requirement rises accordingly. The amount of vitamin E in most multivitamin and mineral tablets should be sufficient. If you want to test the effects of an extra measure, talk to your doctor about a daily supplement of 400 to 600 international units.

The B vitamins

The B complex is a family of eight vitamins, some numbered, some not: B_1 or thiamin, B_2 or riboflavin, B_3 or niacin (or nicotinamide or nicotinic acid), B_6 or pyridoxine, B_{12} or cobalamin, folacin or folic acid, pantothenic acid, and biotin. B-complex tablets vary widely, from formulas that contain a few milligrams of each B vitamin to high-potency pills that deliver at least 100 milligrams of each. The formulas balance the B vitamins, which work together in such a way that taking an excess of one may cause a deficiency of another. Although 113 of our participants take the B complex, too few of them specified any dosage formulation for us to make a recommendation. Their reasons for taking the whole complex include relief of pain or swelling (four participants), less fatigue (two participants), physical flexibility (one participant), diabetes (one participant), and a vegetarian diet (one participant).

B vitamins often come up short in the the diets of people with arthritis, according to researchers at the University of Florida who made an in-depth study in 1983 of the way their patients normally ate. As a group, the twenty-four people with rheumatoid arthritis and twelve others with osteoarthritis were consuming far less than the RDA for folacin, vitamin B_6, and pantothenic acid, as well as these other nutrients: magnesium, zinc, and vitamin E. Some of the foods that are richest in B vitamins, such as liver and kidney, are forbidden for certain people with arthritis. Others that abound in them, however, are *whole-grain* cereals and breads, fish, and green leafy vegetables. These, incidentally, are some of our survey participants' most highly recommended food items. (See Chapter 13.)

In a later dietary assessment study at Albany Medical College, reported in 1987, a group of fifty-two people with rheumatoid arthritis were found to follow diets generally deficient in the B vitamins folic acid and pyridoxine. Some of them were also low in magnesium. The twenty-one women in the study group were getting too little zinc. Interestingly, the researchers found that *most* of the twenty-four patients who were taking food supplements were *successfully correcting* the deficits in their diets.

Methotrexate, an immunosuppressive drug recently approved by the FDA to treat rheumatoid arthritis, can cause a deficiency of folacin. This is a main action of the drug, not a side effect. In fact, some physicians believe that trying to correct the deficiency with folic-acid supplements will undermine the drug's usefulness. Four participants in our survey, however, were taking therapeutic doses (1 milligram) of folic acid on doctor's orders *because* of their methotrexate therapy—to help chase the nausea and other side effects caused by the drug. Practitioners are divided on this question at present; however, studies are under way to settle the issue. Meanwhile, if you are taking **Rheumatrex** or **Methotrexate**, you'll want to discuss your vitamin choices with your doctor, since many multivitamin supplements contain folic acid. The salicylates—aspirin, diflunisal (**Dolobid**), and salsalate (**Disalcid** and **Monogesic**)—can also create a folic-acid deficiency, and your doctor may want you to counteract it by taking at least the RDA of 400 micrograms that are included in most multivitamins and B-complex preparations.

Vitamin B$_6$

Vitamin B$_6$, or pyridoxine, has a long history as a popular lay treatment for a form of arthritis called carpal tunnel syndrome—a debilitating wrist problem that necessitated surgery for eleven of our participants. Now there is scientific acceptance of the idea as well. In 1986, the American Chemical Society gave its highest award, the Priestley Medal, to Dr. Karl Folkers, director of the Institute for Biomedical Research at the University of Texas in Austin, for his painstaking efforts to prove that carpal tunnel syndrome can be treated with daily doses of 100 milligrams of vitamin B_6. There's a catch, though. Not *all* cases of carpal tunnel syndrome can be laid to B_6 deficiency.

Of the fifty-one survey participants taking supplemental B_6, one used it as an antidote for stress, and five noted that it eased their pain. "If I didn't take my 200 milligrams of vitamin B_6 every day," says a sixty-year-old housewife from Indiana, "I would not be able to write, draw, or raise my arms over my head." The RDA for B_6 is just 2 milligrams, but many doctors believe that up to 200 milligrams a day (the amount often used to treat premenstrual syndrome) is a safe dose. More than that can lead to nerve damage.

Vitamin B_{12}

Vitamin B_{12} (cobalamin) is the second most popular B vitamin among our participants. Forty take it, but only four tell why: for more energy (three participants), or because it helps arthritis (one participant). B_{12}, which is not found in any fruit or vegetable, is the one vitamin that strict (vegan) vegetarians can't get from their diets, and so they must rely on a supplement. The RDA for most adults is 3 micrograms. (Vegetarians take note that brewer's yeast contains *no* B_{12}.)

Vitamin B_3

Vitamin B_3 eases pain for at least one of the twelve participants who take it, and imparts a healthy feeling to one other. It has three names—niacin, nicotinamide, and nicotinic acid. Niacin, a student teacher from Utah reports, makes her dizzy. And niacinamide (another form of niacin) is the treatment used for forty-odd years by internist Dr. William Kaufman of Stratford, Connecticut, to relieve arthritis pain and stiffness. The medical establishment rejected Dr. Kaufman's reports of success, however, and balked at the high doses he gave his patients. These ranged from 900 to 4,000 milligrams a day, while the RDA is less than 2 milligrams. Dr. Kaufman has been cited frequently in *Prevention* magazine and in books also published by Rodale Press, *Prevention*'s parent. To his credit, Dr. Kaufman always emphasized the fact that high doses of B₃ were *not* for self-treatment, and must be supervised by a doctor, though it would probably prove quite difficult to find one willing to do so.

Vitamin A

Vitamin A is drawing attention these days as a possible cancer preventive and as an important nutrient for proper immune-system functioning. Only one of the sixty-two survey participants taking it, however, mentioned any special benefit as far as arthritis is concerned. Another fourteen take beta-carotene, a vegetable extract that your body can convert to the active form of vitamin A. Like vitamin C, A can make a healthy contribution to your recovery from surgery. The RDA is 4,000 international units a day for women and 5,000 for men.

Vitamin D

Do you now or have you ever taken corticosteroids? These drugs include prednisone, prednisolone, and cortisone acetate. They are all powerful anti-inflammatories, but they all contribute to bone deterioration, such as osteoporosis (thinning of the bones), osteomalacia (softening of the bones), and osteopenia (loss of bone substance). Rheumatoid arthritis alone—even if you've never had so much as a single dose of any steroid drug—may predispose you to thinning, weakening bones that break easily, and increase your need for vitamin D and calcium. Fifty-five of our survey participants take vitamin D supplements, including a forty-four-year-old office manager from New York, whose rheumatologist has her take 50,000 international units per week, plus calcium.

Doctors at the Royal National Hospital for Rheumatic Diseases in Bath, England, examined a group of elderly women with rheumatoid arthritis. Five of the women had suffered fractures in the long bones of their legs, while the other twelve

women had had no such bad breaks. When the doctors interviewed all the women at length about their diets, they discovered that the ones with broken bones were getting *far less*
vitamin D than the other women. (They ate less margarine, for
example, and fewer eggs, which are good sources of the vitamin.) "This suggests," the physicians wrote in the *British Medical Journal* (November 23, 1974), "that dietary vitamin-D
deficiency was an important cause of the fractures. . . ."

They also noted that the women were poor, and perhaps
could not afford to buy foods rich in vitamin D, so they prescribed an inexpensive supplement containing 300 international units (less than the RDA of 400) a day. Because these
particular women were housebound, too, they weren't even
getting the vitamin D that comes free for the asking by spending twenty minutes in the sunshine every day.

Cod liver oil

This old-fashioned fish-oil folk remedy is largely a combination
of vitamins A and D. Fifty-five of our participants take it regularly—either as a tablespoonful of liquid, or in capsule form,
and sixteen of them say it relieves arthritis pain. The amounts
of the two vitamins vary from one brand of cod liver oil to
another, but most recommended doses contain on or about the
RDAs for vitamins A and D. We've already touched on the
value of these vitamins, but the value of cod liver oil may be
greater than the sum of these two parts. As its name makes
plain, cod liver oil comes from the liver of a cold-water fish.
And some brands contain the omega-3-type essential fatty
acids found in new-wave fish-oil capsules, like **MaxEPA**, which
have recently been shown to be of benefit to some people with
arthritis.

There are important differences between the two fish oils,
however. Cod liver oil comes from the fish's liver, while **Max-
EPA** and the like are derived from the flesh of oily fish. The
liver origin is what gives cod liver oil its store of vitamins A and
D. **MaxEPA** contains very low levels of these vitamins. And so,
while volunteers in research studies have taken as many as
fifteen or twenty capsules of **MaxEPA** every day for weeks on

end—with no known ill effects—an equivalent number of cod liver oil capsules could deliver a *toxic dose* of vitamins A and D. Cod liver oil also contains more cholesterol. "I started taking cod liver oil (my own idea to grease my joints!)," writes a retired NASA secretary from Texas, "and was relieved so much, but when my doctor discovered during an annual physical that my cholesterol level was three points below heart-attack level, I had to stop taking the cod liver oil."

Minerals

Several of the minerals essential to good health are especially important in arthritis care. The same dietary studies mentioned earlier in this chapter, which showed that people with arthritis tend to take in too little of the B vitamins and vitamin E, also showed deficiencies or less-than-ideal levels of magnesium, zinc, and calcium. These, along with iron and potassium, are the minerals that our participants take most often as dietary supplements.

Calcium

In the wake of a national furor over osteoporosis, calcium has become one of the most popular dietary supplements of all time, particularly among women, who are especially prone to the disease after menopause. But most people with arthritis—men and women alike—need lots of calcium anyway. It helps keep the bones strong, along with vitamin D, and may ward off the bone damage from steroid drugs. A New Zealand study tested the value of calcium supplements for people taking these drugs, and the researchers were gratified to discover that 1,000 milligrams of calcium a day (200 milligrams more than the RDA of 800 milligrams) seemed to slow down and even *reverse* the process of bone loss. "The dose of calcium used and its timing require further study, as do its effects on bone density," they report in the *American Journal of Clinical Nutrition*. "Until such information is available, the use of calcium supplements in steroid-treated subjects would appear to have a reasonable basis."

If you are over sixty-five, your ability to absorb calcium from foods is not what it used to be, making it even more unlikely that a healthy diet could fulfill your calcium needs.

More survey participants take calcium than any other mineral supplement, with 270 of them using from 250 to 1,500 milligrams daily. The advantages, they say, include relief of leg cramps for nine of them and relief of arthritis pain or swelling for another fifteen. "I once ran out of calcium tablets and had to wait three or four weeks before my order arrived," says a retired legal assistant who now lives in rural Wisconsin. "After several days of missing my calcium supplement, my hands became very sore. After nearly two weeks without calcium I could hardly use my hands and would awaken in pain and stiff every morning. Once back on calcium, it took a few days, but all symptoms disappeared and have not returned. My daily calcium intake, including the calcium in food I eat, is between 1,500 and 2,000 milligrams."

Very few participants mentioned the brand of calcium supplements they use, but a study reported in 1987 in *American Pharmacy* showed vast differences in the way these products disintegrate and dissolve in the gut. For example, **Potent Calcium 600 mg** from General Nutrition Centers took over an hour to disintegrate when tested, so that only 5 percent of the tablet had dissolved after thirty minutes, while **Calcium Carbonate** from Roxane Labs, Inc., disintegrated in just two minutes and was 100-percent dissolved after thirty minutes. Your best assurance of getting the full dose of calcium in any product is to swallow it with a meal, so that the tablet stays in your stomach long enough to dissolve completely. Splitting up your dosage—500 milligrams with two meals instead of 1,000 milligrams all at once—offers still more assurance of absorbing the nutrient.

Many of our survey participants take prescription or over-the-counter antacids to counteract the stomach upset caused by arthritis medications. But a few of them take **Tums** as an inexpensive calcium supplement, since each tablet contains 200 milligrams of calcium carbonate (or 300 milligrams in **Tums E-X**).

Ask your doctor about taking 1,000 milligrams of calcium a day, or 1,500 milligrams if you are a woman past menopause. You need to take vitamin D along with the calcium to give your body the best chance of putting the calcium to good use. Also remember that what you *do* is as important as anything you take. For no amount of calcium supplements can undo the bone loss caused by inactivity. In other words, exercise is essential. (See Chapter 18.)

Zinc

Zinc was used successfully to treat arthritis in an experiment that involved twenty-four people with rheumatoid arthritis at the University of Washington in Seattle. In one part of the study, half the volunteers took zinc supplements three times a day for twelve weeks, while the other half took placebos. Those on zinc had less swelling, less morning stiffness, and an overall better sense of well-being, according to Dr. Peter A. Simkin's report in the British medical journal *Lancet* in 1976. Since then, other studies have documented zinc deficiencies in the diets of people with arthritis, but there have been no formal attempts to treat the disease with large doses of zinc. (Volunteers in the Washington study took about ten times the RDA for this mineral.) Sixty-one of our participants take zinc regularly, perhaps because news of the zinc–arthritis study was reported in the popular press.

Nutritionists and physicians at Albany Medical College, Cornell University, and New York University, among others, have investigated the effects of arthritis drugs on various essential minerals. The drug penicillamine, for example, which is often used to treat rheumatoid arthritis, is supposed to make your body excrete copper, but it can also cause you to lose zinc.

Iron

Every time you take an aspirin or other NSAID, you may lose a tiny bit of blood. Over time, these little losses can mount into iron-deficiency conditions, and forty-three of our survey participants are offsetting them with an iron supplement. (People with rheumatoid arthritis are often anemic, regardless of their drug therapy, since the disease itself can *cause* anemia.) The RDA for iron is 10 milligrams for men and 18 milligrams for women ages eighteen to fifty (to make up for the blood lost during menstruation). These quantities of iron are more than many people get in their diets, but the amount included in your multivitamin tablet is probably sufficient to make up the difference. If medications and upcoming surgery drive your personal iron needs even higher, though, ask your doctor about an appropriate supplement.

Summary of Vitamins and Minerals

- A daily multivitamin and mineral supplement seems essential to fill the gaps in your diet and make up for some of the nutritional problems arthritis causes, from decreased appetite or cooking ability to incomplete absorption of some nutrients.

- If you have specific vitamin deficiencies, addressing the problem with the proper supplements can help you feel better.

- Surgery may drive up your need for certain nutrients, such as vitamin C, vitamin A, and iron.

- Many arthritis drugs create deficiencies of certain nutrients, by interfering with their absorption, for example, or by hastening them out of your body. The drugs include aspirin (vitamin C), methotrexate (folic acid), penicillamine (copper and zinc), and steroid drugs (calcium).

- Blood loss from chronic use of aspirin and other nonsteroidal anti-inflammatory drugs can lead to iron deficiency.

- Some vitamins apparently play specific roles in relieving arthritis-related problems, such as vitamin C for the bruising common to rheumatoid arthritis, vitamin E for its possible anti-inflammatory action and relief of drug-caused tissue damage, and vitamin B_6 for relief of some cases of carpal tunnel syndrome. Many other possibilities exist but have not been proven scientifically.

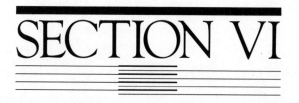

SECTION VI

HOW THE COLLECTIVE WISDOM OF SURVEY PARTICIPANTS CAN HELP YOU ON A DAILY BASIS

My personal experience was a real crisis at first. Even though I had faith in my doctors, I still had a lot of unanswered questions that doctors don't have time for.

—Survey Participant #610, a county sheriff from Kansas

Other people with arthritis are really helpful because they know from experience what works and what does not.

—Survey Participant #232, an accounting clerk from Texas

I think you can learn to help yourself more than anyone else can help you.

—Survey Participant #471, a homemaker from Utah

16

HOW AND WHY TO BUILD A POSITIVE OUTLOOK IN SPITE OF ARTHRITIS

■ How arthritis affects emotions ■ How attitude affects arthritis ■ How survey participants control stress ■ How they lift their spirits

No matter what medications they take or other kinds of help they've received, many of the 1,051 participants in our Arthritis Survey count their own positive outlook on life among their most potent weapons against arthritis. They complain little, although they have suffered much, and they believe that their attitude helps them feel and function far better than they otherwise might.

For although arthritis is a malady of the joints, it can also inflame anger, rain depression, and rob people of their self-esteem.

Arthritis is not *caused* by emotional problems, to be sure, but it kicks up a lot of strong feelings, and it can *respond* to feelings, too. Stress, for example, often makes arthritis symptoms flare, while the relief of stress may drive those symptoms into remission. Even when it comes to medical care, emotional factors seem to tip the odds in favor of benefiting from certain drugs or procedures. For it sometimes happens that two people with the same kind of arthritis, whose X rays reveal identical degrees of joint damage, react quite differently to the same treatment—apparently because one has a positive mental outlook and the other feels beaten before beginning.

In this chapter, our participants will tell you all about their personal struggles, speaking frankly of dreams dashed by arthritis—and new dreams they conjured to fight their way out of hopelessness. We'll add to their comments a few accounts of medical studies showing how important it is to feel in control of your arthritis, instead of controlled by it, and suggesting ways for you to gain that control.

Survey participants will also describe the relaxation techniques they rely on, like imagery and self-hypnosis, to reduce stress and thereby relieve pain. And they're happy to share the things they love to do, from praying to playing piano, that lift their spirits and may do the same for yours.

Emotional Fallout

It should be easy to understand, even from a healthy distance, how losing the ability to do what you've always done could make you furious, or sad, or both. Anyone should be able to see that being in pain is reason enough to get depressed occasionally. Yet people in our survey note that most of their friends and family members do *not* appreciate their emotional turmoil, and definitely do not want to hear about it. Worse, some of their so-called friends imply that arthritis came about as the *result* of their internal upset, instead of the other way around.

Doctors, too, have sometimes been guilty of blaming their patients for bringing on arthritis by virtue of their personality problems. Dr. Martin A. Shearn of the University of California School of Medicine in San Francisco, who has studied and written about the psychological aspects of arthritis, found several early attempts to categorize people with rheumatoid arthritis as being by turns masochistic, self-sacrificing, moralistic, perfectionistic, and inhibited. It has also been said that people develop arthritis because they are unable to express anger and therefore harbor hostility or resentment. But there is no evidence to support these stone-casting ideas. Indeed, as more recent studies have shown (and as you could have told the researchers), there is no personality "type" that distinguishes people with arthritis from anyone else.

"You have to have a good attitude," concludes a sixty-five-year-old former telephone operator from North Carolina, "and be happy, or, believe me, you'll feel worse. I've always been a cheerful person. I try not to get down in the dumps, and find that people like me a lot better for the effort. I try to forget about 'Old Arthur,' as I refer to my arthritis, and still go on trips, go shopping, laugh with friends, and do not complain."

It Couldn't Happen to Me

On first hearing that they had arthritis, some of our survey participants simply could not believe the news. Younger people especially, who tend to think of arthritis as a disease of old age, may *deny* what is happening to them, as a way of dealing with the shock. "When the doctor showed me my X rays compared to normal X rays of someone else's hands and feet," says a twenty-two-year-old college student from California, "I finally started to face the fact that I had a problem."

Denying arthritis means denying its proper treatment as well, and actually making the condition worse as a result. "I was fourteen when I learned I had arthritis," writes a forty-seven-year-old occupational therapist from Colorado. "I did not accept my disease for years, and continued to do activities, including sports, that I had done before, even though I had to take pain medication to get through them. I did a lot of damage to my elbows and feet that way."

Denial, anger, anxiety, and depression are most often *normal reactions* to the challenge of adjusting to living with arthritis. Their normalcy, however, doesn't make them any easier to bear; and some physicians believe that depression and anxiety actually *lower* your tolerance for pain.

Some fifty of our participants sought the help of psychologists or psychiatrists to get them through emotional crises related to arthritis. The college student mentioned above, for example, is in psychotherapy now and finds that it helps her face the fact of her arthritis and consequently take better care of herself. And the occupational therapist reports that a psychiatrist "enabled me to vent my feelings and work on my self-image, as well as other problems. He also prescribed antidepressants that were helpful."*

A Sense of Loss

The majority of our survey participants do what they want to do in spite of arthritis, but some of them feel a tremendous sense of loss. "I have wishes unfulfilled, and poverty due to living on social security and Medicare," writes a forty-six-year-old former proofreader from Oregon who was forced to leave her job in 1985 because of increasing pain and fatigue. "I feel I'm always the watcher, never the participant, and it's sad. But I try to be cheerful because my arthritis also affects those who love me."

Drs. John L. Black and Maurice J. Martin, two Mayo Clinic psychiatrists who wrote about depression and arthritis in *The Journal of Musculoskeletal Medicine,* explain that loss is a frequent cause of depression, and that people must have a chance to recognize and grieve the loss before they can pick up and carry on. The loss can take any form. One person loses sight of himself—becoming a *patient* instead of a *person.* Another loses a job, and with it her whole social network.

"I had a job I loved for twelve years," says a sixty-one-year-old widow from Ontario. "I ran the cafeteria for an import-export company. I did the ordering, cooking, and serving, and in general looked after my extended family every day. I even got to do special luncheons for out-of-town guests. When my knees became really bad three years ago, I had to stop work and go on a disability pension. It has taken me a long time to get it through my head that I cannot go back to work, even when I feel well, and stand for seven to ten hours at a stretch, then ride a highway bus home. But I am learning."

One participant, a forty-five-year-old former insurance

---

*Twenty-two survey participants take antidepressant medications, such as **Elavil** (amitriptyline) and **Tofranil** (imipramine). Some of them take the drugs for depression, and some for pain, since the family of tricyclic antidepressants, to which these drugs belong, has been shown to help relieve arthritis pain. These are not first-choice drugs for arthritis, however, and have their own set of problem side effects.

agent now living in Oklahoma, not only lost her job because of arthritis but her marriage as well. "As I became less able to be in control," she recalls, "our family life deteriorated. My son and middle daughter became unruly and involved in drugs. My husband would not face or acknowledge that I had rheumatoid arthritis. He called me a malingerer.

"On several occasions when I had severe flareups, I was unable to feed myself or the dog, as I could neither walk on the cold kitchen floor nor open a package or can. My husband would not change his lifestyle or buy devices or gadgets that would help me function. This was not because he was an ogre, but because he preferred to deny that I was ill and that I was no longer able to provide him with the services he was accustomed to having me provide. He renewed the lease on our two-story condominium in San Diego in 1982, although I had obvious difficulty climbing the stairs, and by 1983 I could not climb them at all. I slept on the living room couch for the next year and a half.

"My eldest daughter, who was working as a nurse at a hospital, moved back home to become my help and chauffeur, since I could no longer drive a car. My youngest daughter was my cheerful friend. The other two children preferred denial.

"I was building a new way of thinking about life by 1984, and I was encouraged by finally winning the award of social security disability, retroactive to 1982. My twenty-fifth high school reunion came up that June, and with help from my daughter I was able to attend part of it.

"Then I acknowledged the final death of my hopes for my marriage. The social security settlement helped me have the funds, and reading helped me get the information on how to obtain a California divorce without an attorney or physically appearing in court. My daughter did the typing and legwork. The divorce, with alimony and child support, was granted in late December.

"My daughters helped me find things like kitchen gadgets and a hand-held shower attachment that helped me become more able to help myself. We three realized we couldn't afford to live in California any longer, so we made our lists of what we needed, did our research, and decided on a place in eastern Oklahoma. A Golden Retriever dog, a sick lady, a twenty-three-year-old lady, and a fifteen-year-old girl set out on a rainy April day from San Diego on a 1,500-mile, twelve-day adventure in an overloaded station wagon pulling an overloaded tent trailer. It was a *great* adventure.

"We've lived out here in the country for three years now. For beautiful imagery, I only have to look around me."

How Powerful Is Positive Thinking?

Our survey files are full of stories from people who made up their minds, or made a pact with God, to win out over arthritis. There are hospital studies, too, showing that grit and guts are quite effective as pain-relievers.

To test the power of a positive attitude against the pain and disability of osteoarthritis, researchers at the University of Alabama gathered a group of sixty-five volunteers who had arthritis in at least one hip or one knee. They wanted to see whether these people's perception of pain and their ability to carry out everyday activities were influenced more by the extent of their actual joint damage—or by psychological factors such as depression, anxiety, and feelings of helplessness.

First they collected recent X rays from all the volunteers, and had two rheumatologists, who never saw the people in person, judge the severity of each one's arthritis on the basis of the joint damage alone. Then the researchers visited the volunteers at their homes, where they interviewed them about their daily lives and gave them a battery of psychological tests. At the end, they pooled all the information they had on each person to see what they could see. And they saw that joint damage alone does *not* account for the amount of pain a person feels, or for the amount of difficulty anyone has in getting dressed, getting around, or getting on at work. In fact, as the researchers reported in 1988 in *Arthritis and Rheumatism*, attitude and emotions may be *more important.* Depression, for example, is more likely than joint destruction to keep people from taking care of themselves. And those volunteers who scored the highest on tests of "resourcefulness" (the feeling that they could cope with any curve life threw them) were the *least* disabled in terms of doing things, no matter what shape their joints were in.

We are painfully aware, in reporting the results of these kinds of studies, that you hardly need to be blamed for any difficulty you are having in controlling your symptoms or managing your daily activities. Having said that developing arthritis is *not* your fault, we are not about to claim that suffering from it *is* your fault because you aren't cheerful enough or resourceful enough to do better. Instead, we present these studies because they validate our participants' experiences, and because they suggest concrete measures anyone can take to try to improve the outcome of arthritis care. Anxiety and depression, for instance, are conditions that can be treated, whether in psychotherapy, with the help of support groups, or by other means. The elements of resourcefulness can be *taught,* psychologists have shown, by arming you with a series of positive statements you can repeat to yourself in times of need. Ideally, these learned "coping statements" take the place of your old self-defeating beliefs, and give you the push you need to take control of your situation—even if you weren't born with a silver lining in your mental outlook.

A good all-around coping strategy is a combination of attitude and action. You use the positive ideas ("I *can* reduce my pain by staying calm and relaxed.") along with specific self-care measures, which usually include taking medication on schedule, resting, applying heat or ice (or both), exercising, eating well, and practicing a relaxation technique.

"For thirty-four years I have tried to look on the bright side of my problem," says a retired automobile dealer from Massachusetts, who's had rheumatoid arthritis since age twenty-six, and diabetes, too. "I can't run but I *can* walk and ride a bike. I can't ski, but I *can* watch. And when I hurt, I know I could hurt more. Attitude is my *best* doctor."

Handicapped by Helplessness

Because arthritis may begin for no known reason and persist with no known cure, it often engenders a sense of helplessness. This is an understandable but counterproductive reaction— because helplessness can lead to depression and the inability, or unwillingness, to follow your prescribed treatment plan. Indeed, the feeling of helplessness is so common and so meaningful in arthritis that a group of psychologists developed a special test to measure it. Called the Arthritis Helplessness Index, it consists of a series of statements, ranging in outlook from "Arthritis is controlling my life," to "I am coping effectively with my arthritis." By agreeing or disagreeing with the various statements, you establish your score; and that score may well determine how you respond to medical care, according to a recent study at the Vanderbilt University Medical Center in Nashville.

The point of the study was to see whether the Arthritis Helplessness Index could predict how well individuals would fare with their arthritis treatments over time. The researchers mailed the index to several hundred people who all had rheumatoid arthritis for seven years or less. In the course of the two-year study, the 368 volunteers filled out the index five times, so the researchers could chart any changes in their outlook. All the while the participants went on seeing their own private doctors, taking whatever medications their doctors prescribed for them. This was a watch-and-see study, and the researchers made no attempt to work with any of the volunteers to teach them particular coping strategies or educate them about arthritis.

As it turned out, the individual helplessness scores stayed pretty much the same throughout. And the volunteers who felt the most helpless fared the worst with their arthritis, from start to finish. They reported more pain and disability than those who did not feel helpless. In fact, the researchers concluded, a high helplessness score could serve as a red flag for physicians, to help them identify, at the outset of treatment, those patients who will likely need extra attention and assistance.

An Antidote for Helplessness

Let's take a close look at an extremely thorough, well-thought-out program for helping people with arthritis take charge of their pain control and defeat the feeling of helplessness. Psychologist Jerry C. Parker, Ph.D. and his colleagues at the University of Missouri School of Medicine devised this particular regimen, and tested it recently on patients at the Harry S Truman Memorial Veterans' Hospital in Columbia, Missouri.

Compared to a purely educational program, or routine rheumatology care, this combination-treatment approach to arthritis proved to make a substantial difference in the way people felt, in terms of both pain perception and feeling in control of their lives.

To start with, the twenty-nine volunteers spent a week as inpatients at the hospital, where they were tested and treated to a five-day crash course in the following subjects:

- the nature and treatment of rheumatoid arthritis

- theories and facts about pain, including its emotional aspects

- stress management, including relaxation training

- distraction strategies for taking their minds off arthritis pain

- problem-solving techniques

- marriage and family dynamics

- communication skills

Every one to three months over the next year, whenever the volunteers returned to the hospital for a routine clinic visit, they also attended a meeting of a support group, where they talked about using the techniques they'd learned in their everyday lives. As a result, they made great gains in their ability to control pain. When the researchers contacted them a year after the study ended, they reported that they were still applying the lessons, because the strategies were still helping.

"If you break a leg, you know why you feel pain, and you know why it happened," Dr. Parker explained when he presented the results of this study to the national meeting of the Arthritis Health Professions Association in Washington, D.C., in 1987. "With rheumatoid arthritis, we don't understand why one person gets the disease and another doesn't. If a sense of helplessness develops, it often starts a vicious cycle in which pain causes depression, which in turn can increase pain and even the disability. Based on what we've learned in this study, clearly, there are pain relief and quality of life benefits beyond standard medical treatment."

The Art of Stress Management

Fully 670 of our survey participants, or 64 percent of the survey group, find that stress aggravates their pain, whether they have osteoarthritis or rheumatoid. "I have found that stress affects how I feel a great deal," says a bookkeeper from New York. "When I let things get to me, my pain increases, which causes more stress, which causes more pain, and so on, round and round."

A composer from California writes, "My arthritis was pretty much restricted to my finger joints, and fairly mild until about three years ago, when I went back to school for advanced studies, living four hundred miles from my wife and kids, and commuting home every two weeks. It was a high-stress program. My arthritis got *much* worse, I think largely due to stress."

Since controlling stress is tantamount to pain relief for these people, you can bet they take their relaxation seriously. Here are the survey's top ten favorite stress beaters.

Technique	Number of Participants Who Use It
1. Deep breathing	210
2. Avoiding stressful situations, including crowds	128
3. Attention-diverting, including hobbies and reading	127
4. Exercise or other physical activity	116
5. Relaxation technique, including self-hypnosis	88
6. Reducing anxiety through self-control, self-affirmation	87
7. Rest	80
8. Imagery or visualization	71
9. Meditation, including prayer	61
10. Resolving the problems that are causing stress	54

Most participants who practice stress control combine two or more of these strategies. The bookkeeper mentioned above, for example, uses several: "When I feel things piling up, I do the relaxation techniques I learned. I also try to busy myself with things I enjoy—whether it's reading or watching TV or working on a craft. Anything to take my mind off what's bugging me. At work when I feel uptight I get up and take a little walk. I am lucky in that I am free to move about as I please, and if I need a break I can take it. I also make it a point, when I'm stressed up, to go to a quiet, relaxing place for a nice lunch. It allows me quiet time to unwind."

Each technique has its own special virtue.

Deep breathing. Your breathing is the most accessible part of the stress reaction, which also includes a speeded-up heartbeat, tensed muscles, and an outpouring of adrenaline. Gently force yourself to breathe deeply and evenly, and the change of pace will slow down the rest of your body. Deep breathing is the beginning of most formal relaxation techniques. Do it by inhaling through your nose for several seconds as you expand your abdomen. (Raising your shoulders doesn't help.) Hold the breath for a moment or two and then exhale through your mouth. Try to make yourself as comfortable as possible. "I sit in my recliner with my feet up," says a former teacher from Idaho, "do deep breathing, listen to music, and sometimes swear a lot."

Avoiding stressful situations. This works well, insofar as you can manage it. Not all stress is avoidable, but try to identify the people or things you don't have to put up with. "I was under a lot of stress during my marriage," an Arizona homemaker recalls. "Once divorced I got relief and a remission which I have enjoyed for twelve years." A forty-two-year-old former television producer writes: "I have changed my home to northern Wisconsin, where the pace of living is laid back. I have removed myself from a high-powered job, loaded with stress and competition. I involve myself with things I enjoy, and not with things I feel I'm supposed to do."

Attention-diverting activities. These get your mind off stress and pain and can be rewarding in themselves. Many of our participants say that the hobbies they enjoy, including needlecrafts of all description, also provide good exercise for their affected joints. "I go to my workshop and build shelves," reports a retired pharmacist from Illinois with arthritis in his knees and shoulders. "The hammering and sawing help. I probably have enough shelves to open a store!"

Exercise. This often chases tension away in short order. Our participants particularly like exercises that get them out of the house, too, such as walking, swimming, and bicycling.

Relaxation techniques. Those mentioned in our survey include self-hypnosis, biofeedback (see Chapter 8), and audio-cassette tapes that calmly talk to our participants and help them clear their heads and relax every muscle. A retired policewoman from New York explains, "I lie down and tell myself to think of nothing and to feel no pain from my head, then face, then neck, and so on, down to my toes." Some learned their technique from a mental-health practitioner, and some from books and tapes. In any case, becoming proficient at therapeutic relaxation takes practice, and any technique works best when practiced every day. One form of self-hypnosis that has been used successfully by people with arthritis, called "glove anesthesia," teaches you to picture your hands covered with gloves upon gloves, so that your fingers feel no pain or other sensations, and then to think of touching the places that hurt, allowing the gloves to absorb all the pain.

Reducing anxiety through self-control, self-affirmation. This boils down to getting a grip on yourself, and giving yourself as much support as you can muster. "I use lots of breathing exercises, in *fresh* air," says a California housewife, "and remember *I'm somebody important.*" An Army officer uses "positive thinking—envisioning success, accentuating positive factors, downplaying the negative." Many remind themselves, "This, too, shall pass."

Rest. Get the sleep you're entitled to at night, participants advise, and slow down or stop during the day if and when you need to.

Imagery or visualization. Some of our survey respondents use their imaginative powers to surround themselves with beautiful, peaceful scenery, even when they're stuck in a stressful situation. "I visualize some kind of water—oceans, rivers," writes a graduate student from California, "and dissociate myself from the present, if it's impossible to leave." Another approach to visualization is to try to journey inward and see inside your joints or imagine specific healing processes going on there. "I talk to my pain," says a New York health consultant, "or to a specific part of my body to find out why it is hurting. I sometimes get immediate release from pain this way."

Meditation. This combines relaxation with an attempt to focus on a word or phrase that clears your mind of other thoughts. (For some participants, prayer achieves the same deeply relaxing, closed-eyed, totally focused state.) Dr. Joan Borysenko of Harvard Medical School, director of the Mind/Body Clinic at Boston's Beth Israel Hospital and author of *Minding the Body, Mending the Mind* (Addison-Wesley, 1987), offers these basic instructions for meditating.

- Choose a quiet spot, away from all distractions.

- Sit in a comfortable position.

- Close your eyes.

- Relax your muscles sequentially from head to feet.

- Become aware of your breathing without trying to control it.

- Repeat a focus word silently in time to your breathing.

- Don't worry about how you're doing, but take note of where and how your mind wanders.

- Practice meditating every day for ten or twenty minutes.

Resolving problems. Sometimes the only way around stress is to face the situation squarely and deal with the problem causing the stress. "I look inside to see what the problem is," reports a homemaker from Vermont. "Sometimes I write on a legal pad until I feel better and can see solutions." Several other participants also use writing as a means of problem-solving. Interestingly, an experiment at Southern Methodist

University, which required a group of college students to write for twenty minutes a day about traumatic events in their lives, showed that the students' immune-system activity increased as a result of this exercise.

A Few of Their Favorite Things

We asked all our survey participants what they do to lift their spirits, and the answers we got were as varied as the participants themselves. Hundreds of them have a favorite hobby that cheers them. They paint with watercolors, play a musical instrument, sew quilts or clothes, build model ships, trains, and planes, take pictures, make pottery, knit, crochet, and collect everything from stamps and baseball cards to china and dollhouse furniture. Staying busy, most of them agree, is therapeutic. And many of them are still busy with their careers, too, getting a great lift from doing their work well.

They love to get out and go fishing, boating, camping, horseback riding, sunbathing, or bird-watching. Some travel far, but many settle happily for a walk or a car ride just to enjoy the change of scenery.

The physical exertion of exercise does the most good for some participants, who beat out the blues by bicycle riding, for example, or walking, swimming, or practicing judo, karate, or Tai Chi. A few choose sports such as golf or volleyball.

Getting things done around the house is soothing for those who like to make home improvements, fix cars, get absorbed in gardening, clean, cook, or bake.

Some participants find their greatest enjoyment in helping others, by volunteering their free time to church activities, community groups, political causes, mental institutions, hospices, hospitals, and senior centers. Others are buoyed by looking after their children, grandchildren, or pets. "What I have done to lift my spirits," writes a former teacher from Massachusetts, "is to bring home a five-week-old puppy, against my doctor's orders (he was afraid I would trip over her) and against my husband's wishes. My 'puppy' was three years old in July, and weighs eleven pounds, fully grown. She has brought so much pleasure to the family, that even my husband now loves her. When you hold her, you forget about yourself, tension goes down, and you're happy all over. Better than any medicine you can buy. She is a joy and a treasure."

Many participants choose to pamper their bodies with a bath, a massage, or a nap. They may treat themselves to a favorite food or drink, too, and perhaps go shopping just to buy something frivolous but affordable.

There are great rewards for many in the social support of their families and friends, clubs, community activities, and self-help group meetings held by their local chapter of the Arthritis Foundation or Alcoholics Anonymous. Some get-togethers are game times, for playing bridge, backgammon, bingo, chess, or horseshoes.

Entertainments needn't be lavish to be cheering. Many participants are happiest when reading a book, they say, listening to the radio, or watching television. "It's hard for me to go to the movies," notes a former cabdriver from Nevada, "because long sitting periods increase my discomfort. I'd rather rent a movie to watch on my VCR, so I can stop, take a break, and move around from time to time." Other participants can and do enjoy attending movies, plays, concerts, baseball games, and car races.

Some go to museums, some go back to school, or take correspondence courses. They lose themselves in murder mysteries, Westerns, romances, and fantasies, but they also like to read newspapers, magazines, and the Bible. They may meditate to improve their outlook, or daydream, or pray, or bend their minds to some conundrum to keep themselves preoccupied. "I do difficult crossword puzzles," writes a veterinarian from New Hampshire, "or try to work out chess moves, or try to think through complex economic theories."

Sometimes they lift their spirits by giving their emotions free expression. "When I'm really down," confesses a former copy editor from Iowa, "I write limericks and insulting greeting cards." "I really need to cry and yell sometimes," says a homemaker from Virginia, "and if I'm not alone, then I do it in the bathroom with the water running." "I have learned to laugh," counters a nurse from Michigan. "Surprisingly, laughter often reduces pain."

Summary of How and Why to Build a Positive Mental Outlook

Though not caused by emotional factors, arthritis can generate anger, denial, anxiety, depression, and feelings of helplessness.

Addressing the emotional problems associated with arthritis is important because:

- Denial can make you ignore proper precautions.

- Depression may keep you from following your treatment plan.

- Anxiety and depression tend to lower your pain threshold.

- Helplessness may lead to depression, and aggravate your pain and disability.

Treatments for relieving or avoiding emotional problems include:

- Psychotherapy (one on one, or in a group)

- Medications, such as antidepressants

- Programs to teach relaxation techniques, "coping statements," family dynamics, communication skills, and the like

Stress frequently exacerbates arthritis pain. Stress-management techniques that may relieve pain include:

- Deep breathing

- Avoiding stressful situations

- Attention-diverting activities, including hobbies and reading

- Exercise or other physical activity

- Relaxation techniques, including self-hypnosis

- Reducing anxiety through self-control and self-affirmation

- Rest

- Imagery or visualization

- Meditation or prayer

- Resolving the problems that are causing stress

17

THE TWENTY-FIVE
TOP-RATED TECHNIQUES
FOR FAST PAIN RELIEF:
At-Home Treatments You Can Use
to Enhance Your Overall Care

■ Rest ■ Heat ■ Ice ■ Baths and showers ■ Exercise ■ Massage ■ Over-the-counter products ■ Joint protection ■ Biofeedback and more

About 100 of the 1,051 participants in our nationwide Arthritis Survey no longer see a doctor, a physical therapist, or any other kind of practitioner for arthritis treatment. They care for themselves, at home, using the techniques covered in this chapter. The other 900, whether they take monthly gold shots, weekly physical-therapy treatments, or daily doses of a prescription drug, *also* use these techniques to boost the effectiveness of their professional care. These are simple but powerful tools that our participants use for *immediate* pain relief.*

*Our participants also practice a variety of techniques at home for *long-term* improvement, which are discussed in other chapters, such as modifying their diet to lose weight and improve nutrition (Chapters 13 and 14), following an exercise routine (Chapters 18 and 19), building a positive mental outlook (Chapter 16), making their surroundings more comfortable (Chapter 20), and learning how to perform everyday activities with minimum pain (Chapter 21).

The twenty-five pain-relief strategies in this chapter are arranged according to their popularity among our participants, beginning with the ones used by the greatest number of people. Although not all of these techniques are appropriate for all people with arthritis, we'll wager that you'll find *at least* half a dozen suggestions on the list that will work for you.

Rest

Two-thirds of our participants stress the importance of rest for pain relief and prevention. Many of them lead extremely active lives but use rest when and as they need to. "Rest" may simply mean a few minutes of sitting in a comfortable chair or taking a break from an activity that causes pain. "Even though I have to work ten to twelve hours every day," writes a forty-nine-year-old dairy farmer from Missouri, "I lie down and rest my back in midday or the pain becomes intolerable." Rest can also mean ample sleep at night and naps in the afternoon to both relieve and ward off pain. A thirty-eight-year-old mother of three from Connecticut observes, "Rest is *extremely* important, no matter how foolish you feel taking a nap or going to bed early. If you're tired, *you hurt!*"

Warm or Hot Baths

"I love hot baths," says a South Carolina secretary, and so do many, many others. Some like it hot, and some prefer it warm, but the bathtub is where half our participants go every day for pain relief. "Sitting in a tub of warm water, not hot, for a good long time—half an hour, say—twice a day, helps about the best of anything," swears a Wisconsin businessman, comparing his tub to prescription drugs, including steroids. An Iowa housewife rates the tub right up there with one of the most popular forms of professional treatment: "Physical therapy helped my back, but I'm better off with hot baths."

A bath is also an effective antidote for stiffness. "I sometimes have to take a bath the moment I get up in the morning," says a Michigan homemaker, "just to get my body moving." Because of the easier movement the water allows, several of our participants like to do their range-of-motion exercises in the tub. "During my hot soak every morning," writes a cafeteria server from Colorado, "I try to manipulate, rotate, and bend the fingers and toes that are affected, as well as move my ankles, shoulders, and elbows."

A tubful of plain water is soothing enough for most people, but a few like to bathe with salts, oils, or bubbles.

The only thing *wrong* with a hot bath, according to a California shipping clerk, is that you have to get out sometime. After twenty to thirty minutes, a hot bath stops being therapeutic and starts to tire the muscles.

Heat

Whether it comes from a heating pad, an electric blanket, a hot-water bottle, a hydrocollator, a heat lamp, or a hot pack made from a washcloth or towel, heat works to drive out pain and stiffness. "I swear by my heating pad," and "I'd be lost without my heating pad," are typical comments from survey participants. In fact, an electric heating pad is the item most likely to be purchased for arthritis pain relief. It's a good investment, to be sure, but here are some homemade alternatives from participants who use them.

- Iron over a wet towel until it is packed with steam. Place a thin towel on your skin, put the steam towel over that, and cover both with another dry towel.

- Run *hot* water on towels or washcloths, wring out excess, and wrap them around affected areas. When they lose their heat in a few minutes, repeat the process.

An entrepreneur from British Columbia finds great relief for his hands under the wall-mounted electric dryers that replace paper towels in some public rest rooms. In fact, they help him so much that he is thinking about buying one for home use. Most participants who use heat therapy find the *dry* heat from hand dryers and heat lamps to be not quite as soothing as the *moist* heat provided by hot towels and many types of electric heating pads, but this is a matter of personal preference.

WARNING: Do not apply heat to a hot, swollen joint.

Showers

"During serious flare-ups," writes a seamstress from Illinois, "I take about three showers daily. It helps." Most people would rather soak in a tub for pain relief than stand in a shower (or sit on a shower seat), but showers do offer a few unique advantages our participants enjoy: (1) The temperature of the water can be changed instantly to give alternating hot and cold treatments; (2) the force of the water can be focused directly on the painful areas, especially if you have a hand-held shower-massage attachment; and (3) it's easier to get in and out of a shower than a bathtub.

Ice

Some participants favor ice over heat for general pain relief, and some use it only on swollen, inflamed joints. "The joint, if inflamed, is hot enough," reasons a retired nurse from New Jersey, "so I apply ice instead of heat." Gel-type ice packs that can be left in the freezer and then molded to fit the painful part are quite popular, but many people have gotten just as much relief from a well-placed bag of frozen peas or a plastic bag filled with water and ice. "I fill a paper cup with water and leave it in the freezer," says a Washington homemaker. "Then I always have a quick pain reliever ready to rub over the joints."

WARNING: Remember that ice carries the danger of frostbite. If you use an ice pack, put a thin dish towel or cloth diaper on your skin for protection, and don't leave the pack in place for more than twenty minutes at a time. The ice-cup massage is safe for a minute or two on any one area—so long as you keep the cup *moving*.

Exercise

Given that a regular exercise program, faithfully followed, can go far toward controlling pain and improving general well-being, there are also specific exercise movements that can be used for *on-the-spot* relief of pain or stiffness. If housework or office work builds up pain in your neck and back, for example, try doing a few simple *head rolls* from a standing or sitting position. You can even do them lying down. (If you have advanced rheumatoid arthritis check with your doctor before attempting this one, since there's a chance the movement could injure you.) Follow these steps in one very slow continuous motion, breathing deeply throughout:

- Tilt your head all the way right as though you were trying to touch your right ear to your shoulder (but don't lift your shoulder to your ear)

- Let your head fall slowly forward to drop your chin almost on your chest.

- Rotate to the left, stretching to get your left ear near your left shoulder.

- Lean your head all the way back and look at the ceiling; repeat in the same direction, and then go the other way twice.

For low back pain, lean your back against a wall with your feet about ten inches away from the wall; tighten your buttocks and your abdominal muscles until you feel the small of your back touch the wall; release; repeat. Shoulder shrugs, rolls, and stretches, finger curls and spreads, and foot circles are just a few of the many other movements you can do during the day, no matter where you are, whenever you feel the need. (See Chapter 19.)

Keeping Busy

Family life, jobs, education, volunteer work, sports, group activities, and hobbies distract our participants' minds from pain, and then some. "I try to ignore the pain as much as possible," says a machinist from Texas, "and get on with my life. I enjoy everything I do, and do it as much as I can. I was told I had only seven or eight years to walk and then I would need a wheelchair. That was nine years ago."

"I have pets and plants to care for, to need me," writes a forty-two-year-old widow from Montana. "I keep active, and if I can't do the thing I want to do at the moment, I do something else until I feel I can. I don't do things just to show off, only to suffer later for it. I use common sense, but I don't fall into the 'I can't' syndrome."

Massage

It's practically a reflex to put your hands on a painful area and rub it gently to bring relief. The warmth and increased circulation do help chase the pain—a fact that has kept massage in vogue for many centuries. Self-massage is quite effective, provided you can reach the parts that hurt. And if you're lucky enough to have someone else give you a good massage, you can let yourself drift into a state of relaxation that may bring you an even greater sense of well-being. "Massage helps a lot," says a university student from California, "because when my body is relaxed, it makes a world of difference in the pain level, especially for shoulder, neck, or back pain. I also find that a good foot and leg massage after walking or working relieves the stress and pressure I feel in those joints."

Some participants like to electrify their massage by using a hand-held massager, or a vibrator unit that slips over the hand doing the massaging, or by leaning against a massage/vibrator pillow.

Comfortable Positions

Many people have a favorite position that can instantly improve the way they feel. "I have no pain when my legs are stretched out, as when I'm lying on my back," finds a retired salesman from Ohio. A teacher from Indiana likes to be sitting down with her knees bent at a 90-degree angle. And a retired railroad carman from Missouri says he needs to get out of bed every night for a while and sit in a chair for pain relief.

Hot Tub or Whirlpool

Most participants rave about plain baths, because most people have plain bathtubs, but those who own whirlpools and hot tubs have the most to rave about. These minispas can combine the soothing comfort of soaking in a wide deep bathtub with the water-jet action of a shower massager. A few technical differences separate the whirlpool from the hot tub: A whirlpool is a tub of any size with a swirling current of water. A hot tub is also a bathtub with churning water, but it is usually made of wood, usually big enough for two or more, and has a heating element in it. A Jacuzzi could be either of these; it's really the name of the company that manufactures some of the most popular models. A California car dealer gives his Jacuzzi a plus-3 rating—higher than he gave to any of the practitioners who treated him. He spends twenty minutes a day in it at 98 degrees, and finds it the best help of all. Our participants also use portable or "home spa" units that work in any standard tub. "I bought a two-hundred-dollar home whirlpool," writes an executive secretary from Texas, "and it was the best two hundred dollars I ever spent. The whirlpool helps loosen tight muscles and relieves the pain. I use it every day."

We're talking about "at-home" treatments in this chapter, but you don't have to have a hot tub or whirlpool at home to enjoy its benefits. Several participants gladly make the trip to a health club or spa to use one. "No matter how swollen I am or how much pain I'm in," writes a legal secretary from Ontario, "five to ten minutes in a whirlpool gives me almost total relief." And an office manager from California says she has kept a trailer at a county park for the past three years, just so she can use the Jacuzzi there.

Aspirin and Other Over-the-Counter Pills

Just as arthritis isn't "minor aches and pains," plain old aspirin isn't ordinary medicine. It's a heavy-duty drug that plays a pivotal role in arthritis treatment. (See Chapter 6.) However, aspirin and aspirin substitutes have another use—as staples in the home medicine chest. And that is where survey participants who usually get by without drugs sometimes look for pain relief.

If you take aspirin once in a while, try taking it with some food or milk, or even an antacid, so that it doesn't upset your stomach. You can choose plain, buffered, coated, or liquid aspirin, but the brand you use is irrelevant as far as anyone can tell.

The best-known aspirin *substitute* is **Tylenol**, which is made of acetaminophen. Some other brand names for acetaminophen are **Datril, Panadol**, and **Anacin-3**. **Tylenol** is quite popular among our participants and was mentioned at least three times more often than any other brand-name, over-the-counter pill. It relieves pain extremely well for many people, but it does not affect inflammation.

Another nonaspirin formula is ibuprofen—the key ingredient in the popular prescription drug **Motrin**. Ibuprofen is sold over the counter, too, in nonprescription strength, as **Advil, Nuprin**, and **Medipren**, to name a few brands. Like aspirin, ibuprofen works against both pain and inflammation.

WARNING: Aspirin and ibuprofen are related to each other and to all of the prescription nonsteroidal anti-inflammatory drugs. Do not take aspirin or ibuprofen if you are regularly using one of these drugs, such as **Motrin, Indocin, Naprosyn**, or **Feldene**, to name some of the most popular ones. If you do, you may increase the risk of side effects from them. Acetaminophen, however, can usually be used with these drugs because it is not an anti-inflammatory. When in doubt, check with your doctor.

Dressing Right

Many of our participants feel a pain when they feel a chill, whether it comes from a wintry blast, an air conditioner on a hot summer day, or a problem with blood circulation. "Above all keep those joints *warm,*" says an antiques dealer from Texas, who sometimes wears three pairs of slacks in the winter to keep her knees free of pain. A nurse from another part of the state puts her hands in special moist-heat mittens when they ache. "I'm obsessed with being cold," admits a public relations consultant from Ohio. "At home, I always wear knee socks and a flannel and wool dressing gown." Many people say they sleep with cotton gloves on, or socks, or both, to ease pain and morning stiffness. And they stress the importance of choosing shoes and clothing they can put on and take off easily.

Liniments

Ointments, creams, and liquids that our participants rub on their joints give many of them relief from pain, stiffness, and muscle soreness and help them get through the day or sleep through the night. "**Aspercreme** works well at night for a good night's sleep," writes an electronics technician from Minnesota. Most liniments bring a feeling of heat to the area where they're applied, and this effect is enough for some people. "**Ben·Gay** is my best friend," says a dressmaker from Illinois. "I use it for warming up my joints." Liniments may irritate your skin if it is sensitive, however, and you may or may not like their strong smell. A New Jersey homemaker jokingly reports that while **Ben·Gay** was temporarily relieving her joint pain, it completely cleared her husband's nostrils.

The top-rated favorites are **Ben·Gay, Aspercreme, Icy Hot, Heet, Mentholatum, Absorbine Jr., Mineral Ice**, and **Myoflex**, followed by **Tiger Balm, Banalg, Sportscreme**, and rubbing alcohol. Here are a few of the "also-rans" (arranged alphabetically) that got five mentions or fewer: **Aloe Vera Rub, Blue Star Horse Liniment, Deep-Down, InfraRUB, Mobisyl, Musterole, Myodyne, Oil of Wintergreen, Omega Oil, Pronto Gel, Rumal, Sloan's Liniment, Soltice**, and **Triple Liniment**.

For cost or other reasons, a few of our participants prefer their own homemade rubs to any available in stores. A North Carolina church organist, for example, occasionally uses her aunt's recipe—a mixture of one pint of rubbing alcohol and one ounce of **Oil of Wintergreen**, with one hundred aspirin tablets dissolved in it. An Illinois housewife relies on the same basic concoction, made with thirty-six aspirin instead of one hundred, which she rubs on her knees before going out to walk.

WARNING: If you are allergic to aspirin by mouth, don't use **Aspercreme** or its equivalent on your skin. If you are unsure about a particular product, show it to your doctor. (Also see Chapter 6 for more information about liniments.)

Meditation, Self-Hypnosis, and Other Mind-Control Techniques

Believing in the power of the mind over the body, many participants use some formal technique for guiding their thoughts away from pain. "The basic philosophy here is 'Heal thyself,' and 'I can overcome,'" explains a clinical psychologist from Tennessee with arthritis in his back and shoulders. "Self-hypnosis has worked for me," he adds, "and not just as a mask for pain." Some find that the deep concentration required for these techniques serves to distract their minds from the pain in their joints. Others feel so relaxed after practicing meditation or self-hypnosis that they are less troubled by pain, and a few actually manage to think their pain away. This is *not* to say that their pain is imaginary, or so minor that it can be easily quelled. Rather, it seems to reinforce what many medical researchers have shown about the mind/brain's ability to generate its own internal pain-relieving drugs, called endorphins. "I could not function while on painkillers, and I was afraid to start using cortisone at the age of twenty-six," writes a production coordinator from Minnesota. "I found I could control my pain with self-hypnosis, heat, and aspirin."

Participants endorse a wide range of mental techniques, from training in Transcendental Meditation, to seeing a psychologist for instruction in self-hypnosis, to simple visualization exercises that originate in their own fantasies. "I sit or lie comfortably," says a Colorado college professor, "relax completely, close my eyes, and think of favorite scenes, such as my childhood home, sunsets, lighthouses against surf, and trout streams." A New York tennis instructor says, "I focus on my goal to be healthy and visualize in my mind all that good health means to me."

If you would like to try your own form of meditation, give yourself the benefit of solitude and privacy for at least ten or twenty minutes a day. Take the phone off the hook, too. Pick your most comfortable position, so that you'll be able to relax your body. In fact, some people's entire "meditation" consists of consciously trying to relax each body part in order, from the forehead to the toes, or vice versa. Closing your eyes and breathing deeply and evenly are also important. Deep breathing, like relaxing, is such potent medicine for some people that they can feel relief just by focusing their minds on inhaling and exhaling, perhaps repeating a sound or word with every breath. The more you practice meditation, proponents say, the better you get at it, and the better it can make you feel. For some participants, prayer confers the same benefits.

Combining Heat and Cold

Thermotherapy and cryotherapy, otherwise known as heat and cold, can make a great team when used one right after the other for combination therapy. Whatever the heat fails to soothe, the ice anesthetizes. The owner of a small business in Utah writes, "I use a heating pad and ice when I have the worst pain. The alternating hot and cold really helps." Our participants mix virtually every form of heat and cold for this technique, such as taking a hot shower and then turning it into a cold shower, using a hot-water bottle or a heating pad followed by an ice pack, and setting up two dishpans full of water for contrast baths. A bookkeeper from California treats her hands and feet this way, immersing them in warm and then cold water, back and forth every few minutes for a total of thirty minutes.

Walking

Even before walking became a hot new trend, complete with fancy required equipment and magazines and videotapes for its devotees, survey participants knew the therapeutic benefits of walking. A daily walk is part of *most* of the regular exercise programs described by our participants. And many of them head out for a walk precisely when they feel their worst, for relief of both pain and stiffness. "Whenever I get painful joints," writes a New York housewife, "I walk until I feel better. Even if I don't go outside, but just walk around the house, it helps me." A Texas homemaker says that if she is troubled by pain or stiffness during the night, she gets out of bed to walk it off. Walking outdoors, provided you are up and ready for it, has the added advantages of fresh air, a break from other activity, and the mental stimulation of the people and things you encounter on your way.

Cool Soaks and Mineral Springs

Not as well known as warm baths or hot showers, and not as popular as whirlpools or hot tubs, cold baths do hold a place in the hearts of some participants. A machine operator from Washington says they help him more than anything, and several others talk about the virtues of soaking their swollen, painful hands or feet in cool water.

Only four of our participants visited natural springs reputed to have healing powers. They all enjoyed the experience, especially since they happened to have the natural wonders practically in their backyards in Nevada, Oregon, and Hot Springs, Arkansas. A photographer from Massachusetts, who was able to try the hot sulphur baths at the Dead Sea Spa while on assignment in Israel, pronounced them "wonderful."

Joint Coverings

Many a wrist and knee have gone into an elastic bandage for awhile to find relief. The wrapping could be an Ace bandage, an athletic ankle support, a Futuro Knee Thermo Comforter, a Barlow Knee Support, or any product that allows you to put *gentle* pressure on the affected joint. Even Band-Aid strips will do, according to an insurance underwriter from Nebraska who finds them just the right size for the small joints of her fingers and toes. Ace and other elastic bandages are reusable, up to a point. "I keep a supply of several elastic bandages in good condition, with lots of stretch," writes a housewife from California, "and wash them by hand as needed." Some of our participants say they get an added measure of relief by applying a liniment before wrapping the joint.

Under their feet, several participants like the feel of an arch support or cushion insert in their shoes. Some of them use orthotics specially made for them by podiatrists or orthotists. Others shop for inserts at drug, shoe, or department stores, or shoe-repair shops. "I am on my feet an average of twelve hours a day," writes a surgical nurse from South Dakota. "The arch supports I bought at a shoe-repair shop for twelve dollars really help."

Herbal Teas and Other Drinks

Hot caffeine-free drinks, especially herbal teas, are not only good-tasting and relaxing, our participants say, but also help alleviate pain. "I like chamomile or peppermint/chamomile mix or comfrey for soothing and relaxing me in general," says a twenty-two-year-old California student who's had arthritis since she was seven. "Maybe it's more mental than physical, but these help, especially on rainy days." A retired office manager from Oregon who can no longer take anti-inflammatory drugs is now preparing her own teas with dried herbs she buys at health-food stores. "In the past, I've taken **Nalfon, Clinoril,** and **Feldene,**" she writes, "but I can't any more because of a problem with my blood platelets. The only drug I use now is

Tylenol, and I'm drinking herbal teas. Alfalfa with nettle seems to help the overall condition for me, and I'm still experimenting with other combinations." Even when the herbs have no noticeable effect on their pain level, some participants enjoy sipping hot herb or spice tea, or hot chocolate, just for the warmth it brings from within.

WARNING: Although herbal teas seem "natural" and harmless, excessive quantities of herbs used medicinally can cause a variety of toxic effects.

A number of survey participants say they sometimes use a glass of wine, or a cocktail, or a "good stiff drink" as a pain reliever. "I like a glass of wine while I cook supper or after a rotten day at the office," says a Kansas computer programmer, "but too much creates problems of fluid retention and self-recrimination."

WARNING: Alcohol creates many other problems, as well, which are all too well known. Speaking strictly about arthritis, however, we note that more than thirty of our participants have a sensitivity to alcohol and suffer increased joint pain after they drink even a small amount of any alcoholic beverage. (See Chapter 13.) "Don't turn to booze for relief," warns a Virginia nursery and greenhouse worker. "Although it gives some quick relief, I drank myself into being an alcoholic while trying to kill that last bit of pain."

Relaxation and Stress Reduction

With the majority of our participants noting that stress aggravates their pain, it follows naturally that a number of them get relief by reducing stress—or removing themselves from extremely stressful situations when they can. Since that's not always possible, and since no life is free of stress, they also rely on stress-reduction techniques to calm themselves and their pain. Meditation and visualization, mentioned earlier, can be used for stress reduction. (These and several other stress-beating techniques are described in Chapter 16.) Here are some steps our participants like to take for a quick fix.

- Concentrate on your breathing. Take very deep breaths by expanding your chest *without* lifting your shoulders. Inhale slowly through your nose for five seconds, hold the breath for another five, then slowly exhale through your mouth. Repeat until your heart stops racing.

- Let out your feelings. Cry, curse, laugh, pray, or whatever the situation calls for.

- Dive into a good book.

- Repeat some encouraging words to yourself—your own ("I can manage this."/"I know this will turn out fine.") or someone else's (a line of poetry, a psalm, a song).

Although we usually think of stress as being mental or emotional or both, some survey participants cite *physical* stress as their worst enemy. A Wisconsin postal clerk's definition of stress reduction, for example, is to avoid any unusual strain on his body, such as heavy lifting and high reaching. When your body is overloaded, the arthritis pain inevitably increases, so it makes sense to try to control *both* kinds of stress.

Food

Whatever they generally eat or avoid eating because of arthritis, several participants have a favorite food that figures in their pain-relief programs. Here are a few examples.

An Oklahoma bank teller: "When I hurt, I baby myself. I get extra rest, I take warm/hot baths and soak twenty minutes. I take extra aspirin, I dress warm from the neck down, including my feet, I drink hot tea, read, and eat oatmeal."

A thirty-five-year-old artist from Ohio who's had both knees and hips replaced: "I feel better once I've eaten a nice salad, fruit, or vegetables."

An Idaho homemaker: "I notice a lot of what I eat depends on how I feel on certain days. The fresh fruits are so refreshing when you don't feel too perky."

Sometimes the *absence* of food is the therapy. "I find that occasional fasting helps the way I feel," says a newspaper reporter from Tennessee. Several clinical studies by medical researchers have shown that some people with arthritis definitely feel less pain after a fast, possibly because the fasting eliminates whatever food(s) may aggravate their symptoms. (See Chapter 12.) However, not enough of our participants used this technique for us to be able to evaluate it. On the contrary, we can see several good reasons for *not* fasting: (1) If you need to take pills regularly to control pain and need to take them *with meals* to minimize the drug side effects, fasting would disrupt your medication regimen. (2) If your appetite is poor and you have trouble eating, fasting might weaken you further. (3) If you are overweight or have an eating disorder, fasting one day may induce you to binge the next. (4) If you have any other medical conditions, such as diabetes, fasting poses even more serious dangers.

TENS, Biofeedback, and Other Gadgets

Many types of professional pain-treating equipment seen in hospitals and practitioners' offices are also available for home use. On the advice of their physicians and therapists, our participants have bought or borrowed devices that stimulate their nerves electrically (TENS units, for *t*ranscutaneous *e*lectrical *n*erve *s*timulation); make them aware of some internal bodily rhythm (biofeedback); stretch them out (traction); or turn them upside down (gravity inversion). (See Chapter 8 for a more detailed explanation of the way practitioners apply these techniques.)

Sometimes called "electric aspirin," TENS units are small but complex machines that can give a gentle analgesic jolt. The unit itself, about the size of a transistor radio, generates electrical impulses. It attaches to your body via wires and electrodes taped to your skin at certain points, depending on where you hurt. No one knows exactly how or why it works, and the effects vary from one person to the next. "I frequently rely on my personal TENS unit," writes a dental hygienist from Delaware, "since I no longer want to take medication. After almost three years of popping pills—**Dolobid, Feldene, Naprosyn, Parafon Forte**, prednisone, and some others I can't remember—I was tired of them, and tired of the nausea and dizzyness. So now I just tolerate the pain with the help of TENS." TENS units are priced at several hundred dollars, but since you need a prescription to buy one, your medical insurance should cover the purchase price or leasing cost.

The equipment used for biofeedback can be as elaborate as a computer, as simple as a thermometer. More than forty of our participants tried one type or another to learn how to gain conscious control over some ordinarily self-regulating bodily phenomenon, such as their pulse rate or the skin temperature of their feet. In operation, the machinery gives you *feedback*, in the form of light or sound, for example, that tells you how well you are controlling your internal *bio*logy. With practice, an Ohio housewife learned how to decrease her pain by raising her body temperature, and a Mississippi real estate agent found that he could avoid pain and stiffness by using biofeedback to relieve tension. If you want to learn biofeedback, look for a reliable teacher, perhaps a psychologist who is familiar with the technique.

Back or neck traction has helped some of our participants, and a few continue the treatments at home, including this bridge builder with the Santa Fe Railroad: "I have a traction device that hooks over an open door. It has two pulleys and a clothesline rope, with a head-jaw harness on one end and a ten-pound bag of sand on the other. I sit under this occasionally, half an hour at a time, and try to work my crossword puzzle while it pulls apart the vertebrae in my neck."

Only one of our participants, a California nurse, owns and uses the gravity-inversion equipment that was fairly popular a few years ago. It allows her to lie down and then turn herself upside down for ten minutes a day, which relieves the pain in her spine.

WARNING: Don't attempt traction (or inversion traction) on yourself without the direction of a physician or a physical therapist.

Wax

Few things warm and soothe aching hands as thoroughly as a dip in hot wax. Paraffin treatments are a popular offering from physical therapists, but several of our participants treat themselves at home. "It was costing me fifty dollars a visit to see the physical therapist," recalls a retired telephone repairman from New Jersey, "and Medicare only picked up twelve dollars of that. The wax felt so good that I wanted to go three times a week, but couldn't possibly afford to, so the therapist helped me buy my own paraffin bath for about $150. Now I use it twice every day." You don't really need a special machine to try this treatment. Here are directions that a Massachusetts yarn-shop owner learned from her physical therapist.

- *Materials:* 3 packages canning paraffin, available in grocery stores
  tall pot, such as a corn cooker or crockpot
  pint of mineral oil
  plastic bags big enough to fit over your hand
  towel (warmed, preferably)

- Melt enough paraffin in the pot to fill it about halfway.

- Add mineral oil until the pot is three-quarters full. Stir well.

- Remove pot from heat and let cool until a light skin forms over the paraffin. Test the temperature.

- Keeping your fingers slightly apart, dip one hand and wrist in quickly and out again. Letting the paraffin dry slightly between dips, repeat this step ten times.

- Cover your hand with the plastic bag and wrap the warm towel over that, leaving them on for twenty minutes. Keep your hand still, or do your hand exercises in the soothing heat.

- Peel off the paraffin and save it to use again another time.

- Repeat the process on the other hand. When you're finished, massage your hands and fingers with the mineral oil that remains on your skin.

You may want to try the wax dip on your feet, too.

WARNING: The hot wax carries two dangers. (1) If you spill the paraffin or the mineral oil during heating, you could start a fire, so be extremely careful, or get a crockpot to use just for this purpose. (2) To avoid burning your skin, be sure to let the wax cool sufficiently before immersing your hand. You can also burn your hand or arm on the hot pot, so dip carefully. Burn safety is what makes paraffin bath units cost about one hundred dollars. They are temperature-controlled to keep the wax between 126 and 130 degrees, and made of heat-resistant plastic.

Saunas and Steamrooms

The major difference between these two kinds of very hot rooms is their humidity. The sauna, heated with hot rocks, is drier than desert air, while the steamroom, as its name suggests, is extremely moist. (The relative humidity in a sauna ranges from 5 to 25 percent, compared to about 95 percent in a steamroom.) Our participants recommend both for the soothing warmth they provide, but the steamroom has the greater capacity to deep-heat your joints, partly because the steam makes it hard for your own sweat to evaporate.

Time Outdoors

Spending part of every day outdoors is a ritual with many of our participants, who get a general feeling of well-being from fresh air—and a few specific benefits, too. Some find special comfort at the beach, for example, where they can bury their hands and feet in the hot sand. And even though sunbathing to get a tan is no longer considered a healthy pastime, sitting in the sun with sunblock or clothes on just to revel in its warmth still feels good.

A writer from Illinois found a surprising source of pain relief when she went camping in Minnesota. At first, she could barely enjoy anything about the trip because her hands hurt so badly, but when she agreed to go fishing with her husband—and repeatedly washed the bait off her hands by dipping them in the icy water of the lake—her condition soon improved.

Summary of Top-Rated Self-Help Measures for Immediate Pain Relief

1. Rest, including ample sleep at night, naps if you need them, and time out
2. Warm or hot baths lasting about twenty minutes
3. Heat from a heating pad, hot-water bottle, electric blanket, or the like
4. Shower, with special water attention to painful joints
5. Ice to reduce pain and inflammation
6. Exercise—both a daily routine and on-the-spot maneuvers as needed
7. Keeping busy with pleasant activities
8. Massage of painful areas within your reach, or massage by someone else
9. Comfortable positions that provide quick release from pain
10. Hot tub or whirlpool baths
11. Aspirin or other over-the-counter drugs on an occasional basis
12. Dressing for warmth, comfort, and ease of getting in and out of clothes
13. Liniments for the massage they necessitate and the heat they generate
14. Meditation, self-hypnosis, prayer, and other mind-control techniques that activate your own inner healing abilities
15. Combining heat and ice for the best advantages of both

16.   Walking for relief and relaxation
17.   Cool soaks for problem joints and bathing in natural springs
18.   Joint coverings for warmth and protection
19.   Herb teas and other warm drinks
20.   Relaxation and reduction of mental and physical stress
21.   Food, particularly a favorite one that is comforting
22.   TENS, biofeedback, and other gadgets, such as traction devices
23.   Wax dips for your hands or feet
24.   Sauna and steamroom use
25.   Time outdoors, including sun and sand "therapy"

18

THE BEST
FITNESS EXERCISES FOR
PEOPLE WITH ARTHRITIS

*■ Walking ■ Swimming ■ Bicycling ■ Garden-
ing and other physically demanding work*

Believing as they do that "using it" keeps them from "losing it," the great majority of our 1,051 Arthritis Survey participants exercise *regularly*. Most of their workouts are a combination of stretching or strengthening exercises for their affected joints, together with some general *fitness* activity—such as walking or bicycling—that they enjoy over and above its therapeutic value.

Some health experts have looked askance at vigorous exercise for people with arthritis, fearing that it would injure rather than improve their joints, but the latest studies show that physical exertion can actually reduce the symptoms of arthritis, provided it's done carefully, with medical approval, and *not* pursued during an arthritis flare-up. Exercise relieves pain for many of our survey participants. It also increases their joint flexibility and range of motion, offers them some protection from deformity and disability, and improves their muscle tone, which in turn builds strength and guards against contractures and spasms. Some of them find exercise an aid to weight loss.

There are other health rewards, too, that you can reap from regular exercise, although they are unrelated to arthritis, such as lower blood pressure, reduced anxiety, a decreased risk of heart attack, greater mental alertness, and even a longer life expectancy.*

In this chapter, we'll look at our participants' favorite fitness exercises, and see what exercise physiologists say about the relative merits of each. But our most important goal here is to encourage *you* to talk to your doctor about taking up one of these physical outlets if you don't already take time to exercise.

Nothing to Fear, Much to Gain

The fitness boom that filled the streets with joggers may have left you feeling left out. All that running and pounding couldn't be good, could it? And if injuries ground so many people who start out with *no* musculoskeletal problems, what would happen to someone with arthritis who attempted jogging or aerobic dance?

The fact is that many people with arthritis can jog—in waist-deep water. And researchers at the University of Missouri Multipurpose Arthritis Center, who enroll many of their patients in twelve-week exercise programs, say that a modified regimen of aerobic dance can improve the physical function of arthritic joints quite a bit. Even a short walk, if you take one *every day,* can work a substantial increase in your well-being within three or four months' time.

"Exercise takes your mind off arthritis," says a writing teacher in our survey, "and fortifies your body to resist its effects." Indeed, a fitness exercise such as walking can help prevent osteoporosis, because it strengthens the bones. Doctors at Washington University and the Jewish Hospital in St. Louis have found that exercise and calcium supplements can even help prevent osteoporosis among women who are already past menopause.

---

*A continuing study of thousands of Harvard University alumni, reported in 1986 in the *New England Journal of Medicine,* shows that physically active men live longer than those who get no exercise.

"I walk and swim, play Ping-Pong, and do mild aerobics," writes a seventy-two-year-old retired pharmacist from New York who's had rheumatoid arthritis since 1954. "I've had to forgo baseball, badminton, tennis, and golf, though. After one good slam in a tennis match, my shoulder is useless, and a golf swing that really twists my knee sends me right to the club-house. But I try to exercise in some fashion for an hour or so a day, even if it's just gardening or washing my car. Sweating seems to help, and the activity *seems* to 'lubricate' my affected areas."

This may be precisely what does happen. The heat you generate by exercising will warm your joints as well as any heating pad. And the motion of the joint is self-nourishing. As Dr. James F. Fries, director of the Stanford Arthritis Clinic, explains in his book *Arthritis. A Comprehensive Guide* (Addison-Wesley 1985), "The cartilage of the joint . . . does not have a blood supply. It gets oxygen and nourishment and gets rid of waste products by compression—fluid is squeezed into the joint space, then removed and replenished. The health of the cartilage depends on motion, because without motion there is no nourishment of the cartilage."

What kind of fitness exercise should you do? Here's a rundown of the ones our participants like.

Exercise	Number of Participants Who Do It
Walk	572
Swim or other water exercise	228
Bicycle or exercycle	116
Physical work, such as gardening	77
Rowing machine, Nautilus, etc.	21
Yoga	19
Dance (ballet, jazz, or "slowly")	11
Aerobics (low-impact or dance)	10
Run or jog	10
Tennis or racquetball	10
Climb stairs	9
Bowl	7

Exercise	Number of Participants Who Do It
Calisthenics	7
Golf	6
Handball, basketball, or volleyball	4
Exercise class at gym	4
Jump (rope or trampoline)	3
Karate or Tai Chi Chuan	3
Fish	1
Play indoor horseshoes	1
Roller-skate	1
Softball	1

Almost any activity beats being sedentary, but some activities are better than others. Let's consider the favorites, in order of their popularity.

Walking

The oldest and best of the weight-bearing exercises

"We no longer dispense eye of newt," Dr. Gene H. Stollerman quipped recently in his regular column for *Hospital Practice,* "but we certainly should be prescribing shanks' mare." Dr. Stollerman called this exercise "walking therapy," and the 572 survey participants who walk for fitness would probably agree with his terminology.

"I walk for at least an hour a day at a brisk pace," reports a fifty-three-year-old Mississippi real estate agent, "and the exercise seems to relieve the tension that can cause pain and stiffness."

"I walk anywhere from one to six miles a day, depending on the season," says a communications consultant from North Carolina, age fifty-six, who treats herself to high-quality hiking boots. "In the winter I take a daily short walk, but in the summer I build up gradually until I'm ready for my outdoor vacation, when I hike long distances in the wilderness. Activity is an important part of my pain management. If I hike *too* far, my ankles swell and hurt, so moderation is essential. But the improved muscle tone I have from walking helps me prevent falls or other injuries, and adds something positive to my self-image and my outward appearance."

The ideal distance or speed you should walk depends on your overall fitness and the degree of joint damage you already have. This is why experts are always telling you to consult your doctor before you begin walking for exercise, even though you've been walking since age one. The general rule is to start out slowly and build up gradually, always listening to your body and your own common sense. One of our participants is beginning by walking fifty feet a day, confident that if she can do that much now, after being sedentary for years, she'll eventually be able to walk more.

Physicians who study the physiology of walking, including Dr. James M. Rippe of the University of Massachusetts Exercise Physiology Laboratory, point out that anyone can start a walking program, indoors or out, that is easy on the joints and doesn't call for a big investment in fancy paraphernalia. Susanna Levin, an editor at *The Walking Magazine,* ticks off some of the other advantages.

- Walking, especially brisk walking, is definitely a good workout that will benefit your heart as much as your joints.

- Since most people can walk for a longer time than they could run, for example, or play tennis, walking tends to build muscular endurance and burn calories.

- Walking is so accessible and do-able that you're far less likely to quit this exercise regimen than any other you might try.

"Do something!" urges a forty-four-year-old factory worker from Wisconsin. "Don't sit around feeling sorry for yourself. Even if it's only a short walk, you'll begin to feel better. I now walk at least three times a week. I go for about an hour, walking briskly for about two and a half miles. It's true that exercise gives you a sense of 'well-being.' And it *doesn't* increase your appetite. For me, it takes *away* the 'munchies' feeling!"

Swimming

Get the most out of exercise with the water's support

Most of our 228 participants who take to the water do so because of the buoyancy of the element, and the way it cushions their joints from shock. "Swimming is the best exercise," says a Michigan homemaker, "since you don't stress the joints. If you can't swim, just kick your legs and do range-of-motion exercises in the water."

"My rheumatologist at the Mayo Clinic told me to swim every day for the rest of my life," reports a forty-year-old social worker from North Dakota. "I try to, and I've also taken the 'Rusty Hinges' water exercise program at the YMCA. The water exercise is good, since you can move without much stress on your joints."

The stress-free environment that the water provides had pretty much convinced exercise physiologists that swimming couldn't have the same bone-building advantages as weight-bearing exercises such as walking and running. However, researchers at the Veterans Administration Medical Center in Portland, Oregon, say that the exertion of swimming *does* put enough force on the bones to strengthen them. They examined men whose only exercise was swimming, and then they compared the thickness of their bones to those of men who took no exercise. They found that the swimmers had a clear edge over the other men.

"I swim for half an hour, six days a week," says a thirty-seven-year-old home health aide from Florida, "and the only reason I don't swim on Sundays is that the pool is closed. I find that regular swimming *eliminates* pain. I *swear* by swimming."

As much as they rave about the sport, our participants rail about the water temperature of some of the pools they have used. "I used to swim a mile to a mile and a half every day," writes a retired office manager from California, "but now I cannot tolerate the cold water the pool has. I've found a private pool that should be available soon with 80-plus-degree water. Swimming *really* helped me, but the *cold* water only made the pain and stiffness worse."

Swimming and other forms of water exercise are touted as being virtually injury-free, but one of our participants, a retired librarian from Missouri, did run into trouble in the water: "I took a swimming course which was to help arthritics through exercise. This proved harmful because the up-and-down movements we were to make with our wrists only made mine sore, and they swelled more. I stopped going to the class. Swimming on my own, though, was very helpful. I am not an expert swimmer by any means. I learned to swim when I was forty years old, when my doctor told me just to go in the water, even if I couldn't swim. Eventually I learned, and my knee improved markedly."

Cycling

Bicycles and exercycles for indoor or outdoor exercise

"A little over a year ago, I started riding a stationary bike daily," says a secretary from Georgia. "I very much feel this has helped keep me limber." She wheels through two and a half miles by the cycle's odometer before she leaves for work in the mornings, and finds, "I loosen up, I feel better, and I now miss my exercising if I am unable to do it for any reason, because the stiffness returns."

There is some controversy in cycling for arthritis, however. Dr. Willibald Nagler, physiatrist-in-chief at The New York Hospital–Cornell Medical Center and author of *Dr. Nagler's Body Maintenance and Repair Book* (Fireside 1988), says that pedaling puts too much stress on the knees and can cause inflammation. If your knees are affected, check with your doctor before making cycling part of your exercise routine. "I tried to continue riding five miles daily on an exercise bike," reports a housewife from Minnesota, "and ended up with swollen knees."

Exercycles are more flexible than bicycles, since you can

reduce their wheel tension to zero, and with it the force your legs must fight. On the other hand, bicycling gets you out and about, and is therefore more appealing as a pastime, giving you a better chance of sticking with your exercise program.

"Exercising is much more enjoyable when done with others," notes a retired family counselor from California who rides her bicycle for thirty minutes a day. "Establishing a regularly scheduled time and place also helps the maintenance of a good exercise program."

Many participants build variety into their workouts by combining more than one type of fitness exercise, including this retired school superintendent from Massachusetts: "I walk at least two miles a day, or in summer swim a half a mile a day. During the winter months I ride an exercise bicycle and work out on Nautilus machines three days a week for an hour at a time."

Physical Work

You don't have to be a "jock" to get your exercise

The fact that "activity" is now considered the equal of exercise by many doctors is proof that fitness has come home. Not everyone can be a marathon runner, but anyone can make some slight increase in everyday activities that could lead to better fitness.

"I work in my garden for exercise," writes a homemaker from Illinois, "hoeing, weeding, and so on, all of which really helps, for as long as two to three hours a day in summer."

The idea that physical exertion "counts" as exercise is a new one, however, and for every participant who named gardening or housework as an exercise, there were others who explained that they couldn't follow an exercise program because they were too busy doing physical work. "I am a waitress," writes a fifty-two-year-old survey participant from California. "I am on my feet a minimum of eight hours, five days a week. I move. When I stop and relax, the pain starts. I use my hands and my shoulders carrying and serving an average of a hundred customers a day. I have a degree in library science, but I cannot do a job that is not physical. When I am sedentary, I stiffen up and can't move at all. I feel that my job as a waitress keeps me alive and moving."

Here's another person who answered *no* to the question, Do you exercise for arthritis? "I do not exercise in a set pattern," says this retired advertising director from Illinois. "However, I keep a two-story house, paint it inside and out, refinish antique furniture, and do garden and lawn work."

"I try to swim laps two to three times a week, and walk constantly," says a thirty-six-year-old freelance writer from New York who has had two joint-replacement operations. "I also do house, garden, and yard maintenance. Sometimes it's exercise enough trying to live a normal, active life."

Summary of Fitness Exercises for Arthritis

Walking is the best fitness exercise for most people with arthritis because:

- It is weight-bearing (and therefore bone-building).

- It offers an easy start and great room for advancement in terms of distance covered and pace achieved.

- It is low-risk, compared to jogging or other fitness activities.

- It can be done indoors or out, with no special equipment.

Swimming and other water exercises are also excellent because:

- The buoyancy of the water protects your joints from shock.

- The water makes possible many kinds of movements that would be difficult or dangerous on dry land.

- The exercise may be bone-building even though it's not weight-bearing.

Cycling is often an ideal path to fitness because:

- Exercycles and multispeed bicycles offer a wide range of tension settings (or speeds) to accommodate different levels of strength and ability.

- The exercise challenges and builds up the leg bones and muscles, although it may aggravate arthritis of the knee.

Physical Activity, such as gardening, is thought to be good exercise because:

- It confers some of the same bone and muscle benefits as other forms of mild exercise.

- It offers the chance for people who are not athletic to become more active, and consequently more fit.

19

WHERE DOES IT HURT? SURVEY PARTICIPANTS' ADVICE FOR SPOT RELIEF FROM HEAD TO TOE

■Range-of-motion exercises for individual joints ■ Strengthening exercises ■ Tips for jaw, neck, shoulders, elbows, hands, back, hips, knees, ankles, feet

On-the-spot measures for pain relief help the 1,051 participants in our Arthritis Survey give an extra dose of special attention to particularly painful parts. For although arthritis can be an all-over illness, most people find that certain joints typically require more exercise than others, or more protection, or more pampering.

This chapter gives you a complete selection of exercises for stretching and strengthening each of your joints individually, plus pain-relieving and pain-avoiding strategies you can use. These tips, like the exercises, are tailored to *specific* joints. (For *general* pain-relief advice, see Chapter 17.) All the exercises are arranged by joint, starting with the jaw and working on down to the feet, so you can turn right to the information you need most. The tips follow at the end of the chapter.

The exercises are the most-helpful and the least-dangerous ones our participants know. They learned many of the motions from their doctors and physical therapists, and some from their own trial-and-error self-experimenting over the years. Unlike fitness exercises that may call for overall exertion and deliver overall exhilaration (see Chapter 18), these movements are designed to help you preserve and extend the range of motion in each part of your body.

No survey participant does *all* the exercises in this chapter. Each person has his or her favorites. You, too, can pick and choose from the exercises that follow, creating your own special routine to suit your needs and abilities. Here are a few suggestions on how to go about it.

- Pick two or three simple exercises for starters, concentrating on the joints that need the most work. You can add more later.

- Show the exercises to your doctor before you attempt them.*

- As a prelude to exercise, warm up with a bath or a shower, or by applying heat to the areas you'll be working.

- Start out slowly, doing only one or two repetitions of each.

- If you can't complete a certain motion, settle for partial success, and trust that improvement will come gradually.

- Expect to feel some discomfort, but don't push through pain.

- As you gain strength and flexibility, increase the number of times you perform each exercise.

- If you "don't have time for exercise," try to do some of the movements while doing something else, such as exercising

---

*All these exercises have been reviewed by Dr. Willibald Nagler and Dr. Irene von Estorff of the Department of Rehabilitation Medicine at The New York Hospital–Cornell Medical Center, but some of them may be better than others for your particular condition. Consult your physician before starting any new exercise program.

your fingers while riding the bus, or your ankles while sitting at your desk at work. Stretching while you bathe or shower saves time *and* gives your joints an automatic warm-up.

Many of our participants do their stretching and strengthing exercises first thing in the morning. Warmed up by a good night's sleep under an electric blanket, they plunge into their range-of-motion exercises before they even get out of bed. In fact, some of them say, the exercises *enable* them to get out of bed feeling flexible and ready to start the day. (As you'll see, many of these exercises can be done in bed.)

The Exercises

Jaw

A-E-I-O-U Shout. Mouth all the vowel sounds, either silently or with a shout. Aim for gross exaggeration of your facial movements, so as to stretch the muscles of your jaw.

NOTE: In *any* exercise, it's a good idea to count aloud, or say something, to make sure you are breathing normally. Many people tend to tense up and hold their breath while exercising, which is counterproductive.

Neck

Head Pull. Sitting or standing, put your hands on the back of your head and gently pull it forward to stretch the neck muscles. (If you have advanced rheumatoid arthritis be sure to check with your doctor before attempting any of these neck exercises.)

Head Roll. Sitting or standing, tilt your head to the right as though you were trying to touch your ear to your shoulder. (Try not to lift your shoulder.) Moving slowly and gently, circle your head forward, so that your chin reaches down toward your chest. Continue around, leaning your left ear toward your left shoulder. Complete the circle by tilting your head slowly back, and then come up to center. (If it hurts too much to tilt back, or if you're still in bed, just do the forward and side motions.) Repeat the whole maneuver in the opposite direction.

Left-Right. Turn your head as far as you can to the right, as though you were trying to see behind you. (Don't push beyond pain.) Return to center and repeat in the opposite direction. Advanced addition: When you turn to the side, try to touch your chin to your shoulder.

Neck Push. Press the palm of your hand against your forehead while you push your head forward. (Don't *move* either part, but just let the arm and neck muscles work out by working against each other.) Hold the effort for just a second the first time, and try to build up to five seconds. (If your hands can't take the pressure, you can use your forearm, or press your head against the wall.)

Bed Head. Lying on your back in bed, press your head back into the pillow. Hold the position for a moment, and then release the pressure. Reverse by lifting your head off the pillow as high as you can, without lifting your shoulders off the bed.

Shoulder Shrug. Sitting, standing, or lying in bed, with your arms at your sides, shrug your shoulders. (This is a shoulder exercise that also helps strengthen the neck muscles.)

Shoulders

Shoulder Shrug. Stretch your shoulders by shrugging them, either one at a time or both together.

Shoulder Roll. Circle your shoulders by moving them up, forward, down, back, and up again. Circle in the opposite direction. You can do both shoulders together or one at a time.

Shoulder Helper. If necessary, you can put your shoulders through their range of motion with the help of your hands. Put your right hand on your left shoulder and gently lift it as far as it will go, then press it down as far as it will go. In the same fashion, move it as far forward and as far backward as you can. Repeat the motions with the opposite hand and shoulder.

Butterfly Stretch. Clasp your hands behind your neck and try to open your elbows out to the sides as far as you can. Alternate position: Start with your hands on your shoulders, elbows pointing out to the sides. Then pull your elbows back as far as you can.

Cane Stretch. If you use a cane, you also have an exercise baton. Sitting or standing, hold one end of the cane in each hand and lift it as high as possible. (If one shoulder works better than the other, then raise that side of the cane higher than the other.) Lower the cane. Holding the cane in front of you, move it to the right and then to the left. Lift one end of the cane up, then the opposite end up. Also try to raise the cane over your head and then bring it down to shoulder height behind your head. If you don't have a cane, you can do these exercises with a yardstick.

Swinging. Sitting or standing, lean forward and let one arm hang down. Swing it gently to and fro, then round in circles. Repeat with the other arm. (You can also do this exercise while lying face down near the edge of your bed. If you do it standing, use one arm to hold on to a sturdy chair for balance while you swing the other arm.)

Full Shoulder Stretch. Sitting or standing, extend your arms straight out to the sides at shoulder height. Move your arms forward, touching your hands together. Move them out to the sides, then back as far as they will go, and out to the sides again. Raise them overhead and lower them to hang at your sides.

Crisscross Stretch. Sitting or standing, extend both arms straight out in front of you at shoulder height. Move them slowly out to the sides. Lower your arms to your sides and then reach out in back. Try to cross your wrists behind you.

Pulley Pulls. You can make a pulley by hanging a length of rope over an open door, or rig up a real clothesline pulley for this purpose. Sitting, standing, or lying in bed under the pulley, take one end of the rope in each hand. Pull down with the right hand, letting it raise your left as high as possible. Reverse.

Circling. Sitting or standing, stretch your arms straight out to the sides like a child pretending to be an airplane. Try to describe tiny forward circles with your hands and gradually make the circles larger. Then circle in reverse. (You can also do this stretch one arm at a time, if that's easier for you.)

Circle Twist. Get in position to do the circling exercise, above, but make your hands into fists. Circle first with the palm side of your fists facing the floor. Twist your arm, so your palms face the ceiling, and circle some more. (The twist part is also good for your elbows.)

Bodybuilder. Raise your arms straight out to the sides and make your hands into fists. Bring your fists to your shoulders, as though you were showing off your biceps. (This is one way to build them up.) Extend your arms straight up as far as you can, so your fists are overhead. Bring your fists back to your shoulders, and then put them straight out to the sides again.

Weightlifter. Try this strengthening exercise from a sitting or standing position, using a can of tomato soup—or a plastic bleach bottle with a small amount of water in it, or a one-pound box of rice—for a weight. Lift the weight straight out in front of you with one arm. Lower the weight, then lift it out to the side, to shoulder height if you can. Lower it again, and then try to lift it behind you about one foot, or as high as you can without straining. Repeat with the other arm. (Also try the *swinging* exercise with one of these light weights.)

Push-offs. Stand facing a wall, about a foot away, and put your palms on the wall at about shoulder height. (Don't attempt this exercise if you have pain or swelling in your wrists.) Lean in toward the wall as far as you can, then push yourself back to starting position. (If you have access to a swimming pool, try this exercise in the water, using the side of the pool as your wall.)

Elbows

Elbow Limber-Up #1. Sitting, standing, or lying down, extend your arms straight out in front of you at shoulder height. Bend your elbows and touch your hands to your chest, then reach straight out again.

Elbow Limber-Up #2. Sitting, standing, or lying down, put your hands on your shoulders, elbows pointing out to the sides. Straighten your elbows to extend your hands out to the sides and then return your hands to your shoulders.

Wing Tuck. Sitting, standing, or lying down, let your arms rest straight down by your sides, palms facing your body. Bend and lift your elbows as you tuck your hands into your armpits. Also try, from this position, to touch your thumbs to your shoulders.

Chop Wood. Sitting, standing, or lying down, clasp your hands and hold them against your left shoulder. Straighten your elbows and bring your hands down to your right thigh, as though you were swinging an ax—gently. Repeat from right shoulder to left thigh.

Elbow Twister. Sitting, standing, or lying down, extend your arms out to your sides, palms up. Keeping your arms straight, turn your forearms to make your palms face the floor.

Free Hand. Sitting or standing, bend one elbow and lift it straight up, leaving your hand dangling, as though someone were pulling your elbow from above with puppet strings. Then straighten your elbow to let your arm drop slowly back to your side. Repeat with the other arm.

Elbow Builder. Strengthen your elbows by putting each forearm under a heavy table or desk, with your palms up, elbows bent. Push up with your forearms, as though trying to make the table rise. Exert pressure for a few seconds, then relax. (If you don't have the right furniture for this exercise, cross your forearms in front of you, elbows bent, and press one arm against the other, first with the left arm on top, then the right.)

Wrists

Wrist Reach. Sitting, standing, or lying down, put your arm in a comfortable position that gives your wrist room to move. Bend your wrist so that your hand drops forward as far as it will go. Then bend your wrist the other way to raise the hand. Repeat for the other wrist. With assistance: If you can't manage the exercise this way, let your arm rest on a table so that your wrist and hand extend over the edge. With gentle pressure, use the opposite hand to guide your wrist through the maneuver.

Wrist Rotator. With your hand and forearm flat on a table, or on the bed as you lie there, rotate your hand toward you as far as you can to get a sideways stretch in your wrist. Then rotate it back in the other direction. (Your palm should slide on the surface, letting your wrist do all the work.) NOTE: If arthritis has pushed your wrist out of line, exercise *against* the drift. That is, if your wrist angles away from you, do only the part of this exercise that calls for rotating it *toward* your body. The same principle of working against deformity holds true for any other joint that is contracted or extended in an unwanted position.

Figure Eights. Rest your arm on a flat surface with your hand extended over the edge. Put your wrist through its full range of motion by turning and twisting it in a figure-eight pattern. Do the same with the other wrist.

Swaying Palms. Clasp your hands in front of you. Push your right palm against your left, so that the left one bends back. Then stretch in the opposite direction by pushing with your left palm.

Wrist Twist. With your forearm and hand supported on a flat surface, palm facing down, turn your wrist to make your palm face the ceiling. Repeat for the other wrist. Extra Twist: Instead of resting your arm while you twist, try this motion with your arm unsupported, and holding a lightweight saucepan by the handle.

Praying Hands. Strengthen your wrists by putting your hands together as though in prayer, with your elbows out, so your wrists are bent in right angles, if possible. Push your palms together, allowing no movement in either hand, and hold the position for a second or so. (Later, you can increase the length of time you hold your palms this way.)

Wrist Rise. Put your hand under a table, with the back of your hand touching the underside of the table. Press up as hard as you can, as though trying to lift the table. Or, you can achieve the same strengthening action by working against the resistance of your other hand. Put your right forearm and hand, palm down, on the tabletop. Using the heel of your left hand to keep the right one from going anywhere, push up with the right and hold for a second or two.

Hands/Fingers

Finger Spread. Resting your hand, palm down, on a flat surface, spread your fingers as wide apart as you can get them. Then draw your fingers together again, keeping your hand flat.

Finger Curls. Begin with your hand up, as though greeting someone, and your fingers as straight as possible. Slowly curl the index finger down, beginning by bending the joint nearest the fingertip, then the middle joint, until your index finger touches the uppermost part of your palm. Uncurl it in reverse order. Repeat for the middle, ring, and little fingers, using the opposite hand to gently curl each one down and then up again. Try to bend all four fingers at once this way.

Okay All Around. Start with your hands open, fingers straight. Make the "okay" sign by touching the tip of your index finger to the tip of your thumb. Release and touch the tip of your middle finger to the tip of your thumb, then the ring finger, then the little finger.

Finger Lifts. With your hands resting by your sides in bed, or on any flat surface, lift each finger as high as you can, one at a time. For strengthening: Try to lift your fingers against pressure, either by sliding your hand under your buttocks, if you're in bed, or by pushing against your other hand or the underside of a table.

Finger Slides. With your hand resting on a flat surface, slide your index finger as far as it will go toward your thumb. (You may need to move it with your other hand.) Continue moving the middle, ring, and little fingers in this direction. Then slide each one away from the thumb as far as it will go. For strengthening: Use your other hand to *resist* each finger's movements. NOTE: If arthritis has already set your fingers on an exaggerated tilt away from your thumbs (a condition called ulnar deviation), just strive to stretch them back toward the thumbs.

Squeeze Play. Strengthen your hands by squeezing a small rubber ball or some therapeutic putty.

Wall Walker. Stand or sit about two feet away from a wall, with your left side to the wall and your arms at your sides. Slowly "walk" the fingers of your left hand up the wall as high as you can go. (This is also a good shoulder exercise. Try not to raise your shoulder or tip away from the wall, but just let your fingers do the walking.) Repeat on the right side.

Typist's Warm-up. Make a fist and then straighten out your fingers. Wiggle all your fingers at once, so that some are going up while others are going down. Circle your wrists. Rub your hands together, as though you were rubbing lotion all over them, to increase the blood flow.

Back

Pelvic Tilt. Lie on your back with your knees bent and feet flat on the bed (or floor). Tilt your pelvis up by tightening your buttocks and pulling in your abdominal muscles. (You should feel the curve in your lower back flatten out.) Release. Breathe deeply throughout, exhaling as you pull in your abdominals.

Knee to Chest. Lie on your back with your knees bent and feet flat. Bring one knee toward your chest as far as you can. Return your knee to the starting position and then straighten out your leg so it is resting flat on the bed. Wobble your leg a bit to relax it, then return to the bent-knee position. Repeat with the other leg. Advanced extra: Once you've raised your knee as far toward your chest as you can, pull it a little closer with your hands.

Knee to Chest Rock. Lie on your back with your knees bent and feet flat. Bring *both* knees to your chest by clasping your arms around them. (It's okay to pull up your knees one at a time by holding the backs of your thighs.)

Curl your head and shoulders forward and gently rock back and forth in this position.

Bent-Knee Sit-Ups. Lie on your back with knees bent and feet flat. Pull in your abdominals and raise the upper part of your body toward your knees. (It may help you to lead with your raised arms. But don't strain. If you can see your navel, you're going far enough to strengthen your muscles.) Advanced extra: Try this exercise with your arms folded across your chest.

Sit-Downs. Sit on a bench or the edge of your bed. Use your abdominal muscles to help you lean partway back, then come forward again.

Cat Stretch. Begin on your hands and knees, with your back flat. Slide your hands forward, letting your elbows bend and touch the floor. Put your head down and your rear end up. Next, smoothly sink back on your haunches, so that you are almost sitting on your ankles. (Your elbows are straight and your head is still tucked down.) Return to the starting position. Now drop your head and curve your back, like a Halloween cat, by pulling in your abdominals. Release and roll your head back.

Hips

Leg Spread. Lie on your back with your legs straight. Spread your legs as far apart as you can to give your hips a sideways stretch. (If you have back pain, move one leg at a time, keeping the other one bent at the knee, foot flat.) Slide your legs back together. Advanced extra: Instead of sliding your leg sideways, lift it and move it gently through the air as far as you can before putting it down. Lift it again and move it back to center. Repeat with the other leg. (Be sure to bend the knee of the resting leg.)

Knee to Chest. Lie on your back, with your knees bent and feet flat. Bring your knee toward your chest as far as you can. Return to starting position, straighten your leg and let it lie flat for a moment, and return to the starting position again. Repeat for the other leg. (This exercise is also included with the back exercises because it stretches the lower back as well as extending the forward motion of the hip.)

Straight Leg-Ups. Lie on your back, knees bent and feet flat. Straighten one leg and lift it as high as you can. Lower it slowly and repeat with the other leg.

Knee Cross. Lie on your back, knees bent. Cross your right thigh over your left thigh. Press your legs together and tip your knees toward the right side, as though you were going to drop them all the way down. Bring your knees back up and uncross your legs to return to the starting position. Repeat with the left thigh over the right, tilting your knees to the left. Alternate position for people with low back pain: Lie on your left side, legs extended. Bend your right knee so that your right foot slides up near your left knee. Stretch your right knee down toward the surface as far as you can, which will rotate your right hip inward. Then raise your right knee as far as you can toward the ceiling, keeping your right foot on your left leg, to rotate your hip outward. Return to the starting position. Turn over and repeat on the other side.

Liftback. Lying face down, raise one leg straight up behind you as far as you can and then lower it. Repeat with the other leg. Alternate position for people with back pain: Try the liftback standing up. Support yourself by holding on to the back of a chair, lean forward slightly, so you don't arch your back, and then raise one leg slowly behind you. Lower it, and try the other one.

Leg Lifts. Stand with your side to a chair so you can lean on it for support. Raise and lower one leg straight out in front of you. Repeat with the other leg. Facing the chair, lift one leg straight out to the side. Repeat with the other leg.

Hip Strengthener. Stand between a chair and a wall, so you can use the chair for support and the wall for resistance. Lift the leg near the wall out to the side. When your leg meets the wall, a few inches off the ground, keep on pushing. Relax and return to standing position. Turn around and repeat with the other leg.

The Squeeze. Standing, sitting, or lying down, squeeze your buttocks together as tightly as you can. Release. Repeat.

Swordplay. Stand facing the back of a chair, both hands on it for support. Bend your right knee and shift your weight to the right, keeping your left leg straight, like a fencer's lunge. Repeat on the other side.

Hip Walkout. Take a few normal steps. Turn your feet out, à la Charlie Chaplin, and walk a bit more. Turn your feet in, pigeon-toed, and walk on.

Water Exercises   If you have access to a pool or a large hot tub, try these:

Scissor Kick. Sit on the pool steps or the bench in the hot tub. Extend both legs out straight in front of you. Spread them apart and then cross your right leg over your left. Spread your legs apart again, then cross the left leg over the right.

Flutter Kick. Hold on to the side of the pool. Kick your legs slowly up and down. (You need not make a splash, but just work against the resistance of the water.)

Leg Circles. Stand on one leg, holding on to the side of the pool. Make a large slow clockwise circle with your extended leg. Make another circle going counterclockwise. Turn around and repeat with the other leg.

Jumping Jacks. Just concentrate on the lower half of this exercise. Put your hands on your hips and let the water help you jump into a straddle position. Then jump to bring your feet back together.

Knees

Knee to Chest. Lie on your back with your knees bent, feet flat. Bring one knee toward your chest. (You can lift your leg with your hands to pull it close, or just bring your heel toward your buttocks, without ever taking your foot off the bed.) Repeat for the other knee.

Knee Push. Lie on your back, knees bent. Straighten one leg so it rests on the bed. Then keep pushing down with that knee, as though you were trying to bend it inside out. Repeat with the other leg.

Knee Press. Lie on your back with legs extended. Press your heels into the bed. (You can also do one leg at a time, leaving the other knee bent.) Turn over and press your toes into the bed. (If you have lower back pain, put a small pillow under your abdomen when you lie on your stomach.)

Chair Bend. Sitting, bend your knee as far as you can, letting your foot move back underneath the chair. Repeat with the other leg. (The closer you sit to the edge of the chair, the more you'll get out of this exercise.)

Chair Lift. Sitting, with your feet flat on the floor, lift your right foot until your right knee is straight. Slowly lower your foot. Try the same lift on the left.

Feet and Ankles

Ankle Twist. Lie on your back with your legs extended and slightly apart. Rotate your ankles so your toes point in, then out.

Foot Circles. Sitting, standing, or lying down, let one foot hang free. Circle it first one way, then the other. Repeat with the other foot.

Runner's Stretch. Stand facing a wall and lean against it. Extend your right leg behind you, with knee straight and toes on the floor. Try to lower your right heel to the floor, to stretch the Achilles's tendon. Return to starting position, and repeat with the left leg.

Ankle Stretch. Sit with both feet flat on the floor. Raise your heels, keeping your toes on the floor. Return to starting position. Then raise your toes while leaving your heels on the floor.

Side Stretch. Sit with your feet on the floor, knees slightly apart. Rotate your ankles so that the arches of your feet lift up and only the sides of your feet stay on the floor. Return to the starting position. Now rotate your ankles the other way, so your knees touch and only the arch sides of your feet stay on the floor.

Soft Shoe. Sit with your feet on the floor. Raise your heels off the floor. Swivel both heels to the right and bring them down. Then leave your heels down and raise the fronts of your feet. Swivel your toes to the right and bring them down. Repeat the whole sequence to the left, beginning with the toes.

Ankle Builder. Stand holding on to a sturdy support. Rise up on tiptoe. Come down slowly.

Ankle Walkout. Walk on tiptoe. Then walk on your heels.

Foot Roll. Sit comfortably. Work a rolling pin with the bottoms of your feet to stretch and massage your arches. (You may work one foot at a time or both together.)

Toe Curls. Sitting or lying down, curl your toes tightly. Then straighten them and splay them out as much as you can.

Toe Helper. Put your toes through their full range of motion by manipulating each one with your hand. Also strive to strengthen your toes by pushing with them against the resistance of your fingers.

The Tips

Jaw

- If you clench or grind your teeth while you sleep, see a dentist for help with breaking the habit.

- Avoid leaning your chin on your hands.

Neck

- Use a pillow that is just thick enough to keep your head aligned with your spine as it is when standing at ease. Keep the pillow under your head and neck when you sleep—not under your shoulders.

- Sleep or rest on your side, preferably, or your back, but not on your stomach.

- If you need the support, wear a soft neck collar from time to time. You can make one of these by folding or rolling a towel to fasten around your neck.

- When you read or watch television, move your neck frequently to keep it limber.

- If you are tense, try your best to keep the tension out of your neck. Take a moment every few stressful moments to shrug your shoulders and circle your head.

- Dress appropriately to keep drafts off your neck.

Shoulders

- Rest your shoulder, when you need to, by putting your arm in a sling.

- Try using a backpack instead of a purse or a briefcase. The motion of putting it on and taking it off is good exercise, and while the backpack is in place, it serves as a reminder about good shoulder posture.

- If you work in an office, try to request a desk chair with arms that can help you relax your shoulders and elbows while typing or using a computer.

Elbows

- Like your shoulder, your elbow may benefit from resting your arm in a sling occasionally.

- Prescribed splints can help control pain and protect joints.

- Make yourself an elbow-warmer from a cuddly knee sock by cutting off the foot part and wearing the leg part on your elbow, over or under your clothing.

Wrists

- Wrists often take well to support from a splint or an Ace bandage.

- Keep your wrists warm with the terry-cloth bands that tennis players wear.

Hands/Fingers

- Try soaking your hands in a sinkful of very warm water before you exercise.

- Treat your hands to the special warmth of a hot-wax dip. (See Chapter 17.)

- Wear gloves to sleep to help reduce morning stiffness.

- Spare your hands by using them both together whenever possible, and doing some of their work with another part of your body altogether—such as closing a door with your shoulder or your hip.

- Leave lids on loosely.

- If need be, consult a mail-order catalog (see Chapter 20) for various items that can help you button buttons, unscrew jars tops, turn keys, open car doors, and the like.

- Many of our survey participants gain flexibility and strength by doing handcrafts, typing (especially on a computer, with its softer touch), and playing the piano or other musical instruments.

Back

- Be very careful about the way you lift and carry even the lightest load. Squat rather than bend over from the waist to pick up something.

- Sleep on a firm mattress.

- Take some of the strain out of sitting by using a good straight-back chair, made even more comfortable with a back-support cushion and a footrest. You can set up a makeshift footrest at work by opening the bottom drawer of your desk and using it to elevate your knees above the level of your hips.

- Carry things close to your body, or rediscover the wheel, and see how much help a shopping wagon or tea cart can be around the house.

Hips

- Don't sit too long in any position. When you take a long drive, schedule a time to stop, get out, and stretch your hips.

- In lovemaking, support your hips with pillows.

- If you use a cane occasionally to spare your hip, make sure that it is the right height (the top of the handle should be on a level with the top of your hip socket), and that you use it correctly—on the side *opposite* the bad hip. Some of our participants have folding canes that they carry with them, just in case.

Knees

- Sleep on your side with a pillow between your knees.

- If you kneel in your garden, support your knees on a cushioned pad.

- Instead of kneeling down to clean the bathtub, use a long-handled mop.

- If you walk with a cane, hold it in the hand *opposite* the bad knee.

- Pull with your arms if your knees give you trouble walking up and down stairs or getting in or out of chairs.

- If you are overweight, your knees will appreciate your losing those extra pounds.

- Keep your knee aligned, when necessary, with a specially made knee support or elastic bandage, and warmed with leg warmers or a sock cut out for the job.

Feet and Ankles

- If you don't have access to a swimming pool or a hot tub, you can still get the benefit of water exercise by working your feet in the bathtub or a pan of warm water.

- Give your ankles the occasional extra support of an elastic bandage.

- Investigate the value of inserts for your shoes, whether these are orthotics designed to correct a specific problem, or off-the-rack padded insoles to make walking more comfortable.

- Choose flat shoes with good support and a wide toe box. Many styles of athletic shoes can fill the bill without calling attention to themselves.

- Like the hands, the feet can benefit from the special warmth of a hot-wax dip. (See Chapter 17 for instructions.)

- If pain in your foot demands that you use a cane, hold it in the hand opposite the bad foot.

Summary of Participants' Advice for Spot Relief

1. Specific exercises, tailored to the individual joints, can stretch and strengthen your muscles to help you preserve or restore your flexibility.
2. Exercise for arthritis is a lifelong affair. Once you

become proficient at your range-of-motion exercises, work at incorporating them into your everyday activities.

3.   The number of repetitions you assign to any given movement may stop at five or ten, or grow to one hundred times a day or more, depending on your needs and abilities.

4.   Sudden sharp pain while exercising is a signal to stop, but be prepared to tolerate some pain while you work to increase your stretch and build your strength.

5.   Warm up before exercising, whether by sleeping under an electric blanket, taking a warm bath, or applying heat to strategic spots.

6.   Find a sleeping position that makes sense for your specific joint problems.

7.   Most joints benefit from an extra layer of warmth, such as a tennis-type wristband or a sock cut to fit around your elbow or knee.

8.   A cane, a supportive splint or wrap—even a sling fashioned from a scarf—can rest and protect a painful inflamed joint.

9.   In your exercise routine and your daily activities, work against the drift of any deformity.

10.   Balance exercise and activity with rest, especially for joints that are inflamed.

20

HOW TO MAKE
YOUR ENVIRONMENT
MORE COMFORTABLE

*▪ The best mattress ▪ Kitchen conveniences ▪
Chairs and stairs ▪ Bathrooms as home hydrotherapy centers ▪ Workplace changes ▪ Car
comfort*

Every room in your house,
every workplace, every mode of transportation, and every
spot you visit contains something that can become a problem
because you have arthritis: The couch is too soft to sit on comfortably; the toilet seat is too low; cooking and eating utensils
are too hard to hold. But every one of these problems has a
solution, as the participants in our Arthritis Survey have found.

Nearly half of our 1,051 survey group members say they
get along splendidly *without* any special aids or adjustments,
either because their successful treatment plans allow them full
function or because their arthritis has not yet restricted them.
Some participants are planning to make certain changes in
their surroundings, and a few asked for advice on what to do
and how to do it. The other half of the participants, on whose
experience we base this chapter, have met and mastered
countless challenges by modifying their environment—at
home, at work, or on the go. These changes run the gamut

from the simple purchase of a single item, such as a jar opener or a back-support cushion, to major overhauls, such as finding a different job or moving to a one-story home. They can be as cheap as a strip of foam rubber to wrap around a pencil or as expensive as an indoor heated swimming pool. We will present all the alternatives we learned about in our survey—both the general suggestions and the many specific items, whether handmade or store-bought. Most of the items can be found at drug or discount stores, in medical supply outlets, or ordered through the mail from the companies our survey participants recommended. You can use the list of mail-order company names and addresses at the end of this chapter to send for their catalogs.

At Home

When a powerhouse electrician and his wife from Pickwick Dam, Tennessee, built their new house three years ago, they used the fact that they both had arthritis as a basic element of the design. Their home is a model of what good planning can do in the interest of comfort. "We installed a heat pump instead of a fireplace or wood stove. We placed all of the electrical outlets high on the walls where they can be reached without stooping. The bathroom is only ten steps from our bed, and the commode is on a six-inch raised platform for easy on and off. We also installed a large bathtub with a whirlpool. Our bed can be elevated at the head and foot, and has a built-in vibrator. The kitchen is small, with all the storage space placed at a height that requires a minimum amount of stooping and lifting."

About fifty of our participants left a large two- or three-story house for a one-level home, an apartment in an elevator-service building, or a new start in a warmer climate. Others, who stayed within the confines of their existing homes or limited budgets, were quite successful in their efforts to revamp their surroundings, as you'll see. Before we trail them around from room to room for special tips about beds, bathtub railings, and the like, here are a few ideas that could work anywhere.

- Rearrange your cupboards, closets, or other storage areas to make sure you put your most frequently used items within easy reach.

- Arrange your furniture for safe and easy passage through the room. Eliminate unnecessary items as you do this, and you'll also simplify your housecleaning. Where possible, position a supersturdy table or bookcase near the places you like to sit, in case you need some help getting up.

- Find out where the drafts are coming from and eliminate them.

- When buying items that you must carry or push—dishes, iron, vacuum cleaner, etc.—choose the lightest ones you can find.

- Make doors easier to open with lever handles that fit over standard knobs.

- Carpet the floors if you can. At least put a rug or a rubber mat wherever you stand for any length of time—in front of the kitchen sink, for example—but get rid of other scatter rugs before you trip on them, especially if you walk with a crutch or a cane.

- Build up the handles of hard-to-hold utensils or tools with pipe insulation, bubble wrap, or even the foam from a plastic hair curler.

- Equip your home with step stools and long-handled utensils (from shoehorns to feather dusters) that save you the discomfort of reaching up and bending down.

- Replace hard-snapping light switches with soft-touch wall switchplates and touch-on attachments for lamps.

An Ohio artist asked a student from the local vocational school to advise her in rearranging her kitchen to save steps, ease traffic flow, and prevent falls and bumps. ("Knee against table legs—ugh!") Then she used the traffic-flow idea throughout her house, keeping furniture in *small* groupings, and she is well pleased with the results. "I also love my bedroom more," she writes, "since I added pillows, a well-lighted vanity, and soul-feeding things like my own corner and my own art creations."

Bedroom

A good mattress is the cornerstone of comfortable living, although the definition of "good" may vary from extrafirm, which is the survey favorite, to relatively soft. Most participants who stress the importance of a good mattress sleep on a combination of layers—and recommend it highly. They begin with a bedboard or platform bed to give a solid base, put a firm mattress on that, and top off the whole with a layer of eggcrate foam. (You'll know eggcrate foam when you see it, with its flat bottom and convoluted top layer that looks as though it could hold a few dozen eggs.) This arrangement combines the firmness needed for good back support with the right amount of soft padding to cushion painful hips or shoulders. Prices for eggcrate begin at about fifteen dollars for a piece big enough to cover a single bed with an inch or so of padding and increase accordingly for larger beds and thicknesses up to about four inches. The nice thing about eggcrate, our participants report, is that it handles your body gently—as though it were as fragile as an eggshell. Manufacturers claim that it cushions and buffers the body by virtue of its many small pockets of air, keeping pressure off the sore spots. Other kinds of mattress pads, made of dimpled foam, achieve the same results for other satisfied participants.

Some people prefer a mattress made entirely of foam, instead of a standard mattress with a foam pad on top. "I have been sleeping on polyurethane—that's the technical name for foam rubber—for over eight years," writes a retired court stenographer from Massachusetts. "This helps to relieve the pressure on my hips, spine, or legs. Regular mattresses caused me much pain. There is nothing that can compare with foam rubber!"

A luxurious covering for any kind of mattress is a woolen bed pad (sheepskin) or electric mattress pad/bed warmer. The luxury comfort of these items frequently comes with a luxury-level price tag as well, but some participants consider them necessities. Flannel or thermal sheets (preferably flat for easy handling, not tightly fitted) are another, less expensive, way to warm up a cold bed. And over the sleeper, the top choices are electric blankets, followed closely by sleeping bags, down comforters, or other *warm* but lightweight covers. "My electric blanket is a lifesaver," says a New York saleswoman. "It allows me to get out of bed each morning."

A bed board is typically a ¾-inch piece of plywood cut to fit your bed and placed between the mattress and the box spring. Once you get used to the support it provides (for sleeping *and* for helping you get out of bed), you may wish you could carry one along on trips—and several of our traveling participants say they use a lightweight version that folds to become portable.

A few additional words about the bed board: It doesn't work for everyone. "My backbone and yours are *not* a straight line like the bed boards so many swear by," says a mechanical engineer from California. "I don't get their geometry." A glass-maker from West Virginia, who's had both hips replaced, agrees: "Yes, I tried a bed board once, for about two weeks. It caused me more pain, so I quit using it. I do need to change mattresses every so often, though, because even a firm mattress finally wears out."

What *does* seem to work in bed for everyone is an extra pillow, or several extra pillows in a variety of shapes and sizes to raise the knees just so, for example, to give the neck a special cradle, to support the hips during sex, or to keep the blankets off feet that hurt. Participants named a variety of specialized items, including neck rolls, butterfly pillows, cervical pillows, orthopedic pillows, arthritic pillows, leg rests, and bed wedges, but an ordinary bed pillow or a piece of foam cut to your exact specifications can work just as well. "I need at least two bed pillows to prop up my legs," notes a Mississippi homemaker. "I don't just put my feet on them, but push them up under my legs for support while resting."

Thirty-two of our participants mentioned that they sleep

on a water bed, and most of them *raved* about its comfort. "Without my 'Flotation System' water bed I could not sleep for more than three or four hours," writes an assembly-line worker from Wisconsin, "and the good night's sleep I get now works wonders for me!" Only one other water bed was mentioned by brand name, the Semi-wave water bed from National Bedrooms, and the rest were just called "wonderful." Why? "The water bed helps a lot because it gives me firmness and heat," explains a Pennsylvania housewife, "with nothing pressing on the bone spurs in my spine." A few men and women said the water bed was the best boon to lovemaking they had found, and an artist swore that if it didn't wiggle so much, she would stay in it all day in wintertime to do her painting. In fact, the only two complaints we heard about water beds came from women who really had no problem sleeping in them but had considerable trouble struggling out of them in the morning. (A water bed must be kept properly filled to give firm support.)

Any bed, truth to tell, can taunt you getting in and trap you once you're there. Many participants lick this problem by raising their beds to a more manageable height—approximately six inches above the norm, or whatever feels comfortable. Beds can be elevated on wood or cement blocks, or, as one disabled civil servant did, by piling on an extra mattress. Several people purchased or built high platform beds, and then found to their delight that the platform offered even better support than their old box spring and mattress. A platform is the ultimate bed board. Hospital beds are also higher than standard bed frames and have the added advantage of motorized movement to elevate your head or legs as you desire. One such bed, a Craftmatic, cost our participant, a retired broker, $1,200.

Two women in our survey say they've had to stop sleeping in a double bed with their husbands and switch to twin beds. Six participants like to put their mattress or a couple of egg-crate pads right on the floor for firm (and inexpensive) support, and another five prefer, at least some of the time, to sleep in their reclining chairs.

Aside from the ideal sleeping arrangement, several participants make their bedrooms more comfortable with a good chair to sit in while reading, a bedside lamp that turns on with the gentlest touch of a button, and a television set. (Remote control is ideal, if you have it, but at least position the TV so you can turn it on without stooping and watch it without straining your neck or back.) A former insurance secretary from California with very limited use of her hands has replaced the door of her bedroom closet with a curtain, and she uses open shelves hanging from the closet pole, instead of the formal bureau with its stubborn drawers.

"I keep a footstool in the bedroom to help me get dressed," writes a retired salesman from New York. "I'm slightly over six feet tall, and it's a long way down to the shoes these days."

Kitchen

With so much time spent here and so many different kinds of tasks to be done, the kitchen becomes a home's haven for gadgets. The most popular of these, by far, among our survey participants are the ones that let everything but genies out of bottles, cans, and jars. There are electric can openers, of course, in plug-in and portable models, stationary jar openers that attach to the wall or under a cabinet, rubber grippers that fit over screw tops and make them easier to open, plastic molds that hold on to the bottoms of bottles while you turn the tops, hand-held gizmos that adjust to fit every size top or cap and remove them with lever action, "tab grabbers" for aluminum drink cans, and the old standbys—pliers and nutcrackers. It seems as though no one can get along without one of these devices.

The most frequently mentioned aid for meal preparation is not a cooking utensil per se, but a high stool that lets one sit comfortably at the kitchen counter or the sink. A few participants have gone a step beyond the stool and actually changed the height of their counters, either raising them to eliminate a lot of leaning over or lowering them to accommodate a cook in a wheelchair. Appliances, too, can sometimes be height-adjusted. "The stove in my kitchen was too low," says a forty-three-year-old secretary from Idaho. "Raising it just four inches lessened the pressure and pain in my knees." Consider yourself lucky if you have a waist-height wall oven.

Under and over the counters, the cupboards themselves can be made more user-friendly by replacing small knobs or handles with ones that are easier to hold, by raising or lowering the handles, by removing snap locks, or by taking off the doors altogether. Inside, you can arrange your foods and utensils so that the heaviest and most-used items are closest at hand. Revolving shelves, or lazy Susans on the existing shelves, can save a lot of reaching, too.

Cadillac appliances for simplifying cooking are the food processor and the microwave oven. The processor makes short work of dicing and chopping, it's true, but not everyone can afford one. A retired educator from Georgia and an Ohio farm wife have both hit on the same strategy to simplify slicing vegetables by hand. They drove a long nail through a cutting board to keep onions or what-have-you in their place. Some participants say that just *using* a chopping board, rather than cutting foods in their hands as they had always done, makes the work easier. A North Carolina homemaker solves the peeling problem by cooking her potatoes with the skins on, and she reasons that she not only saves herself the aggravation of peeling but adds a few extra nutrients to her family's meals. Participants who insist on peeling, though, prefer bona fide vegetable peelers to paring knives. Some find that a peeler with a U-shaped handle is easier to use than the straight-handled peeling/coring type. Electric peeling wands sell for about fifteen dollars.

As for the microwave, it is the first choice of those who like to cook early in the day for reheating at dinnertime, those who cook huge quantities of food on good days to freeze for bad times, and those who rely heavily on packaged frozen foods such as potpies and TV dinners. Any oven can heat up frozen foods, of course, but the microwave does it faster *and*—even more important to some participants—doesn't require the use of pots or pans. If you're sticking with your conventional oven, you may want to trade in your heavy cookware and dishes for lightweight ones.

The other appliances cited in our survey for comfort and convenience are the large electric mixer with dough hook for those who make their own bread, the dishwasher, and the electric pot scrubber. However, many of our participants don't use the dishwasher even though they have one, on the grounds that a sinkful of warm water and dirty dishes is good therapy for the hands. Several of them say they intentionally leave dishes in the sink overnight, so the chore of washing them first thing the next day can help banish the morning stiffness in their fingers.

As we mentioned earlier in this chapter, almost any utensil with a handle can be made into a custom-fitted tool by wrapping and fattening the handle until it's easier to hold. Here are the materials our survey participants use for this purpose.

- sponges fastened with tape

- foam or rubber tubing, which can be cut to any length, with center holes of various diameters

- foam-type hair curlers

- dish towels or washcloths

- plastic bubble wrap used to protect fragile items for shipping

If none of these works on your kitchen sink, consider trying one of the commercially available tap turners that come in a variety of designs and shapes to fit over any type of faucet. A few of our participants replaced the existing taps on their sinks with flat blade-shaped handles—or a single lever-type faucet that controls both the volume and the temperature of the water.

There are also many specialty utensils manufactured with extrathick, extralight, or angled handles, all available by mail order, as well as lightweight mugs with easy-grip handles, and some with *two* easy-grip handles.

Bathroom

The bathroom is typically the home hydrotherapy center for arthritis self-care. Well over half of our participants turn to it *at least* once a day for the soothing powers of a hot shower or a warm bath. A good number of them say they also exercise while bathing, because the warmth and buoyancy of the water make movement more manageable. Home hot-water therapy is so important to one Illinois lawyer that he installed a special large-capacity hot-water heater in his home to assure himself an abundant supply.

You may find it easier to turn the water taps if you exchange your round or four-pronged faucet handles for lever-shaped ones, or use a cushiony rubber jar grip from the kitchen for this purpose.

For safety, our participants favor some kind of handrail on the tub side, which also eases entry and exit. In the stall shower, too, they say, a rail or "grab bar" makes a good investment. Your tub should of course be equipped with a no-slip bathmat, and for comfort, you might like to try a bathtub mattress or a cushion made of inflatable plastic. The ultimate luxury though, is a home spa unit that churns the bathwater with whirlpool action.

"I found that I was in a hot tub of water so much," writes a hairstylist from Virginia, "that for Christmas I asked for a portable whirlpool. I love it. I use it a couple of times per week, and to me it's worth its weight in gold. The one I have is by Pollinex, and it allows me to adjust the speed and direction of the water flow, so I can let the water pulsate just where I need it—and at different times, I need it at different places. For about $150, I have found my salvation. It was my idea, too, not the doctor's, and it's better than any medicine he has prescribed to date!"

The shower version of the whirlpool bath is the pulsating or massage-type attachment, such as the ones manufactured by Pollinex and Water Pik. Some of these replace the existing shower head, changing the force and flow pattern of the water. Other types attach to the tub faucet, serving as hand-held showers that allow for extra attention directly on painful places.

Our participants also like to shower sitting down, on a homemade or store-bought shower seat. Even those who can stand comfortably choose to use the seat because it helps prevent falls, facilitates washing, and makes it easier to take full advantage of the water. "I use a piece of plywood to straddle the bathtub edges when I shower," says a Pennsylvania masonry contractor, "so I can sit down and give my knees a shower-massage treatment."

A few of our participants, however, find the height of the tub side to be an insurmountable obstacle. A Michigan housewife reports, "We removed our old bathtub, because it was difficult to step high to get into the tub. We now have a walk-in shower with a seat and a pulsating shower head. This is a tremendous help to me." One retired plumber from Wisconsin who had an old-fashioned high bathtub with feet built an elevated platform to help him get in and out of it.

Once you have gone to any trouble or expense to avoid extra stooping and reaching while you bathe, you don't want to be foiled by something as simple as a slippery bar of soap. A resourceful Arizona craftswoman says she crocheted a small mesh bag to hold her soap, and she keeps it tied to the shower head on a long string. Avon and several other cosmetics manufacturers achieve the same end with a "soap on a rope" that hangs conveniently from the faucet or around the bather's neck. A long-handled back brush is another nicety—or even a yardstick with a sponge on the end of it, as suggested by a North Carolina maintenance man.

An extremely popular way to raise the comfort level in the bathroom is to raise the height of the toilet seat. There are several models of raised seats, from specially shaped foam pads about two inches thick to steel-and-plastic additions that elevate the seat level as much as eight inches. Any of them can be installed or removed quite readily, so it needn't be considered a permanent change. In fact, several of our participants say that they have used a raised toilet seat as a temporary measure while recovering from surgery, for example, or during a painful flare-up.

Armrails are also a useful addition to the toilet, whether or not the seat is raised. Some armrail styles automatically raise the seat level an inch or so when installed, and the installation is usually a simple matter of slipping some aluminum rails together and into position.

Several participants like to use an electric toothbrush, not just because of its brushing action but because of its thick easy-to-hold handle. "For myself and for my arthritic patients," says a dental hygienist from Delaware, "I make a special toothbrush by wrapping bubble wrap (bubbles out) around the handle a few times and securing it with strapping tape." Two products mentioned by a Missouri National Guardsman, "Floss Fingers I" by Preventive Dentistry Products and "Floss Mate" by Butler, will let you floss your teeth with one hand, and without the dexterity usually required to floss the back teeth. Pump-type dispensers for toothpaste, soap, and hand lotion may also simplify your washing-up.

Living room

If you do most of your sitting in the living room, you have many options for making that pastime as comfortable as possible. The simplest is to start with what you have and modify it if you have to. A straight-back chair is many people's favorite, because it combines decent back support with a relatively high seat that is easy to reach and to leave. If the chair has arms to aid you, so much the better. If it feels too hard on your hips or doesn't give enough support for your lower back, you can pad the appropriate places. "I have straight-back chairs in the kitchen and the living room," says a retired kindergarten teacher from Rhode Island, "and I use cushions with them." Low chairs cause her so much trouble that she never uses them, preferring to *stand* at friends' houses if no suitable chair is available.

Cushions on chairs also serve to raise them a little higher, which is all to the good. Many styles are portable, and many of our participants do carry a favorite chair cushion wherever they go, whether it's an inexpensive piece of flat foam or a costly automatic lifter seat with spring-action that actually helps them to their feet. It is also possible to raise a chair or a couch from the bottom up—by standing it on a platform about four inches high, on risers or wood blocks, or by replacing the existing legs with taller ones. Some of the mail-order catalogs offer "chair raisers" that attach to furniture legs and raise them three to five inches.

Only a few of our participants felt the need to go out and buy a new chair, but those who did were awfully pleased with the result. The favorite investments were recliners or lounge chairs with footstools, because of the reduced pressure on knees and hips while sitting. Others preferred rocking chairs or posture-control chairs. Some of the armchairs purchased came complete with built-in heating elements for the back, or vibrator/massage units, or both. "My easy chair is the most useful item I've found," writes a retired science teacher from Texas, "and I found it in a department store. Shopping for it was a time-consuming job, as I had to visit many stores in order to get a properly fitting chair. A chair that does not fit properly means only one thing: lots of pain." *Amen.*

Stairways and entryways

"Stairs are my worst enemy," admits a retired nurse from Pennsylvania. In her own home, she avoids them with an electrical lift that carries her up or down the stairs along a steel beam. Other participants, who shared her sentiments but couldn't afford this several-thousand-dollar convenience, either moved or resigned themselves to living on one floor of their homes. "I haven't been upstairs in ten years," says a seventy-five-year-old Kentucky housewife with arthritis in her knees. "The last time was when I went to get Christmas decor no one else could find. I was home alone, without a phone up there. I found what I wanted, all right, but I couldn't walk back down. I finally had to throw a leg over the bannister and slide down. 'Twas fun."

Others, who find stairs difficult but not impossible, say they get by with a good sturdy handrail. They say that handrails are essential on *all* stairways, even the two or three steps that lead up to the front or back door.

A few participants have rebuilt their outdoor stairways so that the individual steps are smaller and easier to climb. Others have replaced the steps with wheelchair ramps, and widened the doorways, too, where necessary. Although a wider entry may sound like a major job for a carpenter, it is possible to expand many doorways by about one and a half inches with offset hinges that swing the door free of the doorjamb.

At Work

More than 90 percent of our survey participants continue to work for a living—or did work until they reached retirement age. They do everything from writing sermons to waiting tables; they manage corporations, assemble automobiles, provide health care, create stained-glass windows, and market cosmetics door-to-door. Most need no special allowances made for them at work, but a few really must modify their activities or change their job descriptions. A North Carolina registered nurse, for example, stopped working in a hospital because it involved too much walking. Now she does private duty nursing, which requires a lot of sitting. "I sit," she adds, "in a straight-back chair."

Changing jobs because of arthritis can be an opportunity for positive growth, as a forty-one-year-old Minnesota woman found when she quit working as a librarian to open her own clothing store and sewing business. "Lifting books and standing on cement floors was stressful to my wrists, hands, and feet," she recalls. "Now I have a carpet in my place of business."

For most of our participants, though, making the work environment more comfortable is a simple matter of adding the right equipment to get the job done.

If you sit at a desk, whether to type letters or design buildings, the key point is to make sure that the chair is a comfortable one. Although it is not always possible to request and receive a new or different chair, you can at least take your own foam seat pad or back-support cushion to work, to make yourself feel at home. Several participants say they are happiest in a secretary-type chair with wheels, because the seat height and back support can be adjusted to suit them. "I put my secretary chair to full use," says an Indiana receptionist, "because I scoot around in it, too." Sitters also like a footstool under the desk, which keeps their knees higher than their hips and thus helps them avoid back pain, a major occupational hazard of sitting at a desk. If you use a typewriter or computer that is positioned at right angles to your desk, you may be able to rig a footstool by opening the bottom desk drawer and resting your feet on it.

Desks and drafting tables can sometimes be height-adjusted, too. A desk with easy-to-pull drawers makes a good co-worker. A few forgo the desk altogether in favor of a podium where they can stand to read and write.

On the desk, our participants prefer electric to standard typewriters, and they like word processors best of all. They select oversize or specially curved pens, preferably with a felt tip because its ready ink flow requires a minimum of pressure to leave bold marks. Those who must use a pencil select the softer leads for the same reason—and electric pencil sharpeners. If the pen or pencil isn't specially designed, they customize it with a plastic triangle or ring, sold in stationery stores, that widens the implement and softens the grip. (Or use the foam curler trick, described earlier.) They use easy-grip, large-handled or loop-handled scissors, or they cut with a newspaper-clipping gadget that they slide along like a razor, without needing to open and close their hands. A smaller stapler, some say, doesn't have to be slammed with a sledgehammer fist. Another convenience is a speaker phone that leaves your hands free, or a lightweight headset that plugs into any modular phone.

Outside the office setting, many of our participants work with their hands for a living or for a hobby. Several have raised or lowered their workbenches for maximum comfort and the safe use of power tools. They also choose lighter-weight machinery, where possible, and get power assistance from gadgets such as the self-charging portable electrical screwdriver, sold at hardware stores. "I like to work in the garage," says a foreman and machinist from Pennsylvania. "A stool with wheels sold by Pep Boys, a national auto supplier, is a big help when working on a car."

On the Go

Cars—with their thumb-action door handles, their crank-up windows, their strangely positioned controls, their oddly angled seats, and the demands they place on the driver's hands, feet, shoulders, neck, back, and hips—are a necessity for most of our participants, who have, by necessity, found ways to make them more comfortable.

You can get past the door-handle problem with a plastic door opener that hooks around the handle and presses that annoying button for you. You can turn the ignition more easily with a wooden or plastic key turner or a small crescent wrench. But once inside you've still got to sit in the driver's seat for some period of time. Make it as comfortable as your other chairs by adding a back support or a folding car seat that offers support for your back and your bottom. Our participants also mentioned gel-filled cushions, inflatable cushions, egg-crate car seats, sacroiliac pillows, massage seats that plug into the cigarette lighter, cervical pillows, and the Posture Curve back support from Body Care, Inc., of New York City. Even if you're driving in the backseat, you'll find that taking some kind of pillow along to wedge behind your back or under any painful area can make the trip more pleasant. A few people prefer to lie down on the backseat, and a former photographer from Illinois has purchased a van so that she can travel lying on a comfortable mattress in the rear.

Several participants say they traded in their stick shifts and clutch pedals for cars with automatic transmission. Buyers beware, however, that the gear-shift lever on many automatics has a thumb button that may be quite difficult to operate.

Most new cars have a host of electronic conveniences and labor-saving designs that could have been custom-made for people with arthritis, from power steering and power brakes to easy-touch buttons that open and close the windows, seats that change position electrically, and more easy-touch buttons that lock or unlock all the doors simultaneously. Cruise control, which can put your car on automatic pilot for long stretches of highway driving, lets you relax your legs and feet at 55 m.p.h., but it's no substitute for stopping the car every hour or so and getting out to stretch.

Large cars are favored for their greater legroom and smooth ride, especially four-door models for ease of getting in or out. "I avoid all cars with bucket seats," says a psychotherapist from New York, "which seem to press on the hip bones and lead to pain."

Once you get where you're going, do you have trouble finding a place to park? Several participants mentioned the value of handicapped license plates or permits enabling them to park right in front of many stores and public buildings. Several others asked us where and how to get them. Since procedures vary from state to state, however, we have to refer you to your local Motor Vehicle Bureau for information on how to apply.

"Don't use the 'Handicapped' parking space if another is nearby," advises a retired engineer from Florida who follows his own advice. "Someone worse off may need it."

Products Available by Mail

Here's a listing of the catalogs our participants mentioned as sources for items to make you more comfortable, more capable, or both.

Comfortably Yours, 52 Hunter Avenue, Maywood, NJ 07607

Aids for Arthritis, Inc., 3 Little Knoll Ct., Medford, NJ 08055

Ways & Means "The Capability Collection," 28001 Citrin Drive, Romulus, MI 48174

Dr. Leonard's Health Care Catalog 74, 20th Street, Brooklyn, NY 11232

FashionABLE for Better Living, 99 West Street, Medfield, MA 02052

Solutions, P.O. Box 6878, Portland, OR 97228–6878

Nelson's Medical Line Warehouse, P.O. Box 20609, Sarasota, FL 34238

Sears, Roebuck and Co. and the J.C. Penney Co. both offer

special catalog supplements for customers who need the kinds of items mentioned in this chapter.

Other catalogs:

Enrichments, Inc., 145 Tower Drive, P.O. Box 579, Hinsdale, IL 60521

Lumex/Swedish Rehab, 100 Spence St., Bay Shore, NY 11706

Summary of Practices and Products to Increase Your Comfort and Safety

Throughout your house

Organize cupboards to keep frequently used products within easy reach.

Arrange furniture for safe passage, minimal clutter, and support when rising from a couch or chair.

Eliminate drafts.

Choose lightweight appliances.

Modify door knobs and handles with easy-open levers.

Use soft warm floor coverings that won't make you slip or trip.

Build up handles for easy gripping.

Let step stools and long-handled utensils extend your reach.

Install easy-touch controls for lamps and ceiling lights.

Bedroom comforts

Good mattress

Foam mattress pad

Woolen or electric bed pad

Flannel or thermal sheets

Sleeping bag

Bed board

Special pillows

Water bed

Raised bed

Hospital bed

Kitchen helpers

Can, bottle, and jar open-
ers
High stool
Revolving shelves or lazy
Susans
Food processor
Microwave oven
Lightweight dishes, pots,
pans

Electric mixer
Fat-handled utensils
Tap turners on water fau-
cets
Chopping board (with
nail)

Bathroom aids

Easy-to-use faucet han-
dles
Tub rail
Shower grab bar
No-slip bathmat
Whirlpool unit
Raised toilet seat
Armrails for toilet

Shower massage
Tub or shower seat
Soap on rope
Bath brush
Electric toothbrush
Dental floss tool
Pump dispensers

Living room

Straight-back chair
Back-support cushions
Chair pads
Footstool

Lifter seat
Chair raisers
Recliner

Stairways and entryways

Electrical stair lift
Sturdy handrails

Modified entry steps
Widened doorways

Office and workshop

Secretary chair
Footstool (or open desk
drawer)

Electric typewriter
Word processor
Fat felt-tip pens

Soft lead pencils
Electric pencil sharpener
Raised (or lowered) work-
    bench
Power tools
Lightweight machinery

Stool with wheels
Easy-grip scissors or clip-
    per
Speaker phone or head-
    set
Small stapler

Car

Car-door opener
Key turner
Car-seat cushion
Automatic transmission
Power steering and
    brakes
Electronic windows and
    locks

Automatically adjustable
    seat
Cruise control
Handicapped plates or
    permit

21

HOW TO GO ABOUT YOUR EVERYDAY ACTIVITIES WITH MINIMUM PAIN AND MAXIMUM EASE

■ Smart tips for joint protection ■ Gadgets that get things done ■ Scheduling activities and rest to help you accomplish more ■ New ways to keep doing what you need to do, what you love to do

Among them, our 1,051 Arthritis Survey participants have racked up some fifteen thousand man- or woman-years of living with arthritis. That's many lifetimes' worth of persevering in the face of pain or disability or both. Through trial and error, these individuals have learned how to go on doing the things they want to do and the things they have to do. Their cumulative experience is an excellent teacher.

No doubt you have devised some of your own methods for handling various chores. Here's your chance to pool your ideas with those of a thousand other people.

The advice our participants offer ranges from general principles, such as "Take it easy," to ingenious specifics, such as, "Tie loops of yarn around the handles of the oven, refrigerator, and kitchen cupboards so they can be opened with the forearm instead of the fingers." It covers everything from keeping house to making love. It includes timesaving tips, work-saving devices, safety precautions, household modifications, and gadgets you can make yourself to make life easier. We have condensed and organized our participants' comments into twenty-five strategies for performing everyday activities in spite of—and without worsening—arthritis pain. We begin with the most frequently mentioned suggestions.

Pace Yourself

Keeping active is extremely important for mental and physical well-being, but finding the right activity level can spell the difference between happy involvement and painful overexertion. Participants stress the importance of pacing themselves to go whatever distance they must cover in a day. "I've slowed down," reports a graphic designer from Oregon, "and in doing so I've found that I have less pain than when I'm in a hurry."

Pacing yourself is as much a mental as a physical activity. It means knowing your own limitations, so you can work within them instead of against yourself. It means exerting a steady flow of energy, instead of erratic bursts. It means, in the words of one retired engineer, "One thing at a time. One day at a time. One life at a time."

Break One Big Job into Several Small Chores

You can do as much as you ever did, in many respects, by taking a different approach to big jobs. Almost any task can be broken into component parts, so you can accomplish each one separately, allowing yourself many small breaks before you reach the final goal. A supervisor in a New York credit bureau plans her housework and laundry so that she does about two hours' worth every night, in lieu of eight hours on Saturday— and she skips the night or nights when her arthritis is most painful. A retired Colorado radio announcer divides up his activities this way: "I clean the house one room per day, working slowly and resting frequently. For exercise, I take three or four short walks per day rather than one long one. But when it comes to making love, there's just no way to do it a little at a time."

Stick to Your Exercise Routine

The vast majority of our survey participants exercise regularly and credit that activity with helping them function better than they otherwise would. "Walking and swimming have given me the ability to continue to live relatively normally and with minimal pain," writes a hospital worker from Michigan. A New Jersey homemaker says that the hand exercises her doctor prescribed enable her to use her fingers better and therefore do more daily chores. Nearly all those who exercise stress the importance of finding and maintaining a routine. "You don't always see immediate results from exercise," explains a retired New York executive, "but you have to keep at it just to stay even." For most people in our survey, exercise is not only helpful but enjoyable in itself, making it a very sweet-tasting medicine: "It improves my mental outlook and gives me an exhilarated feeling," a Tennessee newspaper reporter observes. (If you don't already have an exercise program or a practitioner who can help you create one, please see Chapters 18 and 19 for specific exercise advice.)

Ask for Help If You Need It

"When I need help," a twenty-nine-year-old Texas teacher has learned, "I ask and don't care if they call me a weakling or whatever. I just laugh at their ignorance and let them assist me." Not everyone can be so cavalier about needing the assistance of others, but if you do need help, you owe it to yourself to say so.

The help may take the form of a hired housekeeper, if you can afford one—or can receive the services some other way. A sixty-eight-year-old resident of a low-income high rise in Seattle has a welfare house helper spend twenty hours per month at her apartment, and, she says, "Having the hard household tasks done for me is a blessing." A person to help with the yardwork or odd jobs makes good sense, too, unless you can rely on a little extra effort from members of your own family, as most of our survey participants do. One homemaker, in fact, puts her "sympathetic husband" first on the list of the most useful items she's discovered for people with arthritis. Similarly, a thirty-seven-year-old insurance agent says, "My wife and I work together. She is aware of my condition and helps if needed. No, neither she nor I tolerate pity and sympathy. Understanding is the key in our relationship."

Rest Periodically

Rest, the number-one self-help strategy for pain relief, is what makes it possible for many of our survey participants to accomplish their day's work. They take periodic breaks, either for a short nap in bed or time in an easy chair, relaxing with their feet up—or in some other comfortable position. A forty-seven-year-old California store owner who's had rheumatoid arthritis since childhood says he manages to keep working by being "up and active two hours, prone two hours." Experiment to determine the amount of rest you need, and then do your utmost to make sure you get it. "When I entertain," says a freelance writer from New Mexico, "I tell people *when I invite them* what time I expect them to leave."

Don't Overdo Any Activity

Moderation is the best policy, our survey participants have found, as almost any activity may lead to trouble if done to excess. How do you know when you've done too much? You learn the hard way, at least once, and then you use that experience to guide you in the future. A retired family counselor in our survey group who can't seem to pull herself away from a job unfinished now avoids the overdo syndrome by setting a kitchen timer before she begins any physically stressful task. If she gets too engrossed to stop when she should, the buzzer is there to remind her.

Another way to keep from overdoing one activity is to alternate chores periodically, as this California housewife does: "I avoid several days of repeated activity, like yardwork, or several hours of any uninterrupted, intense similar activities as was my pattern before the arthritis set in ten years ago." Here's how a homesteader in Wisconsin uses a similar ploy: "When I wash dishes I only wash a few, then I dry them and put them away. If I just stay at the sink for a long time, it really brings on the pain."

Listen to Your Body

When something you are doing becomes too physically stressful, heed your body's danger cries right away. Stop, stretch, rest, change activities—do whatever the situation seems to require. If you push through a sudden sharp pain, you may injure yourself seriously. This goes for exercise, too, where the athlete's trendy motto, "No pain, no gain," has been exposed as a foolish philosophy. "In cleaning house or making love," suggests a Pennsylvania salesman, "do only what and how much your body tells you you can do—and believe me, it tells you!"

Use Good Body Mechanics

Be mindful of your affected joints and spare them any undue strain. In daily activities, including your exercise routine, it's best to avoid quick jerky movements that can give your joints a jolt. Try to maintain good posture when standing (not military attention, but a comfortable relaxed stance), and think about your posture when you're seated, too. If you can identify certain actions that tend to bring on pain, try to avoid them or work around them. An aircraft designer from New York says he performs what he calls "motion study" before tackling new tasks. "I don't rush into anything," he explains. "I try to think it out before starting, foreseeing the safest and easiest positions as much as possible."

Participants with special hobbies were particularly inventive on this score. For example, a Kansas county sheriff who loves to build and fix things was having trouble using a screw-driver for a long enough time to accomplish much. Then he discovered that it helped to tighten with his left hand and loosen with his right, so that he was always turning the screw-driver toward his arthritic thumbs instead of away from them.

Try Sitting Down on the Job—or Anywhere Else

Several of our participants live by the credo, "Never stand when you can sit, and never sit when you can lie down." Many of them manage to continue at their regular jobs because they can carry out their responsibilities from a chair. An Indiana factory worker explained, "I am fortunate to have a job where I can sit most of the time and run my machine. This takes the load off my back and knees."

A high bar stool at the kitchen counter is what enables many of our participants to cook for themselves. They sit while preparing food, while ironing, and while doing the laundry. A thirty-nine-year-old Florida housewife has had rollers put on her most comfortable chair so she can sit while vacuuming and mopping the floor. In low-down work such as gardening, a small short-legged stool or a low stool with wheels can be a tremendous help.

Although the majority of our participants prefer sitting, a small percentage of them cannot sit comfortably even for a short time, including a draftsman who works standing at an easel instead of leaning over a table, and a budget analyst who writes while standing at a podium rather than sitting at a desk.

Avoid Heavy Lifting

There are many definitions of "heavy." For a sixty-four-year-old retired typist, "heavy" means anything over five pounds. For a forty-one-year-old registered nurse, "heavy" means a patient's body, as she can no longer lift one by herself. What-ever your definition of "heavy," don't tax yourself by lifting more than you can handle. Here's the strategy favored by a thirty-seven-year-old electronics technician from Virginia: "I lift smaller loads and make more trips, rather than try to lift one large load."

When you do lift, remember to keep the item close to your body instead of holding it with outstretched arms, so as not to strain your back.

Save Steps—and Stairs, Too

With a little forethought, you can save yourself a lot of extra running around that may sap your energy. For example, a Nevada accountant plans his errands by geographical area so he can accomplish several chores at once instead of needing to make repeated, separate trips. An interior decorator from Ohio writes, "When I shop, I stop in the entrance and look over the store, thinking how I can save steps before I venture in. At shopping malls, I sometimes use a wheelchair." Others skip as many trips to the store as they can by shopping from mail-order catalogs.

At home, too, especially if you have stairs to climb, try to plan your activities to minimize the number of trips you make from one part of the house to another. You may want to keep an upstairs and a downstairs supply of inexpensive cleaning and grooming supplies so you'll always have what you need at hand. "I make as few trips as possible to the basement," says a nurse from Michigan, "and once I'm in the basement doing my laundry, I stay there until the wash is finished."

Participants who mention stairs urge extreme caution in using them: Take them one at a time, hold on, and don't fall. If it's easier for you to go downstairs backward, then by all means do so.

Change Positions Often to Avoid Stiffness

Don't get stuck standing or sitting in any one position for too long a time. Try to switch positions periodically, or at least move around from time to time to loosen up. In the car, too, remember to stop *at least* once every two hours on long trips to get out and walk around.

"Taking stretch breaks is the best technique I've found to keep me going," says a thirty-seven-year-old Californian with osteoarthritis. "I have a typing business, and I've learned to get up every hour and stretch, no matter what!"

If only they could follow this rule while sleeping, many of our participants say ruefully, they would be able to start the day with much greater ease. Since they can't, they do the next best thing, which is to find a comfortable position for sleeping. The two favorites are (1) on the side in a fetal position, with a pillow *between* the knees, and (2) on the back with a pillow *under* the knees. Pillows used in these ways help keep the lower back in line. You can find many styles of specially shaped knee wedges and neck pillows, or you can use standard bed pillows, folding or stacking them under your knees to suit your needs. A fifty-eight-year-old Texas woman says the best pillow for between the knees is a child's float ring, covered with a flannel pad.

Here are some other suggestions for smoothing the way out of bed.

- Do some gentle stretching exercises in bed before you try to get up.

- Keep some milk in a thermos at bedside, and set your alarm for half an hour to an hour *before* your wake-up time so you can take your medication, go back to sleep for awhile, and reawaken less stiff.

- Take your medication with a late snack just before you go to bed at night to allay nausea and morning stiffness.

- To rise, position yourself near the edge of the bed, on your side. If you're lying on your right side, use your left hand and arm to steadily push yourself up to a sitting position as you swing your feet down, then stand up.

Relax Your Cleaning Standards a Little Bit

Learning to look past the dust makes housekeeping much easier. Changing the sheets less often helps, too. (And if you have fragile hands, choose flat sheets over fitted ones.) Accepting something short of perfection from yourself, though difficult, comes highly recommended by our survey participants.

"My goal is to be as pain-free from arthritis as I can," reasons a crafts instructor from Ohio, who has both rheumatoid and osteoarthritis, "so housecleaning takes a backseat in my schedule. I do such work when I'm feeling well enough to do so. My family and friends must accept this, as I must accept my limitations."

"I'm less particular about the house," concedes an Iowa housewife. "I do what I can and I don't fret about what I can't."

A soil tester from Wisconsin quips, "If your guests don't like your housekeeping, hand them the broom."

Set a (Flexible) Schedule

Many participants find that arthritis pain or fatigue (or both) ebbs and flows over the course of the day, creating a pattern of can-do and can't-do times, and they schedule themselves accordingly. "I rise early and do almost all my housework and cooking before noon," says a retired teacher from New York State. "By 1 P.M., I am too tired to do much." Accepting of this framework, they figure out which activities deserve top priority, and then try to do those things during their best time of the day. "Early afternoon is the best time for making love," notes a Connecticut homemaker, "after the morning stiffness is gone and before the evening tiredness sets in."

Several participants emphasize the importance of keeping a regular schedule to make sure they get enough rest, take their medications at the proper times, and exercise for a certain number of minutes or hours each day. A well-planned schedule can enhance your self-care program, as long as it *serves* you and doesn't *drive* you. Or, as a retired Florida car salesman put it, "Schedule—and then reschedule when necessary."

Let One Joint Compensate for Another

At the beginning of this chapter, we mentioned the yarn loops tied on cabinet doors that let a North Dakota social worker use her wrists and arms to do what her hands cannot. Many of our participants have found ways to let one joint compensate for the disability in another. For example, you can use your feet to wipe spills from the floor with a cloth or sponge, work an electric can opener with your forearm, and seal the lids on plastic containers with your elbow. You can use your hips, shoulders, elbows, or rear end to push doors open or shut. You can also operate the foot pedal of a sewing machine with your hand. You can pick up your child, as one Kentucky mother does, with your wrists. "Just favor the aching parts," advises a retired electrical engineer from Texas. "They're not always in the same places."

Here's a related rule from a communications consultant in North Carolina: "Never use one hand if you can use two. It reduces the wear." Other participants who follow her advice note that they always use two hands to push/pull the vacuum cleaner, to lift, and to carry.

Speak Out to Spare Your Hands

When someone wants to shake your hand in greeting and you are afraid the contact may harm you, what do you do? Several of our participants say they avoid handshaking altogether, and explain as much to any new acquaintances at the first introduction, as this artist from Pennsylvania does: "When meeting people, smile gently and say, 'I'm afraid my arthritis is acting up.'" If that kind of frankness doesn't appeal to you, there are several more subtle escapes. Depending on the social situation, you may be able to get around a handshake, if need be, with a quick hug, a touch on the arm, or a pat on the back. Sometimes it's friendly and painless to take the other person's hand with *both* of yours.

Many of our participants solve the problem of *hand* writing by using a typewriter or word processer, but some find typing just as difficult as holding a pen. These people keep up their correspondence by telephone or by dictating letters into a tape recorder and sending the cassettes through the mail.

Protect Your Joints from Injury

When you can't avoid using your affected joints, you can guard against injury with many kinds of protective coverings. These range from back braces and cervical collars to splints and simple elastic bandages. Most people who use them do so only at specific times or for specific tasks. A Rhode Island homemaker wears a cervical collar while doing housework, for example; a Tennessee secretary puts splints on her wrists when typing or playing golf; and a California composer with rheumatoid arthritis who is mindful of how he uses his hands all day finds he needs to give them extra protection at night: "I try not to bump my fingers or let them bend suddenly or too far, as it can be very painful. I avoid jobs that require too much flexing, as that also makes the pain worse, and I drop things a lot. Sometimes, I splint a finger before going to bed, because if I roll over and bend it too far, the pain is intense."

Bend from the Knees—or Avoid Bending Altogether

Many of our survey participants who suffer back pain from arthritis say they stoop down rather than bend over when they have to reach to the floor, letting their legs do the work instead of straining their spines. This is sound practice for the back, but if your knees are arthritic—and we counted more sore knees than bad backs in our survey group—stooping may be difficult, if not impossible. Some individuals say they must avoid stooping or bending altogether. "The only thing I have changed is that I can no longer stoop," says a seventy-one-year-old Pennsylvania saleslady who has had arthritis for forty-seven years. "Stooping is very hard on the knees, and once I'm down, it's very difficult for me to get up."

One solution is to use a long-handled spring action tool that extends your arm's reach by about three feet and has a hand with magnetic fingertips that are quite good at picking up dropped coins, paper clips, and the like. Almost everyone who uses this item has his own name for it. Our participants called it by turns a reacher, a gripper, an extender, a long-lifter, a pick-up stick, a grab-it, and tongs, but they all meant the same thing. You can buy one for about eight dollars by mail order (see Chapter 20 for more information) or try to make something similar yourself out of a clothes hanger or other materials: "A helpful homemade tool to reach things too high or too low can be made from a broomstick," writes a seventy-four-year-old copy editor from Oregon. "Cut off the broom and cut the head off a nail. Then pound the nail into the end of the stick." She adds, "You could even clean up litter in the park with this gadget." A Montana ranch wife made her "picker-upper" by screwing a cup hook on the end of a thirty-six-inch pole.

Prepare Yourself for Extra Exertion

Anytime that you're planning on being more active than usual or are about to do something that has brought on pain in the past, you may be able to ward it off by trying a pain-relieving strategy in advance. "When you are going to do something that usually causes more pain," writes a homemaker from Utah, "use medication and precautions *before,* not after the pain starts. Some problems can be avoided or at least minimized by using caution and good sense." Use whatever works for you. Our participants favored two aspirin (or other medication), a warm bath, a nap, or a massage. A Georgia accountant says, "I find that making love *after* a hot bath or shower lessens the pain in my hip."

In Making Love, Strive for Open Communication with Your Partner

Finding a comfortable position for lovemaking takes inventiveness and the willing cooperation of both partners. It also calls for "more talk" and "frank communication," our survey participants say, which may actually enhance closeness and enjoyment. "My husband is so caring and loving," writes a thirty-four-year-old Florida housewife, "that we have a very good sexual relationship, no matter how bad the arthritis is. We do sometimes have to adjust positions depending on where I hurt, but being creative makes lovemaking even more exciting."

Among those survey participants who favor a specific position for intercourse, the first choice is to have the woman on top, no matter which partner is the one with arthritis. In this position, a man need not support his own weight on his knees, wrists, or elbows, and a woman need not support a man's weight. Some couples are more comfortable making love on their sides, either face-to-face or with the man facing the woman's back. "Lying on one's side is easier on the back than the missionary position," explains a California homemaker, "and is quite pleasant to both parties." But the majority of those who comment about sex say that they tend to vary positions from one time to the next. And in *any* position, they avow, the idea is to concentrate on the lovemaking and not on pain and stiffness. "If you don't love your lover," observes a photographer from Massachusetts, "it will hurt whether or not you have arthritis. If you are both crazy about each other, you find ways to please each other and spare yourselves pain." Some of the ways our survey participants mention include more caressing and foreplay, oral sex, and mutual masturbation.

Several of our participants candidly concede that they have to make love less frequently, less energetically, or abstain altogether because of arthritis pain, age, other health problems, or a combination of these factors. "Make love at seventy-five and seventy-eight?" asks a Kentucky housewife with a serious heart condition and a thirty-year history of osteoarthritis. "Well, no pain in saying 'I love you' and kissing him on the nose." Others claim that sex actually has a positive effect on their pain. "Sex is good therapy," says an executive recruiter from Texas who's had rheumatoid arthritis for twenty of his forty-five years. "It releases endorphins—the body's own pain-killers!" A Wisconsin practical nurse writes, "Making love regularly seems to have a carryover effect in lessening pain." And a Michigan factory worker finds, "It limbers up everything and makes you feel good!"

A few survey participants praise their water beds for making sex less painful and therefore more enjoyable. Many more are content with a few well-placed pillows to support their hips or knees during sex.

Meet Life's Little Challenges with the Proper Tools

Elaborate plastic food packages, medicine bottles with child-proof lids, and soft-drink cans with ring-pop tops are just a few of the items that bedevil our survey participants' attempts to carry on with business as usual. They fight back by arming themselves with pliers to open bottles, a crescent wrench to turn the car key, scissors to slit sealed bags, and ingenuity to use everyday utensils in creative ways, such as cleaning the bathtub with a floor mop instead of kneeling down and leaning over to do the job in the usual way with a sponge. If you can't handle the tops on aluminum drink cans, turn them over to your electric can opener, or purchase a "tab grabber" made for the job. If your medication comes in a childproof container, put it in a different bottle as soon as you get it home so you'll be able to get at it when you need to. If you hate the one-finger pressure needed to push the small nozzles on aerosol cans, you can get a spray-handle kit that converts an aerosol can to a spray gun.

Some participants get a lot of help from the cane or crutch that they have to carry anyway, using it to make the bed, to push couch pillows in place, to close the drapes, or open the windows. Most have discovered some small or inexpensive item, from a long-handled shoehorn to an oversize felt-tip pen, that makes a big welcome difference in getting things done. "The feather duster is the greatest invention since the can opener," writes an insurance secretary from Texas. "It helps keep furniture clean and I don't have to rub the furniture with a cloth, move knickknacks around, or worry about bumping my fingers while dusting." (Many other convenience items recommended by survey participants are described in Chapter 20.)

Let Your Furniture Help You Up

When getting out of a chair or up from a kneeling position, use your arms to pull yourself upright—and spare your knees. Several participants say they arrange their furniture with this idea in mind, setting their chairs near something very sturdy, such as a wall divider or solid cabinet, which they can grab hold of to pull themselves up. "I can't get up from a low chair or couch," explains a writer from Texas, "so the low couch that I have—because I can't afford to buy a new one—is close to a table, which I pull up on." Others have installed special grab bars or railings in key locations about the house. And a lithographer from California, disabled by both rheumatoid and osteoarthritis, helps himself up with ropes hung from the ceiling of his apartment.

Stay Warm

Dress for warmth in layers of comfortable clothing that let you keep your body at your ideal temperature as you go through the day. From the comments we received, this rule applies not just in cold climates but to warm ones as well, where air conditioners can create misery-provoking drafts. Many of our participants select soft loose clothes that have elastic waists instead of buttons and zippers. They like long underwear, sweat suits, leg warmers, knee socks, and natural fibers such as cotton and flannel.

Certain painful joints just seem to work better with the

benefit of a special extra layer to help retain warmth. Gloves are a frequently mentioned favorite, and so are socks with the feet cut off to make a cozy knit tube that slips easily over an elbow or knee. "To keep the body heat in my hands at night," writes a sixty-six-year-old home health-care aide from Florida, "I rub on Vaseline and wear cotton gloves to bed." A thirty-nine-year-old housewife from Pennsylvania uses terry-cloth bands (such as the ones tennis players wear) to hold warmth in her wrists, and a sixty-one-year-old motel maid from Ohio frequently wraps her knees or ankles with clear plastic wrap in on-two-hours/off-two-hours cycles.

Everybody hangs pot holders near the stove, but if your hands are extremely sensitive to cold, you need a pair of "oven mitts" by the refrigerator and freezer, too. And when you make yourself an iced drink, try covering the lower half of the glass with an elastic slip-on coaster or a folded washcloth.

Carry What You Need—Comfortably

Big pockets, baskets, tote bags, plastic grocery bags with handles that loop over the wrists—even shirttails, in a pinch—make it easier for our participants to carry miscellaneous items about the house, off to work, or home from the store. Several women note that they have traded in their handbags for a roomy lightweight backpack. This makes sense for basic comfort and is especially useful for those who need to carry a back-support pillow or other special aids wherever they go.

If there *is* an item that can help you do your day's work more comfortably, whether it's a cushion, a splint, or a folding footrest, do find a way to carry it with you so it's there when you need it. For example, a sixty-five-year-old secretary from California says she always wears a scarf, and that way, if her shoulder acts up, she simply ties the scarf into a sling. At the same time, try to lighten your load by *not* dragging along the things you really *don't* need.

Wheeled carts are reliable helpers for toting laundry, groceries, or garbage. And several women say they use a tea cart at home for transporting cleaning supplies or meals from one room to another.

Get a Power Assist

Depending on the availability of human help at your house and the amount of money you can spend, you may want to find a motorized way to accomplish certain tasks. Several of our participants rely on snowblowers to clear their walks, rider mowers to cut the grass, and a host of indoor laborsaving devices, from electrically powered vegetable peelers to self-propelled vacuum cleaners. (Vacuuming, by the way, was cited most often as the chore most likely to cause pain, so a lighter-weight, easier-to-use model may be well worth its cost.)

Although there is a well known power-assist way to take care of dirty dishes, we have more participants who advocate hand-washing than ones who recommend using an automatic dishwasher. "Washing dishes feels *good*," says a retired teacher. "Between the warmth of the water and the exercise of squeezing the sponge, it's practically therapy." (If squeezing a sponge is painful, try flattening it with your palm. You may want to try a mitten-shaped bath sponge that you can *wear* for washing and wring out by pressing against the sink.) Several participants say they intentionally leave their dinner dishes in the sink overnight, because dish washing is the best antidote they've found for morning hand stiffness.

While you're at the kitchen sink, please be careful not to strain your other joints with the position you assume. If your knees or feet bother you, try sitting on a high stool. If it's your back that's the problem, you can (1) spread your legs slightly and bend your knees to relieve the pressure; (2) open the undersink cabinet and rest one foot inside it; or (3) rest one knee on a chair.

Summary of Tips on Keeping Up Your Everyday Activities

Pace yourself.
Break one big job into several small chores.
Stick to your exercise routine.
Ask for help if you need it.

Rest periodically.
Don't overdo any activity.
Listen to your body.
Use good body mechanics.
Try sitting down on the job—or anywhere else.
Avoid heavy lifting.
Save steps—and stairs, too.
Change positions often to avoid stiffness.
Relax your cleaning standards a little bit.
Set a (flexible) schedule.
Let one joint compensate for another.
Speak out to spare your hands.
Protect your joints from injury.
Bend from the knees—or avoid bending altogether.
Prepare yourself for extra exertion.
In making love, strive for open communication with your partner.
Meet life's little challenges with the proper tools.
Let your furniture help you up.
Stay warm.
Carry what you need—comfortably.
Get a power assist.

ABOUT THE RESEARCH

The 1,051 participants in our nationwide Arthritis Survey first learned of its existence from their favorite newspapers and magazines—*USA Today,* the *New York Times,* the *American Legion Magazine, Prevention, Popular Science, McCall's Needlework and Crafts, Field & Stream, Writer's Digest, Mother Jones, Medical Self-Care,* and others—where we placed advertisements and public notices inviting people with arthritis to fill out a detailed questionnaire.

Interested volunteers wrote to us or called our toll-free number to get a copy of the six-page Arthritis Survey questionnaire. In filling out the form, they told us about every doctor they had seen because of arthritis, from rheumatologists to clinical ecologists, and every non-M.D. practitioner as well, including chiropractors, physical therapists, and nutritionists. They answered questions on the effects—and side effects—of a medicine-chestful of prescription drugs, injections, and professional treatments ranging from acupuncture to wax dips. A few of the participants were serving as research subjects in clinical trials of new arthritis treatments, and they gave us a fascinating glimpse of things to come.

They also told us about their operations and the long-term results of surgery. They ran through their exercise routines. They explained the ways they had changed their eating habits and how they had benefited from the change. They reported on over-the-counter treatments they had tried—and under-the-counter ones, too, such as DMSO and bee venom. And they told us what they did for themselves to relieve pain, raise spirits, and generally make life easier. (The text of the questionnaire comprises Appendix A.) In the vast majority of the 1,300-some responses we received, the detailed answers dispelled any doubts about the authenticity of the participants' experiences. However, we did have to reject about 150 questionnaires that were incomplete or otherwise unusable.

As a token of our thanks for the time they spent sharing their knowledge, we sent each participant a check for eight dollars. As it turned out, a few of the checks came back to us, with notes saying that we should put the money toward the research—that participating in the survey had been a welcome chance to reach out and help others.

The money to conduct the survey (to cover advertising, printing, postage, payments to participants, long-distance telephone calls, and clerical help) came from our publisher, St. Martin's Press. This meant that we did not have to seek the financial support of any foundation or manufacturer. We are very pleased that we were able to work independently, without the pressure or influence of any organization's vested interest.

From among the 518 survey participants who volunteered to talk to us on the telephone (in addition to filling out the questionnaire), we chose 100 people to interview at length.

In talking about their complaints, several participants noted that they hate being called "an arthritic" or "an arthritis sufferer," as though they were nothing more than the victim of their disease. They prefer to think of themselves as the people they really are—as husbands, wives, parents, friends, partners, and valued employees. They work, or have worked, as accountants, advertising directors, archaeologists, armed-service members, army recruiters, artists, assembly-line workers, audiologists, auto mechanics, bankers, barbers, bartenders, beauticians, bookkeepers, bricklayers, budget analysts, cabdrivers, cafeteria servers, car dealers, carpenters, cartographers, chemists, childcare providers, chiropractors, choir directors, civil servants, college professors, composers, computer operators, construction workers, consultants, cooks, corporate executive officers, dairy farmers, dental hygienists, dentists, designers, detectives, dietitians, disc jockeys, doctors, dog breeders, draftsmen, dressmakers, dry cleaners, economists, editors, educational administrators, electronics technicians, engineers, entertainers, family counselors, farmhands, fire fighters, food brokers, foremen, forestry technicians, foundry workers, gardeners, guards, home health-care aids, hospital and nursing-home volunteers, househusbands and housewives, housekeepers, insurance agents, interior decorators, investors, janitors, lab technicians, laborers, lawyers, lecturers, letter carriers, librarians, locksmiths, loggers, machinists, maintenance workers, manufacturing representatives, medical assistants, merchant seamen, meter readers, military officers, miners, ministers, musicians, newspaper reporters, nuns, nurses, occupational therapists, oil-field roughnecks, optometrists, painters, paramedics, personnel directors, pharmacists, photographers, piano tuners, pilots, plumbers, police officers, porters, postmasters, printers, proofreaders, psychotherapists, purchasing agents, railroad carmen, ranchers, real estate agents, receptionists, registrars, researchers, restaurant owners, retail buyers, sales clerks, sanitation workers, sculptors, secretaries, securities traders, shipping clerks, shopkeepers, silversmiths, small-business owners, social workers, soil testers, supervisors, tax consultants, tax representatives, taxidermists, teachers, telephone operators, tennis instructors, traffic monitors, travel agents, traveling salesmen, truck drivers, typists, USDA food inspectors, veterinarians, waitresses, welders, welfare investigators, and writers.

Our participants come from every one of the fifty states. While most of them live in the large population centers— California, New York, Florida, and Texas—the Arthritis Survey reached Myrtle Creek, Oregon; Boonville, Missouri; Blue Diamond, Washington; Horse Cave, Kentucky; Iron River, Wisconsin; Hepzibah, Georgia; Ceresco, Nebraska; and Eagle, Alaska. We also had a total of nineteen participants from the Bahamas, Puerto Rico, and Canada. We drew the line there, however, and denied the survey requests we received from residents of Spain, England, Chile, the Philippines, and other foreign countries, because we wanted to focus on practitioners and treatments that would be accessible to North American readers.

The characteristics of our survey group match the national portrait of people with rheumatoid arthritis and osteoarthritis in terms of age and sex. In all, 68 percent of them are in their forties, fifties, or sixties, and 67 percent are women. We counted 416 participants with rheumatoid arthritis, 564 with osteoarthritis, and 71 with a combination of both. (You'll find a summary of the demographics, including age of onset, in Appendix B.)

The participants who answered our ads are "self-selected" volunteers, as opposed to subjects picked at random. A few researchers contend that self-selected participants are somehow special or atypical—that they answer a call for volunteers because they have "an ax to grind," and that this invalidates their responses. However, our earlier survey research project, which was described in our book *Backache Relief* (Times Books, 1985; NAL/Signet, 1986, and a Book-of-the-Month Club Alternate Selection), brought in very few people who had nothing but an ax to grind. Most of the participants in that survey responded because they had found an effective approach to back pain, after years of searching for one, and wanted to share what they had learned. In the Arthritis Survey, too, the respondents wrote in to share their experiences, not air their grievances.

In the hospitals where clinical trials are conducted, research subjects are also self-selected, to a degree. Even though potential subjects literally arrive on the doorstep because illness drives them to seek treatment, their participation in trials is by no means automatic. Researchers must solicit volunteers by approaching each patient who has the disease of interest, explaining the nature of the study and the risks involved, and then getting the patient's consent in writing. Ethical concerns have put an end, thank goodness, to the only truly random selection process in human studies: that of experimenting upon the unwitting or unwilling inmates of asylums, state hospitals, and penitentiaries, or on soldiers, prisoners of war, or the poor.

Advertising for subjects as we did is a well-established research practice. Health scientists looking for appropriate outpatient volunteers to serve as research subjects have used all imaginable approaches to attract them, including newspaper ads, radio spots, posters, press releases, and by making appearances at civic-group meetings. Paying research subjects is likewise standard procedure. Volunteers typically receive free medical care or a direct cash payment for their participation.

Tabulating and analyzing the data from the Arthritis Survey questionnaires was a massive job that took more than six months. It was further complicated, and *greatly* enriched, by those participants who not only wrote all over the printed form but then tacked on a page or two—or eight or nine—of extra details. This was not the kind of material that could be fed into a computer or turned over to research assistants. We read every questionnaire at least three times and began keeping tallies by hand. These eventually filled some four hundred spreadsheets, which we had to tailor-make to our purposes. On several of the popular drug treatments, for example, we often needed as many as thirty to forty columns for the side effects alone.

In addition to the wealth of information from our participants, we also used online medical literature services to give us monthly updates on relevant current research reported in the medical journals. We took each month's list to the medical-school library at the State University of New York's Stony Brook campus, where we read the original articles in their entirety. This helped us explain and augment the information from our participants with the latest research findings from professionals in nutrition, rheumatology, orthopedics, and related fields.

APPENDIX A

Arthritis Survey Questionnaire*

Dear Survey Participant,

Thank you for agreeing to take part in our nationwide Arthritis Survey.

We will use the information you provide as the basis for a new book we are writing about *osteoarthritis* and *rheumatoid arthritis.* In the hope of helping others, we ask you to tell us your experiences, opinions about the treatments you have tried, and tips on how to live with arthritis.

Our first book, *Backache Relief* (Times Books, 1985; NAL/ Signet, 1986), based on a similar nationwide survey, was chosen as a Book-of-the-Month Club alternate selection. The arthritis book will be published by St. Martin's Press in 1989.

You have our word that we will treat your personal information with respect and keep it *confidential.* Your name will not be used in the book or put on any kind of mailing list.

*To save space, the survey questions are printed here in list form—without the blank areas where participants wrote their responses.

Please try to answer the questions with as much *detail* as you can give. If you need more space, feel free to attach extra pages; we are interested in *everything* you have to say about arthritis.

As a token of our thanks for the time you spend sharing your knowledge, we will be happy to send you a check for $8 within 7 to 10 days of receiving your *fully completed* questionnaire.

Name / Address / Age / Sex / Occupation

Check which arthritis you have: osteoarthritis ———— rheumatoid ———— (Other forms of arthritis are *not* included in this survey.)

What parts of your body are arthritic?

How long have you had arthritis? (If less than 6 months, please do not fill out the questionnaire.)

On a scale of 0 to 10, where 0 means pain-free and 10 means intense pain that keeps you from doing anything, how would you rate your condition on average? Circle one number: 0   1   2   3   4   5   6   7   8   9   10

[pain-free]   [intense pain]

PROFESSIONAL CARE

Please list all the *kinds* of practitioners who have treated you. (For example, rheumatologist, internist, physiatrist, chiropractor, osteopath, physical therapist, nurse, Yoga instructor, etc.)

Please look at the list you just wrote and put three plus signs (+ + +) after those who gave you a *great deal of help* that lasted *a year or more.*

Put two plus signs (+ +) after those who gave you *a little help* that lasted *a year or more.*

Put one plus sign (+) after those who gave you *only temporary relief.*

Put a zero (0) after those who *didn't help at all.*

Put a minus sign (−) after those who *made you feel worse.*

In the space below, please comment about the practitioners you have seen. (For example, tell *how* they helped you or made you worse.)

Are you satisfied with the care you are receiving now? If not, what are you planning to do?

What kinds of arthritis diagnostic *tests* have you taken?

(For example, X rays, blood tests, arthroscopy, joint aspiration, etc.)

What would you say about these tests to someone who needed to take them? (Are they expensive, painful, useful, etc.?)

Do you take *aspirin?*

If yes, how much each day?———— Check one: plain—buffered—coated— What does it do for you (pain relief, side effects, etc.)?

TREATMENTS

What prescription drugs do you take? (Some examples are Deltasone, Dolobid, Feldene, Indocin, Motrin, Naprosyn, Oraflex, Orudis, Ridaura, Tolectin, etc.)

Now give (+ + +) to pills that helped you *a great deal* for *a year or longer.*

Put (+ +) after any that helped you *a little bit* for *a year or longer.*

Put (+) after those that gave *only temporary relief.*

Put (0) after the ones that *did no good.*

Please give as many details as you can about your reaction to these pills, including any side effects (dizziness, nausea, etc.).

Please list any *injection* treatments you have had (gold, methotrexate, cortisone, etc.) and tell what they did for you.

Please list other professional treatments you've tried (acupuncture, physical therapy, splints, biofeedback, manipulation, massage, etc.).

Of these, what helped the most? What made no difference? Did any treatment injure you?

SURGERY

Have you had surgery for arthritis?

If no, skip to the section on Exercise.

If yes, please name the joint(s) involved and what was done (total knee replacement, partial hip replacement, wrist fusion, etc.), including the year you had the operation.

If you have an artificial joint and know its brand name (Zimmer knee, Techmedica hip, etc.) please give it:

How long did it take to fully recover from surgery?

What follow-up treatment (physical therapy, exercise advice, etc.) did you receive after your operation(s)?

Please tell the outcome (pain relief, greater mobility, infection, etc.) of your operation(s).

What advice would you offer someone considering arthritis surgery?

EXERCISE

Do you exercise (stretch, swim, walk, etc.) for arthritis? If no, please skip to Other Treatments.

If yes, please tell *what you do* and *how much time* each day you devote to exercise:

How did you learn exercises? (Doctor, book, class, etc.)

What benefit(s) do you get from exercise?

If you have ever been harmed by exercise, please tell what happened:

What exercise advice can you offer other arthritis sufferers?

OTHER TREATMENTS

Please list any over-the-counter remedies (liniments, pills other than aspirin, etc.) you've used for arthritis, and tell what they did for you.

If you have tried any arthritis treatments that most doctors reject (copper bracelet, insect venom, hormone, etc.) please list them and describe what they did for you.

Please give any helpful information (danger, cost, etc.) you can for others thinking of trying the treatment(s) you just named.

NUTRITION

Have you changed the way you eat (avoid some foods, eat more of others, etc.) because of arthritis? If yes, please give details:

What has your doctor told you about nutrition and arthritis?

Does arthritis affect your food shopping and cooking? If yes, in what way?

What vitamins/minerals, if any, do you take, and what do they do for you?

Please give *comments* or *questions* you have about nutrition and arthritis:

SELF-HELP

What things do you do for yourself (rest, warm baths, ice bags, etc.) that give you pain relief?

What do you do to lift your spirits?

Does *stress* make your pain worse?

If yes, what techniques (deep breathing, imagery, etc.) help you reduce stress?

Have you changed your *home* or *workplace* and the things in it (raised toilet seat, bed board, etc.) because of arthritis? Please list the changes:

Please name the most *useful items* you've discovered (homemade, store-bought or mail-order) for arthritis sufferers, and where to get them.

What are some of the ways you've found for doing *common activities* (from cleaning house to making love) without increasing pain or injury?

We are *not* affiliated with the Arthritis Foundation, but we would like to know if that group has helped you in any way (information, support, etc.):

If you would be willing to discuss exercise or practical tips in depth with us, please give your area code and phone number:

Best time to call: AM————PM————

If you know another arthritis sufferer who might be willing to participate in our survey, please give his or her name and address:

THANKS AGAIN!

APPENDIX B

Survey Demographics

The 1,051 participants in our Arthritis Survey are a diverse group of 352 men and 699 women. We knew even before we began soliciting volunteers that we would have more women than men in our survey population, since rheumatoid arthritis affects about three times as many women as men, and osteoarthritis is also more common among women.

	Number of Participants with Rheuma- toid Arthritis	Number of Participants with Osteo- arthritis	Number of Participants with Both Forms
Men	153	188	11
Women	263	376	60
Total	416	564	71

Our participants range in age from twelve to ninety-three, but more than two-thirds of them are now in their forties, fifties, and sixties.

Age Range	Number of Participants in This Age Range	Percent of Total
10–19	7	1%
20–29	44	4%
30–39	117	11%
40–49	165	16%
50–59	224	21%
60–69	325	31%
70–79	144	14%
80–89	21	2%
90–99	1	———
Age not stated	3	———

Arthritis is frequently called a disease of old age, despite the fact that hundreds of thousands of children suffer from juvenile rheumatoid arthritis. Even the two forms of arthritis covered in our survey—osteoarthritis and rheumatoid arthritis—take their toll among the young and middle-aged. More than half of our participants, or 557 individuals, are under the age of sixty *now,* and 450 of them had arthritis before they reached age forty.

Age at Onset	Number of Participants	Percent of Total
0–9	26	2%
10–19	71	7%
20–29	140	13%
30–39	213	20%
40–49	247	24%
50–59	209	20%
60–69	95	9%
70–79	25	2%
80–89	2	———
Unstated	23	2%

Although most of our participants have found relief in a combination of professional treatments and self-help strategies, they have endured their share of pain. Here's how they rate themselves, on average, on our pain scale, where 0 means pain-free at present, and 10 signifies intense pain that keeps them from doing anything.

Pain Rating	Number of Participants	Percent of Total
0	10	1%
1	25	2%
2	53	5%
3	102	10%
4	133	13%
5	209	20%
6	150	14%
7	139	13%
8	111	11%
9	53	5%
10	45	4%
No answer	21	2%

We had to pool and average the answers of those who gave themselves a range-type rating, such as "2 to 4," or more than one answer, such as "4, except during flare-ups, when it jumps to about 9½." Several participants who gave no answer to this question went to some lengths explaining how hard it was to put a number rating on pain. It was simpler, by far, to say which joints were, or had been, painful.

Affected Joint(s)	Number of Participants Affected There
Knees/Legs	634
Hands/Fingers	590
Spine	416
Shoulders	284
Feet/Toes	274
Hips/Pelvis	274

Affected Joint(s)	Number of Participants Affected There
Neck	245
Elbows/Arms	232
Ankles	160
Wrists	150
"Most" or "All" joints	125
Jaw	37
Ribs/Breastbone/Chest	18

We have more survey participants from California than from any other state, followed by New York, Florida, and Texas.

State	Number of Participants	State	Number of Participants
Alabama	16	Massachusetts	15
Alaska	4	Michigan	37
Arizona	18	Minnesota	23
Arkansas	17	Mississippi	4
California	117	Missouri	21
Colorado	15	Montana	4
Connecticut	9	Nebraska	10
Delaware	4	Nevada	6
District of Columbia	1	New Hampshire	5
Florida	64	New Jersey	30
Georgia	14	New Mexico	6
Hawaii	3	New York	87
Idaho	7	North Carolina	20
Illinois	33	North Dakota	1
Indiana	29	Ohio	52
Iowa	12	Oklahoma	12
Kansas	11	Oregon	19
Kentucky	13	Pennsylvania	45
Louisiana	15	Rhode Island	4
Maine	5	South Carolina	7
Maryland	12	South Dakota	13

State	Number of Participants	State	Number of Participants
Tennessee	23	Washington	32
Texas	62	West Virginia	8
Utah	5	Wisconsin	37
Vermont	1	Wyoming	3
Virginia	21		

Other Homes	Number of Participants
Alberta	1
British Columbia	3
Manitoba	1
Nova Scotia	1
Ontario	8
Saskatchewan	1
Bahamas	1
Puerto Rico	3

APPENDIX C

Drug Interactions

Medications used to treat arthritis, whether they are prescription drugs or over-the-counter products, can cause serious trouble when mixed with other medicines. This reference chart is a convenient guide that may alert you to potential problems, which you should discuss with your doctor.

The drugs are listed in alphabetical order. The information is based on the *Physicians' Desk Reference* and *The People's Pharmacy.*

Prescription Drugs

Name	Type	Bad Matches and Their Possible Dangers
Azulfidine (sulfasalazine)	Anti-inflammatory	Digoxin (for heart trouble)—reduced absorption of digoxin
Butazolidin (phenylbutazone)	NSAID (Nonsteroidal Anti-Inflammatory Drug)	Anticoagulants—bleeding Methotrexate (for cancer or rheumatoid arthritis)—increased toxic effects of methotrexate Anticonvulsants (for seizures)—increased toxic effects of these drugs, including loss of balance Aspirin or other NSAIDs—gastrointestinal problems, including ulcers Oral diabetes drugs—extremely low blood sugar Penicillamine—blood and kidney disorders

Prescription Drugs *(Continued)*

Name	Type	Bad Matches and Their Possible Dangers
Clinoril (sulindac)	NSAID	DMSO—reduced efficacy of **Clinoril**; peripheral neuropathy
		Aspirin—reduced efficacy of **Clinoril**
		Aspirin or other NSAIDs—gastrointestinal problems, including ulcers
		Dolobid (diflunisal)—reduced efficacy of **Clinoril**
Cortone (cortisone acetate)		See **Deltasone**
Cuprimine (penicillamine)	Chelating agent/ Antirheumatic	Gold—serious blood and kidney disorders
		Antimalarial—blood and kidney disorders
		Cytotoxic drugs—blood, kidney disorders
		Butazolidin—blood and kidney disorders
Decadron (dexamethasone)		See **Deltasone**

Prescription Drugs *(Continued)*

Name	Type	Bad Matches and Their Possible Dangers
Deltasone (prednisone)	Steroid	Anticonvulsants—reduced efficacy of **Deltasone**
		Antituberculosis drugs—reduced efficacy of both **Deltasone** *and* these drugs
		Aspirin and other salicylates—reduced efficacy of aspirin or other salicylate
		Barbiturates (certain sedatives)—reduced efficacy of **Deltasone**
		Diuretics—depleted potassium stores
		Oral contraceptives—Increased toxic effects of **Deltasone**
		Live vaccines—failure of vaccine to take effect; onset of illness it's meant to prevent
Depen (penicillamine)		See **Cuprimine**

Prescription Drugs *(Continued)*

Name	Type	Bad Matches and Their Possible Dangers
Disalcid (salsalate)	NSAID	Gout medications—reduced efficacy of these drugs
		Anticoagulants—bleeding
		Aspirin and other salicylates—toxic levels of active ingredient, as the drugs are so closely related
		Oral diabetes drugs—extremely low blood sugar
Dolobid (diflunisal)	NSAID	Anticoagulants—bleeding
		Antacids (taken regularly)—reduced efficacy of **Dolobid**
		Acetaminophen—elevated blood levels of acetaminophen, posing threat to liver.
		Indocin (indomethacin)—fatal gastrointestinal hemorrhage
		Clinoril (sulindac)—reduced efficacy of **Clinoril**
		Naprosyn (naproxen)—decreased urinary excretion of **Naprosyn**
		Aspirin or other NSAIDs—gastrointestinal problems, including ulcers

Prescription Drugs *(Continued)*

Name	Type	Bad Matches and Their Possible Dangers
Easprin (aspirin)	Salicylate (NSAID)	Anticoagulants—hemorrhage
		Oral diabetes drugs—extremely low blood sugar
		Insulin—extremely low blood sugar
		Gout medications—small doses of aspirin reduce efficacy of these drugs
		Alcohol—gastrointestinal bleeding
		Steroids—increased risk of ulcers
		Butazolidin—increased risk of ulcers
		Phenobarbital—reduced efficacy of aspirin
		Beta blockers—reduced anti-inflammatory effect of aspirin
		Antacids—changes in **Easprin**'s enteric coating
		Methotrexate—increased toxicity of methotrexate
		Other NSAIDs—Gastrointestinal problems, including ulcers

Prescription Drugs *(Continued)*

Name	Type	Bad Matches and Their Possible Dangers
Feldene (piroxicam)	NSAID	Anticoagulants—bleeding
		Aspirin—reduced efficacy of **Feldene**
		Aspirin or other NSAIDs—gastrointestinal problems, including ulcers
Imuran (azathioprine)	Immuno-suppressive	Allopurinol (for gout)—increased toxicity of **Imuran**
		Alkylating agents such as cyclophosphamide and chlorambucil—cancer

Prescription Drugs *(Continued)*

Name	Type	Bad Matches and Their Possible Dangers
Indocin (indomethacin)	NSAID	**Dolobid** (diflunisal)—fatal gastrointestinal hemorrhage
		Aspirin—reduced efficacy of **Indocin**
		Aspirin or other NSAIDs—gastrointestinal problems, including ulcers
		Probenecid (for gout)—increased blood levels of **Indocin**
		Lithium (for depression)—elevated lithium levels and possible lithium toxicity
		Diuretics (for hypertension)—reduced efficacy of the diuretic; kidney problems
		Beta blockers—reduced efficacy of beta blocker
Meclomen (meclofenamate sodium)	NSAID	Anticoagulants—bleeding
		Aspirin—greater blood loss in the stool than from either drug alone
Medrol (methylprednisolone)		See **Deltasone**

Prescription Drugs *(Continued)*

Name	Type	Bad Matches and Their Possible Dangers
Methotrexate (methotrexate)	Antimetabolite	**Butazolidin**—increased toxicity of **Methotrexate**
		Aspirin and other salicylates—increased toxicity of **Methotrexate**
Motrin (ibuprofen)	NSAID	Anticoagulants—bleeding
		Aspirin—reduced efficacy of **Motrin**
		Aspirin or other NSAIDs—gastrointestinal problems, including ulcers
Nalfon (fenoprofen calcium)	NSAID	Aspirin—reduced efficacy of **Nalfon**
		Phenobarbital—reduced efficacy of **Nalfon**
		Anticoagulants—bleeding
		Anticonvulsants (for seizures)—increased toxicity of these drugs

Prescription Drugs (*Continued*)

Name	Type	Bad Matches and Their Possible Dangers
Naprosyn (na-proxen)	NSAID	**Anaprox** (naproxen sodium)—elevated blood levels of the active ingredient, as the drugs are very closely related
		Diuretics—kidney trouble
		Anticoagulants—bleeding
		Beta blockers—reduced efficacy of beta blocker
		Probenecid—increased **Naprosyn** potency
		Methotrexate—increased toxicity of methotrexate
Orudis (keto-profen)	NSAID	Aspirin—reduced efficacy of **Orudis**
		Diuretics—kidney failure
		Probenecid—inhibited excretion of **Orudis**
Plaquenil (hydroxy-chloroquine sulfate)	Antimalarial	Penicillamine—bone-marrow depression; kidney trouble
Prednisone		See **Deltasone**

Prescription Drugs (*Continued*)

Name	Type	Bad Matches and Their Possible Dangers
Rheumatrex (methotrexate)		See **Methotrexate**
Ridaura (aura-nofin)	Gold (Antirheu-matic)	**Dilantin** (for epilepsy)—increased blood levels of **Dilantin**
Rufen (ibu-profen)		See **Motrin**
Sulfasalazine		See **Azulfidine**
Tolectin (tolme-tin sodium)	NSAID	Anticoagulants—bleeding Diuretics—kidney trouble Aspirin and other NSAIDs—gastrointestinal problems, including ulcers
Zorprin (aspirin)		See **Easprin**

Over-the-Counter Drugs

Name	Type	Bad Matches and Their Possible Dangers
Advil (ibuprofen)		See **Motrin**
Anacin (aspirin)		See **Easprin**
Anacin-3 (aceta-minophen)	Analgesic	**Dolobid**—elevated levels of acetaminophen, posing threat to the liver
Arthritis Pain Formula (aspirin)		See **Easprin**
Arthritis Strength Bufferin (aspirin)		See **Easprin**
Ascriptin (aspirin)		See **Easprin**
Bufferin (aspirin)		See **Easprin**
Datril (aceta-minophen)		See **Anacin-3**
Medipren (ibu-profen)		See **Motrin**

Over-the-Counter Drugs *(Continued)*

Name	Type	Bad Matches and Their Possible Dangers
Nuprin (ibuprofen)		See **Motrin**
Panadol (acetaminophen)		See **Anacin-3**
Tylenol (acetaminophen)		See **Anacin-3**
Tylenol Extra Strength (acetaminophen)		See **Anacin-3**

SELECTED BIBLIOGRAPHY

In the course of researching and writing this book, we read dozens of books, newsletters, magazines, and medical journals. Our survey participants also mentioned particular sources they had read and found useful, although, as one of them remarked, "From the looks of the Arthritis Survey questionnaire, you will be combining a great deal of material that I had to find by reading numerous books."

Following is a partial list of the items we read. The entries are grouped according to general subject area. We make no attempt to rate the books in comparison to each other, although our comments about them are quite candid.

Books

Understanding Arthritis by the Arthritis Foundation (New York: Scribners, 1984). This book discusses the various types of arthritis, including lupus and ankylosing spondylitis, from symptoms to treatment. It is comprehensive but utterly dry and dispassionate. Predictably, it overlooks nutritional and other approaches that are outside the traditional medical model of arthritis treatment.

Arthritis. A Comprehensive Guide by James F. Fries, M.D. (Reading, MA: Addison-Wesley, 1979). This top-selling arthritis book is informative, well organized, and well written. Its author is director of the Stanford University Arthritis Clinic. The text does a good job of explaining a dozen different forms of arthritis, summarizing technical data about arthritis drugs and providing practical tips about reducing pain in joints and getting through daily activities more comfortably. Its failing is its tunnel vision, its unswerving obeisance to orthodoxy: All prescription drugs are useful. Doctors know best. Cooperative patients get well.

The Arthritis Helpbook by Kate Lorig, R.N., and James F. Fries, M.D. (Reading, MA: Addison-Wesley, 1980). This is the practical-applications follow-up to *Arthritis. A Comprehensive Guide.* Based on what the authors taught in lay arthritis classes at the Stanford Arthritis Center, the book's goal is to help individuals become "arthritis self-managers." It provides useful information about joint protection, stress reduction, exercise, self-help aids, and drugs. It is, overall, a helpful and easy-to-follow guide. But, like Dr. Fries's other book, it has a strong medical bias. The coverage of diet and nutrition, in particular, adheres strictly to Arthritis Foundation dogma.

Living with Arthritis by the *National Enquirer* (New York: Pocket Books, 1985). This collection of material published in the *Enquirer* and obtained from the Arthritis Foundation is the best value among mainstream arthritis books—comparable to a blending of Dr. Fries's two books at a bargain price. Like them, it is limited to strictly orthodox thinking. For although the *Enquirer* specializes in splashy headlines about titillating subjects, its medical reporting is tightly controlled and carefully checked by doctors.

Christiaan Barnard's Program for Living with Arthritis by Christiaan Barnard, M.D. (New York: Fireside/Simon & Schuster, 1984). After his career as a heart surgeon was ended by rheumatoid arthritis, Dr. Barnard wrote this book about the disease and his personal battle to overcome it. The writing is a bit patronizing, as Dr. Barnard is his own main interest. One of his most interesting points is that orthodox medicine has its limits, and that doctors with arthritis, like everyone else, venture outside the medical establishment in search of hope and help. Dr. Barnard tried, among other things, a course of treatment with fetal lamb cells at a private clinic in Switzerland, and extract from the New Zealand green-lipped mussel.

The Arthritis Exercise Book by Semyon Krewer (New York: Cornerstone Library/Simon & Schuster, 1981). Krewer, who also has arthritis, is an atomic physicist with an extensive knowledge of physical rehabilitation. His book, based almost entirely on his own personal experience and his readings, is endorsed by important members of the arthritis establishment, from Dr. Fries to renowned physiatrist Dr. Rene Calliet. Indeed, nearly every therapeutic exercise for arthritis is covered here in more than 250 pages. The problem is knowing which of the exercises to do. What's more, we believe that some of the exercises, especially the straight-leg sit-up, are dangerous to attempt—even for people who don't have arthritis.

The Arthritis Book of Water Exercise by Judy Jetter and Nancy Kadlec (New York: Holt, Rinehart and Winston, 1985). Kadlec is an occupational therapist who has used her own personal experience with arthritis to help develop the Arthritis Aquatics Program cosponsored by the Arthritis Foundation and the YMCA. Nonweight-bearing exercises in the water have been shown to be beneficial for many people with arthritis, and this book covers most of them in good detail.

Arthritis: Relief Beyond Drugs by Rachel Carr (New York: Harper & Row, 1981). Indeed, drugs are barely mentioned, except to lament our over-dependence upon them. This is a book of exercises, deep breathing, relaxation, and mind control—the techniques that helped its author overcome osteoarthritis. Some of the movements, such as the pelvic stretch and the straight-leg sit-up, strike fear in our hearts, but most of the program is well thought out and the exercises are well cap-

tured in photographs of average people performing them—
not supersupple models.

Natural Relief for Arthritis by Carol Keough and the editors
of *Prevention.* (Emmaus, PA: Rodale Press, 1983). This interesting book contains copious diet and nutrition advice. Keogh
recommends and reprints the no-fat diet developed by the late
Nathan Pritikin. Although the Pritikin diet rules out several
food items that may be arthritis-aggravating, such as pork and
sugar, it also excludes sardines, mackerel, and other fatty fish
that have recently been shown to be *beneficial* for many people with arthritis.

Arthritis and Folk Medicine by D. C. Jarvis, M.D. (New York:
Fawcett Crest/Ballantine Books, 1962). The subtitle of this
best-seller tells the story: "A doctor reveals the nature secrets
and folk medicine practices of Vermont." Dr. Jarvis is as sin-
cere as he is offbeat. His heart belongs to apple-cider vinegar,
which is the healing hero in most of his anecdotes. Some of Dr.
Jarvis's other theories include the advisability of a low-protein/
high-carbohydrate diet, the avoidance of processed foods, and
the addition of kelp and fish meal to the diet.

The Arthritic's Cookbook by Collin H. Dong, M.D., and Jane
Banks (New York: Bantam Books, 1975). Dr. Dong is a medical
doctor with arthritis who couldn't be helped by orthodox
means. His predominantly fish diet has helped thousands of
other people with arthritis, according to Dr. Dong, but he
offers not a morsel of substantiation. Although the Dong diet
fared no better than a placebo diet in a controlled study
funded in part by the Arthritis Foundation, the results have
spurred both controversy and further research. (See Chapter
12.) The Dong diet is much more restrictive than our Arthritis
Survey diet, as it excludes all fruit and all dairy products. However, some of the fish recipes are excellent.

New Hope for the Arthritic by Collin H. Dong, M.D., and Jane
Banks (New York: Ballantine Books, 1975). This sequel to *The
Arthritic's Cookbook* explains Dr. Dong's dietary regimen in
greater depth and provides more elaborate menus and advice
about meal planning. However, there still are no statistics or

other evidence offered to support his claims for the diet's success among his patients and readers.

The Arthritis Relief Diet by James Scala, Ph.D. (New York: New American Library, 1987). The byline on the dust jacket of this book reads "Dr. James Scala," and it is only by reading inside that we discover the author is not a physician but a biochemist. His research and his reading of other people's research led him to promulgate his diet plan, which he offers with this incredible promise: "All you have to do [to achieve arthritis relief] is make a personal commitment to follow the diet revealed in this book." The diet spells out the virtues of fatty fish as modern science understands them, but includes such entries as "Glazed Duck with Peanut-Rice Stuffing" and "Rabbit with Red Wine."

Dr. Mandell's Lifetime Arthritis Relief System by Marshall Mandell, M.D. (New York: Berkley, 1985). The basic premise of this book is that arthritis is caused by allergies to foods and environmental chemicals. Detailed instructions are offered on how to identify the offensive agents and eliminate them from your home and place of work.

The People's Pharmacy by Joe and Teresa Graedon (New York: St. Martin's Press, 1985). Although the information is not limited to arthritis treatments, this book does a good job of painting a realistic picture of the up and down sides of drug treatment, including extremely useful charts on drug interactions.

The Pill Book of Arthritis edited by Lawrence Chilnick (New York: Bantam Books, 1985). This text is no more informative than any all-purpose drug reference book, but it *is* convenient to have all the arthritis-relevant material in one place, with color photos of the pills. Conspicuous by their absence are **Orudis, Methotrexate, Ridaura**, and a few other pills that came on the market after this book was published.

Minding the Body, Mending the Mind by Joan Borysenko, Ph.D. (Reading, MA: Addison Wesley, 1987). Arthritis is never mentioned in this book, but the author, who directs the Mind/

Body Clinic at New England Deaconess Hospital, does an admirable job of providing clear instructions for meditating, relaxing, deep breathing, and breaking destructive patterns of thought and behavior. All of the advice is aimed at helping readers achieve control over their illnesses and their lives.

Love, Medicine & Miracles by Bernie S. Siegel, M.D. (New York: Harper & Row, 1986). This highly acclaimed book has its usefulness for people who are open to the attitudes and techniques espoused here. Bernie, as the author says he likes to be called, makes his most valuable contribution when addressing other doctors, urging them to overcome the barriers that separate them from their patients as people—to speak and touch freely, to stop acting like a god and just relate to fellow human beings. The message offered to people with chronic illnesses is potentially less benign, however, because the philosophy of "You can heal yourself" can be inferred to mean, "You brought the illness on yourself. Your pain, like your failure to get well, is your fault."

Bees Don't Get Arthritis by Fred Malone (Chicago: Academy, 1979). This is a loosely organized and loosely written diary of one man's experiences with bees, beekeepers, arthritis, and various other people and things he encounters on his "32,000-mile odyssey discovering the curative powers of honey, pollen, propolis and bee stings." In any given chapter, you may discover as much about the conditions of this or that roadside camping ground as you do about the lore of the honeybee in the treatment of arthritis.

Newsletters

HealthFacts published monthly by the Center for Medical Consumers, Inc., New York. Although it is inexpensively produced, with no photos or fancy graphics, this is simply the best newsletter we have seen in its class. Each six-page issue provides in-depth coverage of one featured topic, plus other brief news items, all based on recent reports in the medical literature and interviews with physician experts. The writing and editing do a good job of digesting complex issues in such a way as to help people make informed decisions about their own health care.

Health Letter published monthly by the Public Citizen Health Research Group, Washington, D.C. Dr. Sidney M. Wolfe, the outspoken editor of this courageous publication, is the self-appointed guardian of the public health. His attacks on various actions of organized medicine and on specific drugs make for twelve pages of fascinating reading and provide much helpful advice. Although Dr. Wolfe sometimes appears overzealous in his charges, we wouldn't want to see anybody cramp his style.

Harvard Medical School Health Letter published monthly by the school's Department of Continuing Education in Boston, Massachusetts. This is a very carefully researched and well-written eight-page newsletter that examines current health issues for general readers, from the doctor's perspective. The physicians who edit the newsletter aim to *inform* the public *without* providing personal medical advice.

INDEX

ABOUT THE AUTHORS

Husband and wife writing team Dava Sobel and Arthur C. Klein bring two entirely different perspectives to their consumer-oriented medical books.

DAVA SOBEL was born in New York City in 1947, into a family with a strong interest in science and medicine. Her father is a doctor; her mother worked as a chemist; and her two brothers are a doctor and a dentist. She was graduated with honors from the Bronx High School of Science and holds a bachelor's degree from the State University of New York at Binghamton.

Although she has spent most of her professional life as a freelance science writer, contributing regularly to *Omni* magazine, *Science Digest, Good Housekeeping, Ladies' Home Journal, Harvard* magazine, *Vogue,* and others, she took a full-time job with *The New York Times* science news department in 1979. As a *Times* reporter, her beat was psychology and psychiatry, and her efforts were recognized with a National Media Award from the American Psychological Foundation in 1980.

ARTHUR KLEIN was born in 1940 in Port Chester, New York, and studied marketing and psychology at Lehigh University in Bethlehem, Pennsylvania, graduating in 1962. He combined his talent for writing with his interest in marketing at Prentice-Hall, then moved to J. Walter Thompson, where he handled accounts such as Eastman Kodak, Citibank, and Carte Blanche.

Beginning in 1969, he worked as a promotion manager for *The New York Times* Company, researching and helping to create new educational and reference materials. Later, as head of his own direct marketing agency, he constructed surveys and questionnaires for clients including Scholastic, Macmillan, and Merrill Lynch. In addition, he wrote essays and social commentary that appeared in *National Review, The Village Voice, Harper's Weekly, Philadelphia* magazine, and *Los Angeles* magazine, as well as a series syndicated by *The New York Times.* He became a member of the American Society of Journalists and Authors in 1976, and the American Medical Writers Association in 1985.

Arthur and Dava met in 1977 and were married within a few months.

Arthur's *un*satisfying experiences with doctors during a bout of debilitating pain in 1980 gave him the idea for their first book, *Backache Relief.* (His "back problem" was eventually diagnosed as a mild form of muscular dystrophy.) Frustrated by the lack of help for his own situation and the bewildering array of specialists professing expertise about back problems, he conceived of a plan to turn the experiences of fellow back-pain sufferers into a source of user-friendly information and advice.

Long before he won a publisher's support of these efforts, he undertook the first nationwide survey of people with back pain by placing advertisements in national newspapers and magazines. He devised a questionnaire that elicited facts about practitioners, treatments, and self-help strategies. The pooled information from nearly five hundred respondents identified one type of medical specialist—the physiatrist, or doctor of physical medicine—who was little known but proved far more effective than either orthopedists or chiropractors in treating a variety of back problems, from low-back syndrome to sciatica. This and other surprising findings, including the news that most drug treatments for simple back pain are remarkably *in*effective, generated tremendous media interest, including a spot on ABC's "World News Tonight" and a cover story in *New York* magazine. *Backache Relief* was chosen as a Book-of-the-Month Club alternate selection.

Almost immediately upon completion of *Backache Relief,* the couple decided to write a second book, because the back pain survey had raised several intriguing questions about arthritis. Some one hundred of the participants attributed their back pain to arthritis. In most cases, they had significantly more pain than the other respondents, and considerably more anger about some of the treatments they'd received. There was a clear sense that many practitioners did not "take arthritis seriously." Also, the complex nature of arthritis was simply beyond the scope of the back-pain survey, and needed to be addressed in a separate study.

Backache Relief was based entirely on survey participants' comments and books written by leading back practitioners, as there was no substantive body of research that addressed the questions Arthur and Dava were trying to answer. In researching the arthritis project, however, they went *first* to the medical literature—to understand the types of medical and surgical procedures that were available and to see what experimental approaches were being tested. Here they encountered their first big surprise, learning that serious researchers were investigating the importance of nutrition in the treatment of arthritis, while the vast majority of practitioners were telling patients that diet played absolutely no role in their disease.

The Arthritis Survey questionnaire that Dava and Arthur devised elicited information on everything from aspirin to zinc supplements, from rheumatologists to acupuncturists, from prescription drugs to over-the-counter pills and rubs, from orthodox treatments to quack remedies, from exercise to eating habits, from surgery to self-help. And the responses from the more than one thousand participants shaped the book you're holding.

In addition to *Backache Relief* and *Arthritis: What Works,* Dava and Arthur have produced two children, Zoë and Isaac, ages eight and five.

HOW TO SEND
YOUR COMMENTS TO
THE AUTHORS

The authors would love to hear from you if you have any comments or experiences to add to the information you've read in *Arthritis: What Works,* or if you have any questions about arthritis you would like to see answered in subsequent editions of this book. Please address your letters to:

Dava Sobel and Arthur C. Klein
c/o Arthritis Survey™
St. Martin's Press, Inc.
175 Fifth Avenue
New York, N.Y. 10010

(Books are available in quantity for promotional or premium use. Write to Director of Special Sales, St. Martin's Press, 175 Fifth Avenue, New York, N.Y. 10010, for information on discounts and terms, or call toll-free (800) 221-7945. In New York, call (212) 674-5151.)

Rodale Press, Inc., publishes PREVENTION, America's leading health magazine.
For information on how to order your subscription,
write to PREVENTION, Emmaus, PA 18098.